ADVANCE PRAISE FOR
DYING AT THE MARGINS

"In his work, *Dying at the Margins: Reflections on Justice and Healing for Inner-City Poor*, David Wendell Moller uses the genre of narrative medicine to usher the reader into the lived experience of persons living and dying on the outskirts of society, bereft of social connections, economic resources, and political empowerment. This work cries out for a preferential option for the poor and vulnerable and represents a call to radical solidarity of mind and heart with our fellow human beings living on the edge and dying on the margins of American life."

—**Beverly Rosa Williams, PhD**, Medical Sociologist,
Associate Professor of Medicine,
University of Alabama at Birmingham,
Birmingham, AL

"All Americans risk dying on the 'end-of-life conveyor belt,' where non-beneficial, high-technology interventions are tried, one after the other, until the patient has died. But, as Dr. Moller explores in *Dying at the Margins*, marginalized communities suffer more than the rest of us in death. This book is a much needed call to action for healers, caretakers, and all in the medical profession, who are perfectly positioned to right this wrong. The compelling stories contained in this text reveal that by opening to the suffering, and the humanity, of disadvantaged patients, we can help heal the world, one person at a time."

—**Jessica Nutik Zitter, MD, MPH**, Author of *Extreme Measures:
Finding a Better Path to the End of Life*

"Through engaging and vivid stories—not bloodless data or social science jargon—Dr. Moller and his collaborators convey a message that medical professionals need to hear: the bitterly ironic reality that the poor, if given the choice, often prefer to continue receiving technologically intensive "heroic" care that socioeconomically advantaged patients and families have been increasingly educated to forego near the end of life. Intimate, powerful, and timely, *Dying at the Margins* explores why the poor make this seemingly odd choice, while also shining a light on the clear cash incentive authorities may have behind depriving the poor of expensive technical care."

—**Theodore Brown, PhD**, Professor of History and Public Health Sciences,
University of Rochester, Rochester, NY

"*Dying at the Margins* brings together essays from leading thinkers and practitioners in palliative care to address an important—though at times neglected—aspect of medicine: care for the urban dying poor. This work gives voice to those dying at the margins of society, who are all too often neither seen nor heard. While the book deals with weighty matters, including the negative impact of racism and poverty on how poorly people of marginalized populations die, it also provides an inspiring way forward for those who have "eyes to see and ears to hear." May those who read this book learn from its insights and heed the call to action contained herein."

—Patrick T. Smith, PhD,
Associate Research Professor of Theological Ethics and Bioethics,
Duke University Divinity School and Kenan Institute of Ethics, Durham, NC

Dying at the Margins

Dying at the Margins

Reflections on Justice and Healing

for Inner-City Poor

Edited by David Wendell Moller, PhD
Chief of Clinical and Organizational Ethics
Anne Arundel Medical Center
Annapolis, MD

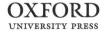

OXFORD
UNIVERSITY PRESS

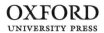

OXFORD
UNIVERSITY PRESS

Oxford University Press is a department of the University of Oxford. It furthers
the University's objective of excellence in research, scholarship, and education
by publishing worldwide. Oxford is a registered trade mark of Oxford University
Press in the UK and certain other countries.

Published in the United States of America by Oxford University Press
198 Madison Avenue, New York, NY 10016, United States of America.

CIP data is on file at the Library of Congress
ISBN 978-0-19-976014-5

1 3 5 7 9 8 6 4 2
Printed by Sheridan Books, Inc., United States of America

"And here is the radicalism that infused that show: that the child is closer to God than the adult; that the sick are closer than the healthy; that the poor are closer than the rich and the marginalized closer than the celebrated."

—David Brooks, reflecting on the TV show "Mister Rogers' Neighborhood"

Despite being at the other end of the lifespan upon which Mr. Rogers' show was focused, the folks whose stories are told in the pages of this book would not only be most welcomed 'in the neighborhood,' they would be celebrated.

In memory of my brother, Bill
(William E. Moller, December 11, 1934–March 8, 2008)
You lived imprisoned within your body
. . . now you are soaring on the wings of angels.

CONTENTS

PREFACE

AN INVITATION TO WITNESS (AND RESPOND)

David Wendell Moller

As he lay dying, Joe Noble spoke of his father. "He was a great man," he reminisced. "I worshipped him."

The greatness of Mr. Noble, Sr., did not reside in economic or social success, however. He lived poor, sacrificed much for his family, and ultimately died of black lung disease. What made him great in the eyes of his son was his unwavering devotion to his family, which persevered in the midst of poverty, exploitation, and deprivation. "He gave up his own necessities so he could support us. While he never said, 'I love you,' I never doubted his love and affection," Joe affirmed.

Blessed with great physical strength, Noble Sr. immigrated to the United States from Russia during his teenage years. Despite being illiterate, he was of great interest to potential employers because of his robust, strapping physicality. For this reason, he initially found employment in a north-woods logging camp, where he worked under dangerous and difficult conditions for years. "He would sleep outside under the horses, with the manure and them urinating on him," Joe lamented. "It was real bad during the winter. Winters were so cold that it took years after leaving the camp until he was able to feel warm again." As Joe was speaking of this, I could not help but think of the World War II veterans who survived the Battle of the Bulge and how many of them had the same post-traumatic response to living through extreme and frigid conditions. They often spoke of how difficult it was for them to feel warm again, of getting past the sensation of being chilled to the bone. Their struggle, despite being so much shorter in duration than Mr. Noble's, is imprinted and honored in the American narrative, becoming the stuff of storytelling and movie-making. Because of their feats, but also because by the way they are embraced and portrayed, they are celebrated as heroes. Nobody, on the other hand, is embracing or honoring the lives of the people whose stories form the basis of this book, namely, those who struggle and suffer at the economic, racial, social margins. Certainly, Hollywood is not making movies about them for the most part. To the contrary, these are people who are often disparaged and ridiculed, despite possessing qualities that make them wonderfully human and authentic. Perhaps it is even fair to suggest that they are heroic themselves, as they are able to navigate debilitating life circumstances in ways that many more fortunate individuals would be unable. (I imagine myself in their circumstances and fully believe I would not have the resilience to cope with the same dignity that they displayed. As you read their stories, I invite you to do the same.) Their strength, courage, and essential goodness is the essential substance of real heroes. Yet, unlike the "honored" heroes of American history, whose stories are proudly told, they remain invisible and a matter of indifference in the mindset of the broader culture.

Mr. Noble Sr.'s life ultimately led him to the coal mines of western Pennsylvania. He had worked as a laborer in various other endeavors, always struggling to earn enough to provide for his family. Seeking a better opportunity, he was convinced by an acquaintance that there was money to be made in the coal mines. So he pursued that opportunity. Yet, once there, he found nothing but continued hardship. "My father became a slave again," Joe recalled with obvious bitterness. "He was able to reach $4,000 annual salary only two times and that was only because of all the overtime he put in. He supported his wife, five kids, and his wife's mother on that income until he was retired by the mine in 1958 at the age of 65."

Joe's dominant feeling toward his father was love and gratitude. He applauded his father's work ethic and sense of duty to the family. "I loved my father. I miss him so," Joe would often say. He spoke with great admiration of how his father would go to work hungry at times so as not deprive his family of sustenance. Joe never resented that he was born poor or the fact that his father's financial struggles ultimately set the foundation for his own life of financial difficulty. Joe was open and direct about his plight. "Yeah, I've struggled financially all my life. Yeah, we experienced hardships because of my background. Adele [his wife] came from a poor family, too, you know. And then things got worse when I was disabled for a lot of years."

He had been working as a respiratory therapist for 13 years. One day, racing to a code, he slipped and fell, injuring his back and winding up on workman's compensation. After losing his disability insurance, he struggled to find work and bounced around from job to job. His wife worked for near-minimum wage as a certified nursing assistant, so financially things were very tight. As Joe put it, "Our children did without, and thank God, we lived thrifty. We both had poverty in our youth . . . and our children grew up as we did. We had no status or prestige. We felt discriminated against but we never discriminated."

Poverty was the only life he ever knew. And like so many other people who live and struggle at the margins, he got sick, very sick, and at a very early age. His cancer was particularly bad. It was invasive and spread throughout the stomach, intestines, and bowel. There was no possibility of surgery as it had spread so widely. Chemotherapy had done little to quiet the cancer's growth, and his fate was that he was to die in his mid-50s. Ironically, the strapping physicality possessed by Mr. Noble Sr. had been passed on to his son. While desperately sick, he was also very strong, and that physical strength enabled him to extend his battle against the disease. He lived with debility and excruciating pain for months. Although his medical treatment extended his life, and for that he was grateful, it also prolonged his suffering, which grew to be intense at times. "This would be over by now, if I wasn't so strong," he cried out in the emergency room one Friday afternoon. Tears were streaming down his cheeks from the pain. One of the nurses in the ER compounded his suffering when she responded to Adele's plea for more morphine by snapping, "He just had some." His pain and suffering were undeniably severe but relieving them and comforting him was not a priority, at least for that particular nurse. He was released from the ER later that night with the somber news that there was nothing that could be done except to try and help him get through the episodes of severe pain.

Within Joe Noble, despite his being raised poor, living poor, and suffering greatly with an insidious disease, resided a remarkable dignity. As he journeyed through the dying process, he fought back anger and resentment, seeking a higher path. And on this path, which Robert Frost once described as the "less-traveled" one, he exalted life. "It's so precious," he would declare. What made it precious was not material success or social status. That he did not have. Instead it was a deeply meaningful sense of spirituality that included an appreciation of the beauty and the joy that can be found in nature. In addition, primary and foremost for him, it was love of family that gave him meaning and purpose and sustained him throughout his struggles.

He thought about you often, I am sure: The reader who would learn a bit of his story at a time in his life when he would not appear at his best. He consciously thought about what he would like to say to you and what he hoped for you to learn from him. His message was not one of despair. Though if it were that would be understandable. Instead, it affirmed the beauty of life and the importance of love to the human condition. When I asked him directly what he would like for you to learn from him, he said:

> . . . tell them that *dying sucks.* It is impossibly, unimaginably difficult to die. Oh, to never see the pear trees again; to know that I am not going to have another Christmas; not to be able to fish anymore; but most of all never to see Adele and the kids again. It's all too hard.

The grief that was striking at him had less to do with his impending death and far more to do with the fact that death would forever separate him from his beloved family.

> I hate it. I just hate it. Dying takes me away from everything that is precious. . . . It is the farewell that is the bitch. It sucks. I love this world. I love the people I am going to leave behind. Adele, the children, that's the hard part. If I could take them in my hand, put them in my pocket and take them with me, then I would be ready to go. It's just so ridiculous having to go.

In many ways, there is a shroud of silence and denial that surrounds the experience of dying in America. Mr. Joe Noble's words break that silence. They are not easy words to hear. Nor is his physical state of being comforting to envision. Instead, they are haunting and distressing. They disturb. They express the depth and rawness of his suffering, both existential and physical.

His story also points to his own recognition of the absence of social worth or status, and hints at the stigma that defined him and his family because they lived in poverty. Additionally, it illuminates how very difficult it can be to go through the dying process. Despite how troubling his words and experience may be, however, they are authentic and carry important lessons about life—if we are willing to listen. They urge us not to take life for granted. Not to pretend that our lives will never end. But instead, to live each day with a sense of urgency and purpose, knowing and accepting that our lives are finite and there are no, 'do-overs.' He prods us not to become lost in trivial pursuits or the allure of material success but to seek enrichment of our humanity through relationships, the love of others, and finding peace within living purposefully.

At this very moment, there are people of all ages and types throughout America who are facing the end of life. Many of them are enduring enormous physical suffering tinged with existential fears, anxieties, and worry. Some of them, like Joe, are also socially estranged and living at the margins. Joe urges us not to ignore those folks because they live at the margins and in the shadows. He urges that we not become dismissive of them and their needs as human beings. He warns that by taking refuge in the comfort of denial and avoidance we abandon them, increasing their isolation by our own indifference to their sufferings. He also cautions against excessive clinical focus and professional detachment that sometimes guide the way physicians and other healthcare professionals deal with the dying persons. While a clinically-detached approach may be successful in containing the messiness and raw emotions that surround the experience of dying, it also leaves patients and families feeling deserted and not optimally cared for. The more humane response, he asserts, is to openly acknowledge their struggles and tend to their sufferings with respect, skill, and mindfulness.

Thus, in the midst of all he was enduring, he confirmed the essential importance of the work of caring for the sick and dying:

> . . . to relieve suffering and help comfort me while I am dying, I cannot imagine more important work.

His message is simple and straightforward: (1) Dying is unfathomably hard, and (2) providing comfort and relieving suffering near the end of life facilitates healing for patients and loved ones in transformational ways. He reminds us that dying is something a person does only once in life and that it is an especially difficult thing to do. He asks that we recognize how hard the process is for both patients and loved ones, and that we remain patient in our interactions with them despite the frustrations they may create. He also stresses the need to deliver our care with conscious awareness of the unique backgrounds of our patients, doing so with humility and cultural sensitivity, which requires an awareness of our own biases and stereotypes whether they be unconscious or otherwise (Figure I.1).

It is unimaginably difficult to die.

He goes on to offer,

> Just remember that human compassion and contact is what life is all about. It is the caring, the emotions, the sharing, and sensitivity. You could do it with a simple smile. You could do it with the kindness of just saying "Good morning" when you walk into a patient's room. It is just acknowledging that they exist and sharing that moment.

Joe knew how hard it is to suffer through the dying process and the courage it takes to face death steadily. He knew this in the most direct way. For this reason, he suggests that patients and families, in their state of vulnerability, may become very dependent

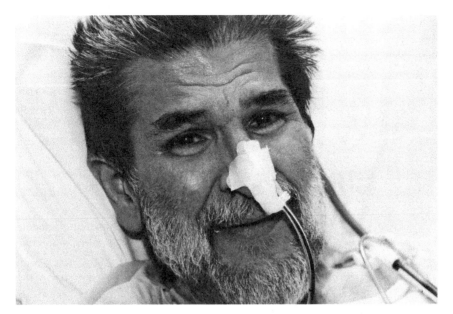

FIGURE I.1 "Tell them how important the work they do is," Mr. Nobel requested.

on their doctors, nurses, and other caregivers. They often will turn to them for answers, guidance, relief, and comfort. He asks that we accept this fact as a privilege and solemn responsibility:

> This is where the compassion comes in. . . . Never lose it in your occupation, your prestige, your wealth, your goals, and your ambition. Never lose it, because if you do, you've lost your soul. You've lost your humanity. . . . It's very, very important. It's the most important part of medicine. So please, I beg of you. Please practice it. Make it a priority.

There is elegance in the way Joe managed his dying. He displayed a certain bravery in facing death with such dignity. Kind of like the dignity with which he sought to live his life, despite its tribulations. His life was never easy. He always struggled because of financial hardship. He endured the social ostracism that comes with being poor in a culture that values consumerism and affluence. Ironically, perhaps it was the hardiness that sustained him through the travails of a life in poverty that also provided a foundational resilience that enabled him to confront death with grace and nobility.

His story is a powerful one, but it is not unique. Like both Joe Noble and his father, in inner cities across America, people live and die at the margins of economic stability and social acceptance. They are poorly understood and suboptimally cared for. These are individuals and families who are physically present with us, but remain far off the radar screen of social visibility and cultural concern. In a certain way, they are "**with** us but not **of** us;" their lives and sufferings often remaining "hidden in plain sight." Joe pleads with us, as he shares his story, to bring these people to attention and visibility. To fail to do so, in his view, would be neglectful. On the other hand, if we do commit to deepening our capacity to understand and serve the most vulnerable among us, we not only would promote the virtues of the healing professions, but we would also become a kinder society.

The struggles of the Noble family revolved around class divisions and associated lack of opportunities. As much as Americans are ill at ease discussing class and the existence of inequality, we are equally uncomfortable discussing the role that skin color plays in our cultural life. Racial prejudice and discrimination, along with gross disparities in economic status are not pretty things. They are also stains upon the belief in American exceptionalism. But the reality is that race does matter, and racism and discrimination are inseparably tacked to the bulletin board of American history. From slavery, to Jim Crow segregation, to the Civil Rights Movement, and on to the continuing struggle to address institutional and cultural racism, the political, economic, and social impact of skin color in America is undeniable. It influences peoples' lives profoundly, including how they live, where they live, and how they are judged and treated by others. Despite the pervasive role that race relations has played throughout American history, there is scant understanding of the actual impact of race on the lives of people. For the most part, the struggles that surround being black in America, especially in the inner-city context, are poorly understood. In large part this is because there is a lack of interest in historical remembrance and developing understandings about what racism (and its similarly sinister twin, poverty) means for people who are subjected to it. This not only reflects disparagingly on the soul of our nation, it serves to perpetuate the harms and injustice associated with bigotry and racism. It is not stretching too far to suggest that there is a universe of disconnect between white experience and black experience as well as a lack of understanding across the racial and economic divide. I think the point can be effectively made by asking a question posed by Senator Bill Bradley decades ago to the American people:

> When was the last time you had a conversation about race with a member of a different race?

The point he was getting at was that such conversations are not regularly a part of American discourse. In fact, they are more than likely to be avoided as they elicit shame and discomfort, and may escalate tensions, resentment, and guilt.

I used to think I knew quite a bit about race in America: that is, until I sought to understand it better by listening to the stories of people living in the inner city. I began by reaching out to them in their homes and communities. Once there, my realization of how little I actually knew came quickly. It began starkly one day when I met Mrs. Black in the cardiology clinic of a safety-net hospital for the first time. I was hoping to secure her participation in the *Dancing with Broken Bones* project and had reserved time to introduce myself before her appointment. After an exchange of pleasantries, I asked her to tell me about herself and her life. Her immediate response was, "I had two sons killed in the violence, she stated matter of factly." It was clearly important to her that I knew this fact about her life. "*The violence,*" as she described it, was a term of familiarity within her world, but not mine. It shaped much of social and personal life in her neighborhood. It took the lives of a number of men, and always hovered over the community as a threatening, dark cloud. It was associated with the fact that gunshots were commonly heard, especially at night; that drug deals were taking place, and that the streets were not the safest. It also portrays that the state of things in this ghetto, like many others, was such that death by violence was not a startling or earth-shattering event. To the contrary, while sad and regrettable, violence happened with such frequency as to "normalize" it in a sense. In this regard, it was especially notable that when she spoke about "the violence" in her world, she did so regretfully, but also with a sense of dispassionate acceptance.

My learning continued when I visited her at home for the very first time. Upon arriving, I felt as if I were entering a foreign country. On two opposite corners down the block there were gatherings of men who were hanging out and appeared less than welcoming to my arrival. I felt a stabbing fear getting out of my car and, at the same time, wondered why her home, which was also on a corner, had no one hanging around in front of it. I put my unease aside, walked up, and knocked on the door. Upon entering, I was struck by how neat and clean everything was and noted to myself the discrepancy between the untidy and disheveled neighborhood outside and the order that she maintained within.

As we sat on a sofa to begin our conversation, I observed how the torn and frayed fabric was held together by duct tape. During our conversation, she told me again about the death of her sons. She described how one was shot and killed while sitting on the front stoop to her house. This murder took place less than ten feet from where we were sitting and talking. Another son, she went on to relate, was gunned down while sitting in a car at a red light. This took place just a few blocks away in a drive-by shooting. Both murders were drug- and gang-related.

Mrs. Black also spoke with great sadness that day about an additional son who was in prison for drug-related offenses. His parole had recently been denied, and she was deflated in her spirits about his continued imprisonment.

> I had two sons killed in the violence, she stated matter of factly.

During this visit, she introduced me to her daughter and her granddaughter. Her daughter was her primary caregiver. As I got to know each of them, I saw how devoted she was to her mother. I was particularly struck by the story of her 13-year-old granddaughter, Phoebe. Phoebe had been struggling at school and was in trouble more often than not. As Mrs. Black described it, "She was running the streets all hours of the night and flunking in her grades." Being the matriarch of her family, and reeling from how her sons had succumbed to the pressures of street life, Mrs. Black obtained custody of her. She was fighting for a different kind of life for Phoebe. She moved her into her house, asserting discipline and high expectations. It took a while, but F's were giving way to C's and B's in school. And, most importantly, Phoebe was safe at home under the caring and loving watch of her grandmother. I was very impressed by how polite and well-mannered Phoebe was in relation to her grandmother. Clearly, her mannerisms and positive spirit were a product of Mrs. Black's influence.

Mrs. Black talked at great length about her life as an African American woman and recalled the prejudice she suffered. She and her family, like so many from her background, sought to rise from the ashes of tenant farming by migrating northward. But, again, like so many, she was unable to escape the impact of prejudice, racism, and blocked opportunity. Thus, she continued to live extremely poor and raised her children in the confines of urban poverty. Her regret in life was not the fact that she lived in poverty and endured the ravages of racism personally. She spoke almost matter-of-factly about how she would be prohibited from sitting at the "white-only" lunch counter at a local department store. She seemed to take it in stride that there was extreme racial segregation that prohibited her from living or shopping in the "nicer areas," even if she could afford to do so. And when she came home one day to find all of her family's belongings on the sidewalk because the rent was overdue (again), that was taken as being par for the course of her life. Instead, her deepest regret was that these facts of her life ultimately became sources of injury that she could not protect her children from. As a kind and good woman, she felt disempowered and helpless in guiding them to avoid and rise above the pitfalls of ghetto life. She suffered their failures, "poor choices," and serious consequences thereof deeply and regretfully.

My relationship with her began at a time when she was very sick and had been diagnosed with congestive heart failure. Her illness revealed another fact of life for African Americans; namely, disproportionate morbidity and mortality. Despite the fact that she was only in her 60s, her disease was advanced. She constantly struggled for breath and strength while coping with swollen ankles and legs that made it difficult for her to get around. On one particularly bad day, when she was very weak and short of breath, she put together a plan for going to the hospital. (Like many urban poor, she relied on the emergency room as a primary site for healthcare, as she did not have a primary care doctor's office to call and seek advice.) Rather than going immediately, however, she purposefully delayed calling 911. She needed to secure overnight coverage for Phoebe first, as she knew she would be admitted to the hospital. She was not quite in crisis yet, so she knew she had a little bit of time before things became critical. She filled me in about her previous experiences with the emergency department and her firsthand knowledge of when a better time to arrive would be. Although she was not feeling well, she was drawing upon her inner resources to preside over the decision-making that day. It was important that she be the one in charge of the time of her departure, not her disease, or even her daughter, who was encouraging her to go immediately. She had a plan, and she would go according to her own timeline. Her spirit of self-determination and resilience seemed impressive. It is fair to view her desire to plan the timeline for calling 911 as one means of staying in charge, of her controlling at least a bit of her destiny. Her emotional strength seemed good and she acted so poised in dealing with her challenges. As best as she could, she was managing things on her own terms.

Mrs. Black was a strong woman. She sought to remain empowered as a person, patient, mother, and grandmother, despite the existence of external forces that constantly threatened to disempower her. I learned, as I got to know her, that the reason the neighborhood men did not hang out in front of her house was that she confronted and berated them every time they would. She engaged in a battle of wills with them. And she won. We talked about how these people were a nuisance and threat to the neighborhood. But she also went on to assure me that I and my car would be safe. She noted that because I was visiting her, they would not mess with me in any way. And she was correct. I never encountered any problems. They honored, I suspect, her steadfast commitment to protecting her home, and they simply never would hang on that particular corner. It probably just wasn't worth the hassle, and perhaps they respected her as a sort of matriarch of the community. She spoke with pride and satisfaction about how she achieved that victory, instructing that it is important in life to stand up and fight for what is right.

When I asked her what gave her strength to face her illness with such dignity she replied, "Faith. I pray every day." She then showed me her Bible. It was placed on the coffee table next to her phone. She described how she was part of a community that would pray by telephone every day at an assigned time. She described this with purpose and appreciation. She felt that as long as she was true to God that God would have her back, and there could be nothing that she could not face.

Another thing that gave her joy, a secular pleasure this time, was working the jigsaw puzzles. Mrs. Black had quite a collection. "I get them at the second-hand store," she explained beaming with pride. "I can't afford to pay full price. Sometimes I can get one for as little as 60 cents. . . . But there will always be pieces missing." The missing pieces never deterred her as she would trace their shape onto the cardboard cover of the box, cut it out from where the color matched, and place it into the puzzle. One would never notice the difference because of her meticulous devotion to detail. For her, they were not just jigsaw puzzles; they were exquisite pieces of art. She took great satisfaction in showing them to me, and I thought to myself how many in mainstream society would ever have to face the challenge of finding something that gave them such great delight for 60 cents.

Mrs. Black spoke often of her granddaughter, doing so with a mixture of sentiment. She loved her and was proud of her for the progress she had made in turning her life around. Yet she also worried deeply about what was going to happen "when Grandma is no longer here." Mrs. Black was a realist and understood how sick she was, and was not secure in her attempts to put together a plan for Phoebe's future after she was gone. Mrs. Black also worried that one day she might die at home and that her granddaughter would have to suffer the shock of finding her dead body while she was alone and no one else around.

The experience of Mrs. Black is not only formed by chronic, intergenerational poverty, as was the life and death of Joe Noble; it is also shaped by being black in a society wherein racism and discrimination play a significant role in beleaguering people and undermining their worth. The deaths of her sons. The imprisonment of another. The struggles that Phoebe faced. The fact that her life was ending prematurely. These are all intrinsically associated with the experience of living as a black woman in one of America's urban ghettos. Her sufferings, real as they were invisible, were truly connected to race and poverty (Figures I.2 and I.3).

The conclusion of this brief snapshot of her life captures how unkind and cruel her life could be. Mrs. Black did die at home from congestive heart failure, and one of her greatest fears came true: the day she died, Phoebe, going into her grandmother's room to wake her up for the day, found her dead in bed.

To this day we don't know where Phoebe is or how she is doing.

Despite major institutional and political efforts to redress the historic injuries of racism, prejudice and discrimination against African Americans still persist. Their history is defined by pervasive trauma related to slavery and segregation. Presently, it is characterized by disproportionate poverty, social breakdown, continued bigotry, excess illness, and early death. There can be little debate that overall the black experience in

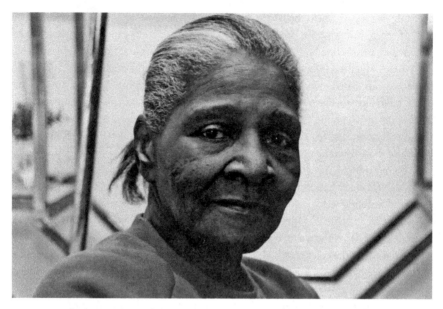

FIGURE I.2 The dignity of Mrs. Black.

America has been filled with tragedy and injury, resulting in harmful oppression and burdens that are difficult to comprehend unless one has suffered them personally.

When people are challenged in life by racial and economic barriers, those obstacles result in real hardship, as Mrs. Black's narrative reveals. In particular, many African Americans and urban poor live in a heightened state of alarm and apprehension in their daily lives. They are exposed to experiences that are unrecognizable in affluent areas of America—such as the terror of early death by drugs or violence that haunts a mother raising her children in a ghetto. This population is also especially susceptible to the early onset of disease and premature death, and commonly encounters limited access to healthcare. They get sick more often, more seriously ill, experience excess mortality, and receive suboptimal care.

While poverty and racial antagonism impact tens of millions of people, the actual harm they inflict is, more often than not, concealed from public awareness. The essential point is that there is, no matter how invisible it may be, enormous difficulty surrounding the lives of people who live at the margins of economic and racial exclusion. Ours is a culture that hesitates to recognize their struggles. Thus, to a large degree, they and their circumstances remain a matter of avoidance and insignificance.

> Few outside their world can imagine their challenges.

The experience of dying while living at the margins is influenced by many factors. First off—generally speaking, we live in a death-denying society. Dying and all that surrounds it are largely hidden from social perception. Heroic technological efforts are used to combat and prolong dying. Lengthy or public expressions of mourning have become

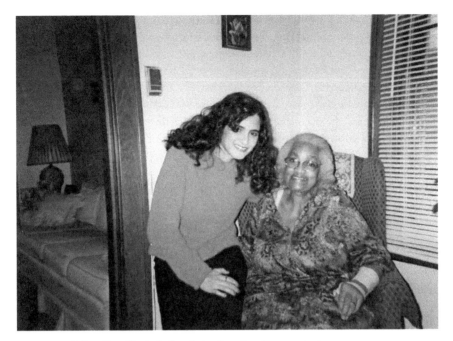

FIGURE I.3 Cultural humility is the foundation for culturally-competent care.

taboo, the experience of grieving becoming private and socially "invisible." In addition, the sufferings encountered by people throughout the end-of-life experience are hidden and not generally visible in daily life. Dying people generally are sequestered in private settings, such as a hospital or nursing home, disconnected from the interactions of main-stream activity in the broader culture. It is not only hard for dying persons and their immediate loved ones to face the realities that surround serious illness, their circumstances are discomforting for others to witness. This widespread unease adds to the unpleasant-ness that characterizes the contemporary dying experience and leads to it being pushed away from public conspicuity. The result is that dying persons and their immediate loved ones are at heightened risk for social isolation. In this framework of cultural denial, death is often fought against by aggressive technological interventions, which in themselves can exacerbate indignities and prolong suffering.

When the struggles that people face in the process of dying intersect with obstacles or obstructions related to racial and economic disengagement, the experience of dying can become even more difficult. If poverty and racism create difficulty throughout life, it only makes sense that they will create unique difficulties throughout the dying experience. Simply expressed, poverty, race, and dying are not hopeful or pleasing to think about. Therefore, it should not be surprising that the dying poor, and all of the issues that they are dealing with, are pushed to the margins of social awareness.

People—generally speaking, but especially in 21st-century America—prefer to sur-round themselves with things that are pleasant, enjoyable, and uplifting. There is a nat-ural aversion to dealing with that which is distasteful, makes us feel bad, or is difficult to observe. Confronting the realities of poverty, racism, or dying certainly doesn't uplift or inspire. So it is easier not to think about the suffering of people or why and how some people suffer unjustly in life, throughout sickness, and onto death. It really is an "out of sight, out of mind" approach to the problem, unawareness becoming a protective shield in this process of denial.

But this approach has consequences. When the lives of the dying poor are pushed to the periphery of social concern, their indignities and sufferings become broadly irrelevant. This detachment creates widespread unawareness of the poor's sufferings and difficulties, leaving their needs significantly unaddressed. It also deprives us of the opportunity to get to know them better, not just in their difficulties but in their strengths. When we do have the opportunity to enter into their lives we ourselves can become enriched by witnessing the amazing qualities they possess, qualities that provide resilience and enable them to get along in very harsh circumstances. By engaging their stories we arrive at a better appreciation of the richness and humanity of their lives. Listening to them and getting to know them a bit can increase empathy and compassion, despite the social and economic divide that separates them. It enables us to develop an appreciation of who they are beyond the stereotypes, gaining insight into their needs and how to better care for them.

Most of us see the poor only from a comfortable distance. Few outside their world can imagine their daily challenges. Social distance and separation obscure not only their sufferings, but the deep humanity that runs through their lives. In this disconnection—social, cultural, residential, as well as economic—their remarkable human qualities inclusive of their spirit, courage, and determination are hidden. But if we open ourselves to understanding the poor as human beings we learn to appreciate who they are with renewed understanding. When we listen to their stories, we observe a faith among many that is unshakable and how it serves as a source of guidance through difficulty in living and dying. We also notice the power of love being displayed in the most artful of ways. Despite being poor and suffering greatly because of it, many live a very rich life. In their stories, we see how faith and community become sources of strength for dealing with difficult situations. In this way, getting to know these folks up close and personal through "story listening" becomes a catalyst for generating insights we would otherwise not arrive at. Thus, as we gain exposure to them by bearing witness to their stories, we come to a greater regard for their lives.

In short, the suffering of the poor is exacerbated by inattention to and dismissal of their needs. On the other hand, if we take notice of them by paying attention to their stories we are led to an appreciation of their soulfulness, their humanity, and become observers of the fundamental goodness that defines much of who they are.

The purpose of this book is to provide a voice and face for these people who otherwise are often "voiceless" and "faceless." A further intention is to advance understanding of their unique needs and promote development of better practices in caring for them. Specifically, this book will connect the voices of the dying poor to the voices of leaders in end-of-life care. Throughout the various chapters, these providers will discuss issues that confront patients and loved ones, offering insights into improving their care and quality of their lives.

Their discussions will revolve around actual experiences of patients and family members as described in my previous work, *Dancing with Broken Bones: Poverty, Race, and Spirit-filled Dying in the Inner City*. The narratives in that book will be discussed with an eye toward deepening understandings about the needs of vulnerable populations, advocating for them, and developing best practices in caring.

My hope is that the concerns of patients and families will be amplified through this effort. Our collective goal is to stimulate deliberation, dialogue, and a call to action among healthcare providers and those in the broader society as well; a deliberation and dialogue that will lead to enhanced interest in serving the needs of those who live, struggle, and die at the margins.

If this book is successful, it will ultimately engender a sense of connection, perhaps even a sense of "oneness," between patients and their loved ones and ourselves. Theirs is a special story. Although filled with hardship and suffering, it yet is graced with spirit, courage, and resilience. I have no doubt that these patients and their loved ones will become our teachers if we are willing to let them. What they will teach is both disturbing and hopeful. On the troubling side, their stories illustrate a darker and more onerous reality of American life, one that is lived daily by tens of millions. They reveal the full range of struggles that the urban poor confront while dying, including pain, suffering, and indignities that are uniquely exacerbated by poverty. They expose the insidious afflictions of racism, and how its harm is intergenerationally transmitted. On a more hopeful note, however, they also illuminate strength and dignity, and profile the courage of people who live creatively and meaningfully in burdensome circumstances. It is this side of the story that gives understanding to why Mother Teresa once observed "The poor, I do not tire of repeating this, are wonderful." In her writings, she also goes on to warn against judging the poor because of how ugly and deplorable their lives may seem to us. She suggests that if we become distracted by the repellent aspects of their external lives, we will have little time left for understanding and loving them as people of a common humanity. Consistent with her teachings, my aspiration is that this book will also serve to unveil and reduce stereotypes, diminish harsh judgments, and cultivate compassionate concern for those who live at the margins of acceptance and desirability.

The innovative work of Robert Coles advances a framework of arriving at understanding of others and their lives. His method is grounded in active listening to their stories. Its cornerstone is letting the stories speak for themselves *au naturel*, so to speak, as opposed to employing organized interview techniques and methodologies that elicit structured responses. It is through attentive and mindful listening to stories, he advises, that we learn how to observe others with empathic understanding. Consistent with this approach, my intent is to advance "special observations" of and empathic connection with those marginalized in life and death by focusing attention on their narratives. It is a call to bear witness to them. It is to promote the proposition that, if we are to become truly serious about caring for the marginalized in life and death, we must begin by understanding the moral, social, and spiritual sensibilities of patients and loved ones as they are experienced within the social, cultural, and economic context of their lives. And that understanding must begin by listening to them describe their lives.

Speaking now together with my collaborators, our aspiration in this effort is that we all will join together in fueling discussion and development of innovative practices in caring for those near the end of life whose lives are impacted by poverty, discrimination, and injustice.

In his autobiography, William Carlos Williams once wrote:

The poem springs from the half-spoken words of . . . patients.

May the poetry that flows from the stories of the patients and loved ones as told in *Dancing with Broken Bones* and illuminated throughout this book, capture our attention and spark compassionate concern. May the insights contained within this work inspire us toward developing more kind, humane, and effective ways of caring for those living and dying at the margins.

While no book is the sole product of an individual author, that is especially true here. Without the collaborators' tireless dedication to advance the field of hospice and palliative care along with their concern to serve the under-served, the book you are now holding would never be possible. Deepest appreciation is extended to each and to all, as well my as admiration for their great work.

One's journey in life is never solitary. It is shaped by the guidance, mentoring, support, and love of others. I would like to acknowledge and embrace:

Aimee Yu—My Mickey Mantle: a great teammate.

Jan Clemons—For her relentless searching for the virtuous path and her courage to travel on it.

Mitch Schwartz and Barbara Jacobs—None of what we are doing would be possible without you.

Terry Walman—In admiration of you as a lifelong learner.

Barry Meisenberg—A luminary.

George Samaras—An exemplar of the art of caring for patients, and a doctor's doctor.

Mark and Joy McPhee —In memory of the sacred moments we shared.

Mary Sayres—May Red Sky shepherd you safely toward your dreams.

Dawn and Dewey-boy, Jessie and King Leo, and Valpolicella—For kindling my joyful spirit and capacity to laugh. We make one beautiful, dysfunctional family.

Brother Richard Connors—With gratitude for the indelible imprint you have made on my life.

Bobby and Bunny—You are loved.

Bink—Still.

Frank (Frankie-boy) Misiti—To the great times and amazing memories of a lifelong friendship.

Kenny-boy—Just because.

Bob Schwab—For your support and in honor of the possibilities for male friendship.

Tammy Wheeler—For her dedication to keeping me on track and for her success in doing so, most of the time.

Joyce Miller—In gratitude for your enduring love of books and a life of service in relation to them.

Pat Czapp—In honor of your devotion to serving the under-served.

I would also like to thank the team at Oxford University Press for their patience and devotion to the project.

And,

For those who shared their stories with me so as to make *Dancing with Broken Bones* possible—You live in my heart.

—David Wendell Moller
Annapolis, Maryland
July 2018

CONTRIBUTORS

Terry Altilio, LCSW, ACSW
Social Work Coordinator
Palliative Care Team
Mount Sinai Beth Israel
New York, NY

Robert Arnold, MD
Professor of Medicine
Chief, Section of Palliative Care and
    Medical Ethics
Director, Institute for Doctor–Patient
    Communication
Medical Director, Palliative and
    Supportive Institute
University of Pittsburgh, School of
    Medicine
Pittsburgh, PA

F. Amos Bailey, MD
Professor, Internal Medicine
Director, Master of Science in Palliative
    Care/Interprofessional Palliative Care
    Certificate
University of Colorado School of
    Medicine
Aurora, CO

Kimberly Curseen, MD
Associate Professor, Internal Medicine
Emory University School of Medicine
Emory Palliative Care Center
Atlanta, GA

Rachel Diamond, MD, MS
Assistant Professor, Palliative Care
Assistant Professor, Pediatric
    Palliative Care
University of Rochester Medical Center
Rochester, NY

**Betty R. Ferrell, PhD, MA, FAAN,
FPCN, CHPN**
Director and Professor
Division of Nursing Research and
    Education
Department of Population Sciences
City of Hope
Duarte, CA

Rev. Robin Franklin
Director, Chaplaincy Services
University of Rochester Medical Center
Strong Memorial Hospital
Rochester, NY

Gregory P. Gramelspacher, MD
Professor of Medicine
Associate Director, Hospice and Palliative
    Medicine Fellowship
Indiana University School of Medicine
Director, Palliative Care Program
Eskenazi Hospital
Indianapolis, IN

Richard Gunderman, MD, PhD
Professor and Vice Chairman
Department of Radiology
Indiana University School of Medicine
Indianapolis, IN

Diane Meier, MD
Professor, Geriatrics and Palliative Care
Icahn School of Medicine at Mount Sinai
The Mount Sinai Hospital
New York, NY

Shirley Otis-Green, MSW, MA, ACSW, LCSW, OSW-C
Founder and Consultant
Collaborative Caring
Toluca Lake, CA

Richard Payne, MD
Professor of Medicine
Esther T. Colliflower Professor Emeritus
Affiliate of the Duke Initiative for Science
    and Society
Member of the Duke Cancer Institute
Duke University School of Medicine
Durham, NC

Tammie E. Quest, MD
Director, Emory Palliative Care Center
Woodruff Health Sciences Center
Associate Professor
Department of Emergency Medicine
Division of Geriatrics and Gerontology
Emory University School of Medicine
Atlanta, GA

Timothy Quill, MD
Georgia and Thomas Gosnell
    Distinguished Professor of
    Palliative Care
Professor of Medicine, Psychiatry,
    Medical Humanities, and Nursing
University of Rochester School of
    Medicine
Rochester, NY

Christian T. Sinclair, MD, FAAHPM
Assistant Professor
Division of Palliative Medicine
University of Kansas Health System
Kansas City, KS

Stacie Sinclair, MA
Senior Policy Manager
Center to Advance Palliative Care
New York, NY

1

STRANGERS AMONG US
POVERTY, RACE, AND THE END OF LIFE

David Wendell Moller

Do not forget to show hospitality to strangers, for by doing so some people have entertained angels without knowing it.
—Hebrews 13:2

URBAN POVERTY AND MARGINALIZATION

Poverty is the worst form of violence.
—Mahatma Gandhi

I had just finished giving a talk at a national conference. The topic at hand was what it is like to live and die in urban poverty. Drawing on the oral and photographic narratives that appear in *Dancing with Broken Bones,* I crafted a portrait of the "invisible" world of the urban dying poor. The presentation described the tension-filled realities that shape their daily lives. It included descriptions of:

- The harsh and unrelenting indignities that surround living in poverty;
- The unique indignities that surround dying in poverty and intensify suffering for patients and loved ones;
- How anger, suspicion, mistrust, and poor communication often create a divide between providers and their inner-city patients;
- How and why some patients are especially grateful for the care they receive in the safety-net system;
- The sources of social support that sustain patients through the most difficult of circumstances;
- The power of faith in assisting patients and loved ones to face their struggles with unwavering resilience;
- How the "mindful presence" of a palliative care team that is dedicated to serving marginalized populations successfully transforms dying from a bleak and dismal experience into one of peace, comfort, and meaning.

My presentation concluded with a description of the end-of-life experience of "Cowboy." A major figure in *Dancing with Broken Bones,* Cowboy had lived as a "homeless" person for three years. I place "homeless" in quotes because if he had ever heard me refer to him as homeless he would have responded: "What you talkin' about? This tunnel under the bridge, which I call *'the cave,'* is where I live and **it is MY HOME.**" Okay, lesson learned: Cowboy, like many others throughout urban America, was at home on the street, and the street was his home. Referring to him as homeless was defining him from a stereotypical view that failed to understand who he was as a person within his world.

This part of the talk described how his intense sense of anger, that defined much of who he was, had its roots in the racism and poverty he endured as a boy in the Deep South. It also noted that his rage and irritability, ubiquitously expressed throughout his life as a coping mechanism, were fading as the love and patience of the palliative care team showed him another way. Rather than shutting down and rejecting them before he would be hurt, as was his pattern in dealing with people, he opened himself up to their caring presence. As a result, over the several months of his dying, he was finding a previously unknown sense of peace and meaning. And, for this, he became very grateful.

His spirit of gratitude was conveyed to the audience during the presentation. I explained that if Cowboy were still alive, he would express that appreciation directly to them and explicitly honor the work they do. He would tell them about its importance and how difficult it can be. He would also advise them not to lose themselves in the work and to "never forget to dance." As part of that appreciation, he would sing them some of his "favorite tunes," as he would put it. This tradition of singing in thanks for the care he received started one day in the coronary intensive care unit (CICU). He had suffered a heart attack in the middle of the night, and in the darkness, he crawled on hands and knees the length of "the cave" and up to street level for help. He was taken by ambulance to the safety-net hospital, where he was stabilized in the emergency department and then admitted into the hospital. The palliative care social worker, Linda, was a regular visitor to him while he was there, and he would sing her some of his favorite songs along with her requests.

I have no doubt that if Cowboy were alive and able to speak to the audience that day, he would have concluded his remarks by singing for them in a spirit of thankfulness. Since that was not possible, the next best thing would be for me to play a recording of him singing to Linda that day in the CICU, which I did. The sound quality of the tape recording was less than perfect. Yet his voice was melodic and soulful, clearly resonating with appreciation and love.

As the songs came to a finish, the final slide containing the words of Cowboy was displayed:

Thank you and thank you for what you do.

These were the words he would often say to the members of the palliative care team and to medical students and resident physicians who were his regular visitors in multiple settings: at the cave, when he was in the hospital, and then later on in the nursing home. So it was fitting for those to be the words that concluded the presentation.

After a moment of quiet, I turned to the audience for thoughts, questions, and reflections. A person in the back row raised his hand, identifying himself as a physician, and stated: "The poor you will always have with you."

Recognizing that this is a passage from the Bible, I anticipated that he was going to speak to the need for compassion and concern for the "least among us." To my surprise, he went in a very different direction. He went on to describe that many people from other countries have come to America, and by dint of hard work, have pulled themselves up by their own bootstraps. His point was that they became successful in building quality lives for themselves by drive and ambition. He spoke with enthusiasm about their ethic of personal responsibility and applauded them. Bringing his commentary back around to the presentation, he criticized the people portrayed in *Dancing with Broken Bones* as lacking ambition and moral character. He stated clearly and directly that these folks lived in the circumstances they do because of personal choice, bad decision-making, and irresponsibility. He was definitive and adamant in this view.

> The disadvantages of being born into and living in poverty make it especially difficult for the poor to rise above their circumstances by merely "pulling themselves up by their bootstraps."

I tried to explain that it is misguided to think that, like simply choosing one's favorite ice-cream flavor at Baskin Robbins, the poor "choose" the dismal circumstances of their lives. The last time I had checked, no one has ever desired to be born into poverty, whether it is in an inner-city ghetto or barrio or in sub-Saharan Africa. For people who are born into poverty—that is simply the hand that they have been dealt. I often describe this as their being "losers in the reproductive lottery of life." Why one child is born in the ghetto while another into the privilege and advantage of affluence is something we will never understand. But what is understandable is how the forces that surround a life begun and lived in poverty are both powerful and debilitating. The people in *Dancing with Broken Bones* experienced the incapacitating harm of poverty in both the rural and urban settings of America. These forces had a real impact on them, causing hardship from birth, throughout life, and on to dying.

I think it is fair to hark back to the words of Mother Teresa, which were noted in the Preface. They urged us to open our hearts with compassionate understanding of the poor rather than making severe judgments about them. This physician's words were, in my view, judgmental and regrettable; they seemed spoken with a lack of empathic understanding, let alone compassion.

Of course, individual choices in life do matter. But that physician's view misses an important point; namely, that poverty is an intractable social ill that does real harm and is embedded in the organization and structure of society. And it is the values, practices, and institutional arrangements of society that allow poverty to be so widespread and impair the lives of the people it touches.

There is no hiding the fact that wealth disparity is real, shockingly so. There are all kinds of statistics, tables, and charts that illustrate the disparity. But the actual harm of economic marginalization cannot be explained by statistics. Rather, it lies in its impact on actual human beings, whereby otherwise good and decent people are damaged by the life conditions that surround them. So, it does raise the question of why the disparity exists and how people wind up living lives of poverty-caused desperation in such an affluent country. Do we as a society on the whole just not care enough about them? The fact is that America has one of the highest rates of wealth disparity among all the advanced societies, and the poor continue to be present in substantial numbers. The corresponding reality is that the poor, including the one-in-five children who live in poverty, have become weaker and more disempowered in recent decades and there is relatively little concern for their plight in mainstream social or political dialogue. Their lives and associated sufferings are off the map, so to speak.

One of the most reliable predictors of success in life is the level of affluence one is born into. The connection between parental income and child success is strong. If one is born into poverty, it is likely that one will live out one's life in poverty. It is no secret that children and youth from lower socioeconomic backgrounds do poorly in school. They perform badly on standardized tests, are less likely to graduate from high school or college, and are less likely to develop skills that will make them competitive economic earners. In many ways their chances in life are severely damaged before they even start. The result is that those who are born into poverty are quite likely to remain in the bottom income bracket throughout their lives and thereby are 'destined' to suffer the hardships of life in poverty.

Putting it simply, the disadvantages of being born into and living in poverty make it especially difficult for the poor to rise above their circumstances by merely "pulling themselves up by their bootstraps." On the other hand, the practical and material ease that accompanies being born into affluence provides an automatic foundation for building a life of achievement and advancement. It provides a clear head start in life. The affluent life may not be free from pressures that strain and stress. But those pressures are far removed from the struggle to survive and get along in everyday life. Few can imagine the overwhelming difficulty of living as a family of four on under $25,000 a year. Or, how about an individual struggling to survive on $15,000 a year? Even with the assistance that is provided by government and private programs, the struggle to keep things together is enormous. It creates worry and insecurity. It haunts. It impels people to find relief and escape; sometimes doing so in less than healthy ways. It compromises development of the whole person and correspondingly decimates self-esteem and wellness for both individuals and families.

> The poor do not choose to be born into their circumstances. Who would?

From a moral and humanitarian perspective, the suffering and struggle that are a part of living in poverty are tethered to social injustice. While the physician at the presentation might be correct in noting that the poor will always be with us, it is important to note that, in so many ways, the poor, while **"with us"** are not **"of us."** They live cast aside into a disenfranchised netherworld of hardship and daily struggle that Michael Harrington defined decades ago as "the other America."[1] Frankly, and from my perspective sadly, that physician's view is consistent with the majority of Americans' thinking about the poor; namely, that the poor are lazy, irresponsible, alcohol abusers, drug seekers, and living contentedly off the welfare system. This view is one that declares that the poor are poor because of their own personal deficiencies. So, shame on them. And an unexpressed corollary to this view is "let them suffer, it's their own doing!"

An essential counter point is that we cannot separate poverty from the prevailing structures which control our economic, social, and political system; a system that does permit, and dare I say, even promotes inequality. Thus, in this view, living poor is not a matter of preference or personal deficiency. It is directly tethered to class, culture, and opportunity structure. These are the core factors that create and perpetuate the circumstances of the poor's lives. The prevailing cultural view, however, often cultivates a negative, stereotypical, and judgmental view of the poor and "how they live." While this is exactly the perspective that was expressed by the previously noted physician, clearly he is not alone in his view. He was stating an attitude about the poor and poverty that is commonplace. Perhaps it is also one that is self-serving in that if the poor are to be blamed, then the rest of us remain blameless and guilt free, "off the hook," so to speak.

Again, I want to reiterate: the poor do not choose to be born into their circumstances. Who would? They do not wish upon themselves the restricted opportunities that are present from the moment of their birth. They are not desirous of the hopelessness, broken spirit, or blocked opportunities that create their adverse childhood experiences and literally have a fracturing impact on body, mind, and soul.

Are some individuals fortunate enough to overcome being born into poverty? Yes, of course they are. But the point to be made is that *most cannot and do not*. It boils down to the issue of control of one's destiny. For most people who live in poverty, it is unrealistic to expect that they will be able to control their future the way more-affluent people do. Pulling oneself up by the bootstraps is an attractive platitude that resonates with the longstanding American value of self-reliance. But those boots in reality are far more likely to be mired in the quicksand of restricted and unequal opportunity than they are of travelling on a pathway out of poverty. Surviving the day is the immediate concern of the poor. Enduring the harshness, boredom, and dismal environment of daily life often leads to a focus on immediate circumstances, not long-term planning. Sometimes the immediacy is shaped by making hard decisions between providing for food, or medical care, or housing. Other times it may be driven by the desire to find a temporary escape from the misery. But the reality is that an empowered sense of control over the future is not readily a part of the opportunity structure of living poor (Figure 1.1).

Thus, for most people who are born into poverty, it is unrealistic to expect that they will find a way out. Horatio Alger–type narratives of rags to riches are popular in that they make us feel good about things. They allow a victim-blaming ethos to explain away the poor's unfortunate circumstances. They blame them for being poor and cultivate a stereotype that they remain poor because of personal deficiency and deviance. This perspective identifies the source of the problem as being within individuals and families, who are said to lack the ambition and personal qualities that would enable them to succeed. They themselves are to blame for their inability to move out and on up. That is the way the story goes—in part because it makes the rest of us feel better about the existence and ugliness of poverty. This view also reduces the perceived need for huge efforts in re-structuring our society to make it fairer and more just, which serves to the status quo and the vested interests that it serves.

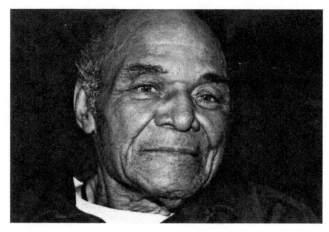

FIGURE 1.1 A lifetime of struggle against poverty and racism never dampened Jessie's spirit or love of life.

In this framework, feel-good stories of those who climb out of poverty and do miraculous things with their lives are touted as a measuring rod for all the poor. "If they can do it, you can, too," the criticism charges. It is comforting to hear the stories of those who climb out of poverty into success. These stories become captivating and inspirational and are synchronistic with the American value of rugged individualism. The danger, however, lies in the tendency to establish these individualized success stories as the backdrop and standard by which all those who are born into poverty are judged. This attitude, however, fails to recognize the existence of obstacles that weigh the poor down and for the most part keep them there.

> While the poor are "with us" they are really not "of us."

Two interrelated points are critical here: (1) The poor have a startling and disproportionately tiny part of America's income, and (2) correspondingly, they have little control over their lives. As a result, every day they confront conditions that make it impossible for them to walk the same path as the rest of us[2] and for the rest of us to have capacity to walk in their shoes as well. The latter point becomes a seedbed for misunderstanding and indifference, which has consequences for how the poor are treated not only throughout life, but also during the illness experience.

In this regard, the poor truly are strangers among us. Simply stated, to be poor in America is not only to be disadvantaged. It is to be different in a negative way.

For this reason, the more we can develop understanding about the tribulations of living in poverty, the more empathy and sympathy we will have for the poor. Many of the conditions that affect their lives each and every day are hard for the non-poor to relate to. For example, it is difficult for those who are more empowered and affluent to understand the impact of what the poor face regularly:

- Lack of private transportation and utter reliance on public transportation to shop, get to work, go to the doctor's office, etc.[3,4] And if private transportation might be available, it is often unreliable, subject to regular breakdown, and a drain on finances;
- School systems that are inadequately staffed, chaotic in daily operations, produce few marketable skills, and lead to disproportionate rates of dropout and "functional illiteracy;"[5]
- Persistent underemployment, unemployment, and discrimination during job searches;
- Sub-optimal access to healthcare;
- Inaccessibility of chain supermarkets in the inner city where healthy foods—fresh fruits, vegetables, fish, etc.—can be found. Instead, fast food choices are abundant, along with ever-present access to liquor stores. Lack of options for exercise prevail;
- Neighborhoods that are filled with substandard housing, which are often unsafe, and in which children go to sleep at night hearing the sounds of gunshots and are socialized into a culture wherein drug use is pervasive.

It is fair, once again, to ask: who would ever choose to be born into these circumstances?

In fact, the contrast between this America and the America that is not poor is striking. Consider the advantages of being born into a world of greater affluence and empowerment, which include:

- Private transportation and multiple cars in many families, often equipped with the latest technology for safety, comfort, and reliability (not to mention status!);
- Schools that are strongly supported by the local community. Many school districts become selling points for people moving into particular neighborhoods and communities. These schools are far more resourced than inner-city schools, the benefit of a better education accruing to the students;
- Access to the best doctors, hospitals, dentists, and other health-promoting practitioners such as chiropractors, acupuncturists, yoga instructors, and massage therapists;
- Prospects for living that, even during times of financial downturn as experienced in the beginning of the 21st century, are never threatened nearly as much as the daily lives of the poor are. During times of economic upturn, the disparity is especially glaring; opportunity for employment is demonstratively greater;
- Options for healthy living abound in more-affluent neighborhoods. Green space and parks are available for exercise. Grocery stores stock healthy foods and dot the neighborhood landscape with the freshest and healthiest possible choices;
- Neighborhoods that are safe and are filled with homes that are comfortable and pleasant to be in.

This is a night-and-day contrast. The benefits of being born into more affluent circumstances are obvious and provide an instant advantage in the so-called competitive footrace of life, while being born poor not only creates disadvantage, it systematically beats people down.

Although poverty in the United States is not as extreme as in some other parts of the world, America's poor do suffer disproportionate hardship. One critical indicator and consequence of this hardship is the ill health of the poor. It is well documented that the more affluent a person is, the more likely they are to be healthy and live longer. On the other hand, the less income people have, the more likely they are to get sick, get seriously sick, and die prematurely. The data are well established and document that disparities in health related to income hold true for almost all risk factors, diseases, and causes of death. These income-related disparities even persist within ethnic and racial groups.

In particular, poor people are more likely to have risk factors such as smoking,[6] obesity,[7] and sedentary lifestyle.[8] Several factors are of special interest here. One is the notion of "food insecurity." When one faces deprivation in life related to poverty, unemployment, and low household assets, access to nutritional food as noted is restricted, creating nutritional vulnerability. The prevalence of this situation, which has been called food insecurity, throughout the nation is significant. In 2014[9]:

- 48.1 million Americans lived in food-insecure households, including 32.8 million adults and 15.3 million children;
- 14% of all households (17.4 million) were food insecure;
- Households with children reported food insecurity at a significantly higher rate than those without children;
- Food insecurity exists in every county in the United States.

In addition, poor Americans are less likely to go to the doctor or have an annual health screening, the result of which is that they are more likely to wind up in a health crisis that sends them to the emergency department and for subsequent hospitalization.[10] In short, people who live in poverty have higher incidence of disability, chronic illness, mental distress, and excess death than those in higher income groups.

Poverty is significant on a personal level, causing hardship in the lives of those it touches (Figure 1.2). It is also significant on a societal level in terms of incidence and

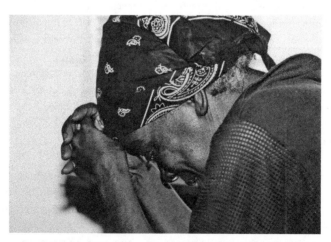

FIGURE 1.2 Despite living poor, Ms. Lilly approached the end of her life with unfaltering faith and dignity.

prevalence. This means that the issue we are discussing is not an isolated factor in American life affecting just a few. So, for example, again in 2014[11]:

- 46.7 million people lived in poverty;
- 21.1% of children lived in poverty;
- 10% of all seniors over 65 lived in poverty.

This is a lot of people. Especially given that America touts itself as the most advanced, prosperous, and exceptional country in the world. In an address before the US Senate Finance Committee, Warren Buffet, the second-wealthiest man in the United States behind Bill Gates, described this situation as the emerging dominance of dynastic wealth and the associated decline of equality of opportunity.[12] In simple terms, this means that wealth is highly concentrated in a relatively few hands: the top 1% control about 35% of America's wealth and the top 2% own a total of 80%. This leaves a staggering reality that a mere 20% of the total wealth of the nation is distributed among the bottom 80%.[13-15]

The point is that inequality is entrenched in the American landscape. Yet, despite the widespread presence of the poor, the poor are not especially visible throughout the culture. They are part of the "other America," not just because of a general lack of spatial proximity. Rather, their "otherness" also lies in cultural estrangement. This estrangement often leaves them "faceless" and "voiceless," and their needs reduced to a regrettable level of societal indifference. As suggested previously, while the poor are "with us," they are not really "of us." That is to say, they may be physically present, but they remain culturally and socially marginalized. Their presence in terms of numbers is large, and their sufferings are undeniably harsh. Yet, despite the prevalence of poor individuals and families, authentic interest in them and their circumstances remains disproportionately small. It is fair to say that this cultural disconnect inevitably leads to inadequate understandings about the poor, who they are, why they are poor, and what their needs are.

The poor, "ever with us but not of us," invite our attention in often negative ways. They inspire complicated feelings that include pity, fear, guilt, shame, revulsion, and anger. These feelings often lead to uninformed judgments, negative stereotyping, and blaming them for being and remaining poor. All of these factors push poverty and the individuals who live in it to a place of social obscurity.

That is not to say that the poor and their circumstances are entirely disregarded. There are pockets of discussion, interest, and concern for their difficulties and some concern about the broader social problem of poverty. For example, there were many points of chaos that defined the presidential primaries and general election for president in 2016. But one especially unanticipated development was the resonance that the voice of Senator Bernie Sanders gained in declaring how the gap between rich and poor has grown to unprecedented size. It is also fair to point out that the worth of the poor is not entirely disparaged in American culture. In some important ways, they have provided fertile foundation for literary creativity. Gems such as Steinbeck's *The Grapes of Wrath* and *Cannery Row,* Walker's *The Color Purple,* Sinclair's *The Jungle,* and O'Henry's *The Gift of the Magi* provide memorable descriptions of the inhumanity of poverty. On a grassroots level, in particular, inventive programs have been established to minimize the impact of poverty. These achievements have been the result of the dedicated efforts of individuals who care about social justice and the human suffering it generates. Ironically, as the poor serve as a constituency for some social and political advocacy groups, they also serve as a source of income for those who work in the social-services sector. Furthermore, the poor, and this includes many undocumented immigrants, perform menial tasks for minimum pay that add to the profit of business owners and insure that unpleasant but necessary work gets done.

This said, however, the poor for the most part remain off the radar screen of the broader society and are largely relegated to a place of cultural "invisibility." There is a natural human and cultural tendency to look away when we are confronted with distasteful and discomforting things. So it is not unusual that a significant part of American society "looks away," averting eyes to avoid seeing the poor and their struggles. For example, we drive past "bad" neighborhoods with windows up and doors locked, typically giving little thought to the people who live in them. When avoidance becomes impossible and the poor do become visible, they can often become a source of exasperation and annoyance. Part of the irritation that they elicit may very well be rooted in how poverty violates core American values such as equality of opportunity, the ethic of hard work, freedom of choice, materialism, and individualism. For this reason, the poor are not just denigrated as economic failures but also as moral failures. In this regard, as previously noted, they are viewed as the cause of their own predicament.

It is striking how little effort is exerted toward fighting poverty, but it is understandable. In a culture that defines the poor as morally inferior, it makes sense in a sad way that interest in addressing their problems would not be a societal priority. So, the dominant tendency is to disengage as much as possible from the realities of poverty through an attitude of general indifference. It is critical to note that the prevailing societal view toward the poor stands in stark contrast to claims of American exceptionalism and the Judeo-Christian values of civility, compassion, and respect for life. To be plain spoken about it, there is nothing compassionate, respectful, civil, or dignified about poverty's pervasive existence in a land of abundance; nor is there kindness in the harsh and pejorative view that stigmatizes and diminishes the human worth of the poor. In short, it is not pressing too far to suggest that the widespread and unabated persistence of poverty in America is far more a moral failure of society itself than the individual moral failings of the more than 46 million people who are subjected to living in it.

Thus, as long as the poor are continued to be judged as moral failures, and that view is perpetuated by Horatio Alger–type exceptions, they will remain fixed within boundaries that separate them from mainstream culture—economically, socially, and politically. As a result, the poor, ever with us, will remain isolated and outcast as "strangers among us."

WORLDS APART: THE PERSISTING RACIAL DIVIDE

I wish I could say that racism and prejudice were only distant memories. . . . We must dissent from the indifference. We must dissent from the apathy. We must dissent from the fear, the hatred, and the mistrust. . . . We must dissent because America can do better, because America has no choice but to do better.
—Thurgood Marshall (Liberty Medal acceptance speech, 1992)

Race is another factor that shapes and marginalizes the experience of people in life and in dying. It is not the biologically determined facts of race that are relevant here. Rather, it is the socially-crafted patterns of prejudice and discrimination that dehumanize people because they belong to a particular race. In many ways, as Americans tend to turn away from facing the injustices associated with poverty, the insidious consequences of racial hatred are also avoided and pushed to the periphery. Although Americans are aware of the historical realities of slavery and segregation, there is little enthusiasm for examining the ways in which racism continues to be a social problem. Justice Marshall spoke the opening words of this section during his Liberty Medal acceptance speech in 1992. Decades later, it is fair to ask in reflecting upon his lament: Have we meaningfully dissented, and is America doing better? While the history of race relations in America is complicated, and reflects meaningful progress in social policy and law, race remains a divisive and fracturing element of life in America today. Racial antagonisms continue to hold an incendiary place in cultural life, and continue to create real harm for real people. For sure, the manner in which both race and poverty injured the patients whose end-of-life stories are told in *Dancing with Broken Bones* suggest that the answer to Justice Marshall is not really, or at least not entirely. Racial divide continues to disunite Americans, creating a different experience for what it means to live as a white and black person.

The first slaves arrived on American soil before the creation of this country. They came against their will over 400 years ago, arriving in Virginia in the year 1619. They were exploited in brutal fashion for economic gain, their humanity being systematically obliterated by their owners and the system that permitted them to be owned as property. Two hundred and forty years later, the Confederacy was formed, the Southern states seceded to protect the sovereignty of the system that protected their "right" to own slaves and to fight against the repression of that "right," and the Civil War began in 1861. Two years later, in 1863, Lincoln's Emancipation Proclamation declared, "all persons held as slaves . . . shall be then, thenceforward, and forever free." While there was strong cultural and political resistance to the freeing of the slaves, Lincoln's proclamation established formal legal freedom that, to this day, has not been fully accompanied by freeing black people from the pain of bigotry and racial hatred. Sometimes this pain is experienced in subtle and nuanced ways. Other times it is egregiously obvious. In either case, it remains a part of the black experience in American society.

Thus, although the Civil War led to the abolishment of slavery, its aftermath was defined by a long, winding, contentious, and conflict-ridden struggle in which America sought to reconcile the historical existence of slavery, forge a new identity, and find its soul. Just a select and brief overview of this journey illustrates how difficult and torturous that process was and remains even today, further confirming Justice Marshall's observation that racism and prejudice are not a vestige of times past but also play out contemporaneously in American life. They are relevant in deep and life-impacting ways to the experiences of so many African Americans—as they made their ways from slavery, to tenant farming, and on to northern migrations where they faced continued racism and blocked opportunities.

It is worth taking a moment to look at a historical snapshot of the tension-filled journey to define the soul of America around race, paying attention to how the evolution of American society was clearly and deeply influenced by racial antagonism (Box 1.1).

Box 1.1 Institutional Progress on Race: A Timeline Snapshot of Uneven Progress and Cultural Resistance

- 1808: Congress bans the importation of slaves from Africa (though the practice continued);
- 1839: Slaves being transported on the ship *Amistad* revolt;
- 1849: Escaped slave Harriet Tubman becomes a leading figure in the Underground Railroad;
- 1857: *Dred Scott* Supreme Court decision declares Congress cannot ban slavery and that slaves are not citizens;
- 1865: Southern states enact postwar "black codes," the purpose of which was to restrict the activities of "freed" blacks and coerce them into poorly compensated labor;
- 1868: The XIV Amendment is passed and gives full citizenship to ALL citizens born in the United States (nullifies the *Dred Scott* decision);
- 1870: Blacks are given the right to vote by the XV Amendment (most Southern blacks remained disenfranchised by state-imposed obstacles such as voting fraud, poll taxes, and literacy tests);
- 1881: Spelman College is founded as the Atlanta Baptist Female Seminary in the basement of an Atlanta church;
- 1896: *Plessy v. Ferguson* upholds the doctrine of "separate but equal," declaring the constitutionality of racial segregation and setting the foundation for the development of Jim Crow laws (Jim Crow was not a person but was a character in a minstrel show, and was used as a term that referred to a wide-ranging set of laws ranging from the later 1800s to mid-1960s that oppressed and repressed black Americans);
- 1924: The number of active members in the KKK is estimated to be between 5 and 6 million;
- 1932: "The Tuskegee Study of Untreated Syphilis in the Negro Male" begins;
- 1947: Jackie Robinson is signed by Branch Rickey of the Brooklyn Dodgers, breaking the color barrier in major league baseball;
- 1947: Penicillin becomes standard treatment for syphilis. Participants in the Tuskegee Experiment are NOT offered the treatment;
- 1948: President Truman officially integrates the US armed forces (blacks had been serving in every major war prior to integration);
- 1952: Malcolm X officially is confirmed as a minister of the Nation of Islam and goes on to become an influential leader and agitator for black rights and empowerment;
- 1954: *Brown v. Topeka Board of Education* declares racial segregation is not constitutional;
- 1957: The Southern Leadership Conference is established by Martin Luther King and several others;
- 1960: The "Greensboro Four" begin a sustained sit-in at a segregated Woolworth's lunch counter in North Carolina. Six months later, they are served lunch at the same counter, as sit-ins and protests spread to other towns throughout the region;

- 1963: Martin Luther King is arrested and jailed during an anti-segregation protest and pens his famous "Letter from Birmingham Jail" advocating for nonviolent protest;
- 1964: President Lyndon Baines Johnson signs the Civil Rights Act;
- 1965: Malcolm X is assassinated;
- 1967: Race riots decimate Detroit and Newark;
- 1968: Thurgood Marshall is appointed to the Supreme Court, becoming the first black Supreme Court Justice;
- 1968: *Loving v. Virginia* is a landmark civil rights decision in which the Supreme Court invalidates laws prohibiting interracial marriage;
- 1972: The Tuskegee Experiment ends after 40 years of unethical practice;
- 1982: Race riots sweep across Los Angeles after white police officers are acquitted in the Rodney King beating incident;
- 1995: The O. J. Simpson trial illustrates how deeply divided Americans still are along racial lines;
- 2001: Colin Powell becomes the first African-American Secretary of State;
- 2008: Barack Obama become the first African-American President of the United States;
- 2014: Racial protests sweep across Ferguson, Missouri, after the grand jury refuses to bring an indictment in the killing of Michael Brown. Racial antagonisms surface throughout the nation;
- 2016: Racial protests and violence spread around the country as killings in Dallas, Baton Rouge, and Minnesota renew visibility of America's racial divide. Racial unease persists and Black Lives Matter becomes a unifying and divisive force in the continuing American struggle with racism;
- 2017: Donald Trump becomes president of the United States;
- 2017: Charlottesville, Virginia, erupts in racial conflict wherein the KKK, white supremacists, and neo-Nazis gather in solidarity to protest the removal of a statue of Robert E. Lee;
- 2017: The cover of *Time* magazine (August 17) carries the title "Hate in America," and inside, various essays describe the persistence of racial bigotry in the country.

It is also important to keep in mind that this history continues to impact African Americans throughout the nation in both urban and rural settings, and in profound ways that are both privately and publicly experienced.

Every time I review the history of race in America, I am stunned by how cruel and epic the journey of black people has been. It is important to remember that real people—individuals, children, families—were subjected to the most inhumane and cruel practices. There was real and extreme suffering for countless numbers. I find it interesting that sometimes America's fascination with the Civil War—the battlefield recreations, the elevations of generals to hero status, the memorabilia, the memorials that have been erected—has been oblivious to how deep and agonizing that suffering was for so many. It is also critical to point out that although laws have changed the role of race in society, especially in regard to the way institutions function, moral injuries and wrongdoings of racism continued to persist. In any kind of survey of the state of race and race relations in America, it is hard to escape the conclusion that America is still steeped in pain, anger, frustration, confusion, and chaos in grappling with racial issues.

There is also fundamental disagreement about whether race matters. On one hand, there are those who deny that skin color is a matter of consequence anymore. Despite the existence of tremendous inequalities, they reject the idea that racism against blacks still holds sway over American attitudes and behaviors. They might even point to a swinging of the pendulum that provides preferential treatment to racial minorities, through affirmation action or preferential admissions for college. On the other side are those who point to the actual existence in society of prejudices, stereotypes, and unequal treatment. This latter view can be readily gleaned from the narratives in *Dancing with Broken Bones*. They illustrate how the injuries stemming from racial prejudice and discrimination, particularly when they intersect with poverty, are in fact passed on from generation to generation. These stories have their roots in slavery and tenant farming, but also show how the legacy of America's racial maleficence remains relevant in the 21st Century. The practices of hatred and discrimination, which eviscerated the human worth of black people throughout history, still take a toll on the psychic identity of individuals, families, and communities. Simply put, they elicit negative judgments of a human being based upon skin color, affecting the way people are treated.

> Have countless white people laughed at jokes that denigrate and humiliate black people? (Have you? Regrettably, I must admit that I have.)

Thus, there is no denying the fact that black experience in America today is shaped by the legacy of slavery. There is no escaping the historical memories of the Ku Klux Klan, lynchings, the anguish of being defined as less than fully human, the realities of poverty that overwhelmed individuals, families, and communities, and the culturally-induced stereotypes that belittled black people.

The institutional and cultural history of America is clear: America came to economic greatness and political power in the midst of structural racism and inequality. While it is easier to think of America's racist tendencies as an artifact of history, the undeniable reality is that racial disconnect continues to exist throughout American society. Pondering a few simple questions, I believe, illustrates the point:

- Is it different to be black in America?
- Do African Americans have a heightened fear and mistrust of the police?
- Are blacks more likely to be judged or thought of differently because of the color of their skin?
- Are blacks thought of and judged by stereotypes?
- Is an African American more likely to arouse suspicion while driving or shopping in a department store, for example, independent of personal and professional achievements because of the color of his or her skin?

- Have countless white people laughed at jokes that denigrate and humiliate black people? (Have you? Regrettably, I have to admit I have.)
- Are people who are African American more likely to be feared because of their skin color?
- Does racial profiling exist?
- Does white privilege exist?
- Is the existence of violence against blacks visible on cell phones and social media across the nation and do these images heighten fear throughout the African-American community?
- Do the history and present-day realities of violence against African Americans negatively affect their well-being and their capacity to trust in the "system?"
- Is being black in America associated with negative outcomes for health and mistrust of the healthcare system?
- Does mistrust of the healthcare system impact end-of-life experience for African Americans?

It is hard, dare I say even impossible, to honestly answer these questions in the negative. The continuing reality is that race matters and suggestions that it doesn't misrepresent the realities that impact the everyday life experiences of African Americans. In crafting a single declarative statement summarizing what is represented here, I would offer something like this:

African Americans have a differentiated experience in American society, wherein they are judged because of their skin color. Historically and presently, black people are seen and judged as less than fully human or worthy. (At their core, racist jokes belittle their humanity, don't they? And perhaps the word "n*****" does it most injuriously of all, whether being used in joke telling or the spewing of hate. It is, after all, a word designed to cut people off at the knees and diminish their worth.) These perceptions underlie racial profiling, which leads to heightened fear of the police along with widespread mistrust and anger within black America. The experience of being black is associated with negative consequences for well-being and health. It also associates with less-than-optimal peace and dignity near the end of life that is in part connected to a deeply rooted mistrust of the medical system.

The health disparities of African Americans are well established. While there is no simple explanation for the disparity, the following data declare how significant it is. To be black in America is to have[16]:

- 60% increase in prevalence of diabetes;
- 2.5 times the rate of maternal death;
- 9 times the prevalence of HIV; 8 times the associated mortality rate;
- 2 times the rate of prostate cancer;
- 40% increase in mortality from breast cancer;
- 40% increase in mortality from stroke;
- 30% increase in mortality from heart disease;
- 40% increase in prevalence of obesity;

- 2 times the rate of infant mortality;
- 2 times the prevalence of sudden infant death syndrome (SIDS);
- 73% increase in prevalence of obesity in children;
- 30% increase in rate of attempted suicide among high schoolers.

There are myriad factors which contribute to these disparities. They include genetics, environment, income disparities, lifestyle, and cultural factors. While it is beyond the scope of the effort here to engage a comprehensive discussion of the factors that underlie health inequality among African Americans, an important take-home point is that there is unmistakable increase in morbidity and mortality for African Americans and that this race-based health disparity is exacerbated when it commingles with poverty.

In summary, the simple point to be made about a profoundly complex issue is that those challenged by racial and economic barriers are more likely to get sick, become seriously sick, and die sooner than those who are not similarly challenged. And they are less likely to receive the kind of healthcare that could improve the quality of their lives.

ANOTHER UNMENTIONABLE: DYING IN A CULTURE OF DENIAL

Death remains one of life's greatest mysteries. For centuries, theologians and philosophers have sought to provide insight into the human encounter with death and to demystify it. These attempts have offered explanations that range from nihilism to existentialism, and on to religiously and spiritually constructed belief systems in an afterlife. On an individual level, whether confronting one's own mortality or witnessing that of a loved one, death variously provokes wonder, fear, worry, hope, and anxiety. Even among the most faithful believers in life after death, the prospects of dying and being dead often elicit dread and fright. This fear has both instinctive and sociocultural roots.

Indeed, it is the capacity to reflect upon death, becoming self-aware and expressive about it, that is a uniquely human ability. The desire and need to find ways of explaining death—to make some sense of it—may be innate to being human, but the ways in which that is done are variable and reflect the prevailing folkways of a given historical era.

In some immutable ways, humans are pre-wired to avoid death. Anyone who has been in a close-call accident situation is familiar with the overwhelming sensation of fear that automatically arises. This instinctive fear of death is also reflected in the terror experienced by soldiers going into battle, the sense of alarm that accompanies the onset of a heart attack, or the disquiet aroused by a cancer diagnosis. It is safe to say that this fear is both ancient and primal. From an evolutionary perspective, it may be viewed as functional in that it has a chilling effect on participating in life-risking behaviors. Ironically, in this regard, the fact of death itself may be seen as life-affirming. But on an individual level, the fears that surround death and dying can become a source of extreme psychological distress related to:

- Fear of the unknown; of not knowing what is on the other side of earthly life;
- Fear of not being, of non-existence, of personal extinction;
- Fear of loss and physical devolution;

- Fear of pain and unrelieved suffering;
- Fear of punishment in an afterlife;
- Anger over separation from life—its beauty, its pleasures, and its joys;
- Worry about what will happen to loved ones afterward;
- Regret for the way one has lived; of wishing for a second chance or a "do-over" to get things right.

The point to be made is that facing the end of life is a huge and difficult thing for humans to do.

Denial of death is also embedded in the prevailing folkways of everyday life.

Ernest Becker connects the human capacity for awareness of mortality to beliefs and practices that seek to deny the inevitably of death. He specifically explores humanity's fear of death and describes how societies create "defense mechanisms" to cope with that fear. His main contention is that death is so threatening to human equanimity that societies construct elaborate mechanisms of denial in order to cope with the disruption of the "serene and ordinary" which is brought about by death. The fear, he argues, is so deep and powerful that it gives rise to the development of personal and societal constructs of denial. As he notes:

> the idea of death, the fear of it, haunts the human animal like nothing else; it is a mainstream of human activity—activity designed largely to avoid the fatality of death, to overcome it by denying in some way that it is the final destiny for man.[17]

His take on the issue is that the terror of death is universal and is intrinsically and instinctively etched into humanity and the fact of being human. As a result, the fears surrounding death lead to denial as a protective defense mechanism. The essential point is that the terror of death prompts systematic denial of its inevitability and/or ultimate power to end life. It was La Rochefoucauld who commented that neither death nor the sun can be looked at steadily. To be human is to desire to live and be well. Death heartlessly eliminates life. In its wake it leaves humans unsettled, trying to find ways of explaining, adapting, and coping with loss. So, it is in the midst of fears that humanity seeks transcendence. According to Becker, we do so by creating cultural symbols and practices aimed at denial in one form or another. Denial becomes a means of coping with the "uncopable." He defines these practices of denying death as "heroic," inasmuch as they offer a means of transcendence and control over the ultimately uncontrollable. After all, in a sense, the hero is one who summons the strength to stand up to death and does not quiver in its presence:

> We admire most the courage to face death; we give such valor our highest and most constant adoration; it moves us deeply in our hearts because we have doubts about how brave we ourselves would be. When we see a man bravely facing his own extinction we rehearse the greatest victory we can imagine. And so the hero has been

the center of human honor and acclaim since probably the beginning of specifically human evolution.[18]

Who is the hero in this view? On an individual level, it is the person who steadfastly looks death in the eye and does not flinch. This may be the soldier who serves magnificently in battle, setting aside his fears for the sake of the mission. Or it may be a deeply religious or spiritual person who is calm and peaceful on her deathbed, comforted and sustained by an abiding belief in that she will live eternally after physical death. Modern medicine and its curative abilities may be relied upon by patients and families in a hope that technology can reverse or postpone death in "heroic" fashion.

Speaking about a broader context of societal denial, Becker describes the existence of what he terms "a hero system." This is the institutionalization of personal heroism; that is to say, a normative or societal standing up to death—through folkways, rituals, and institutional practices. Each society, in its own unique ways, establishes such systems, in ways that are consistent with its own culture. While different in form and style, these hero systems all aspire to mitigate the threat of death and to help secure social and personal stability during its occurrence.

It may be that the system is formed by practices that are magical, primitive, or religious. On the other hand, it may be modern, secular, and scientifically grounded.[19] An example of the former would be religiously based beliefs that promise an afterlife. These beliefs, and the rituals that support them, ease the sting of death by denying its finality. It asserts a view supported by organizational doctrine and dogma that promise life everlasting. And it is through this system of beliefs and practices that death is "defeated," as it is rendered impermanent and gives way to resurrection. This religiously based transcendence offers a means of maintaining hope and strength in the face of loss. It asserts that death has no final power over us and questions, "O Death, where is thy sting?"

Secular forms of heroism can be found in advanced medical technology or cultural practices that render dying "invisible" in daily life. In the high-technology setting, the armamentarium of modern medicine is used to fight against and stave off death. The all-too-familiar stories of battling against disease in intensive care units (ICUs) across America, sometimes at every stage of the disease and at great human and financial expense, are reflective of a cultural practice relied upon to combat death or at least delay it. The appeal of using technology to fight against death is found in the popularity of TV doctor shows, in which aggressive life-saving procedures are commonplace. It is interesting to note, for example, that on TV CPR is far more successful in saving lives than it is in real-life medical encounters. But such successes, even though not a part of real life, become a standard by which the general population evaluates the effectiveness of it and other aggressive, life-sustaining technologies. In this way, these fictitious medical scenarios both are part of and enhance cultural belief in the power of high-tech interventions to overcome death. In doing so, they subtly encourage a view in which death is defined as an enemy to be defeated, not one in which it is seen as a natural and inevitable part of life. And, in this framework, the best defense against death is to put it on the defensive through a full-court press of high-tech treatments.

Denial of death is also embedded in the prevailing folkways of everyday life, as the "unpleasantness" that surrounds dying, suffering, and death is often kept in a deep freeze of silence. As a result, death and dying are not very discernible in daily life. In this way, denial may assume the form of a cultural avoidance supported by the structure of everyday language, images, and daily activities. This reflects a "let's not think about, let's not talk about it, and avoid it as much as possible" kind of mentality. While such avoidance may be sustainable for a while, it is effective only up until the point that death becomes no longer escapable. No matter how much we may avoid thinking about or recognizing death in daily life, sooner or later that avoidance becomes impossible. Death will come sooner or later, to our loved ones as well as ourselves. When it does come knocking on one's own personal doorstep, denial and avoidance become more difficult. Thus, in an environment of avoidance and denial, when dying presents itself the result is a state of crisis and disbelief as people are not prepared to deal with it. In the throes of crisis, it is not unusual for them to rely on technology to prolong life, demanding aggressive treatment and for "everything to be done." This situation plays out normatively in ICUs each and every day.

So, whether it is in the form of cultural avoidance, religiously-based doctrines of eternal life, or the waging of medical battles against disease and death, these human constructions have one thing in common: In their own way they each attempt to say NO to death.

The take-away point is that fear of death is not uncommon and that humans have sought throughout history to find ways to cope with their fears. Some of what is at play here is an instinctive disposition to repudiate death as being inevitable, which creates a certain pressure for both individuals and societies to find ways of coping with the facts of death, when it becomes unavoidable.[20] As noted, the ways in which humans have dealt with mortality are reflective of the folkways and social structures of a given time and place. Despite variations in form, throughout the ages humans have created social practices designed to provide protection from the threat of death. The existence of these practices is as universal as the instinctive fear of death itself.

Upon examination, it is not difficult to see that the ways people die have changed dramatically over the centuries and that death today is not what it used to be.[21] While people are certainly living longer, the experience of dying in 21st century America has become especially miserable and suffering-filled. But this was not always the case. Looking particularly at Western civilization, it is clear that for millennia death held an important and meaningful place in the life of the community. In what might be described as the *traditional pattern of death*, suffering and dying were faced with the support of rituals, ceremonies, and elaborately-constructed meanings that helped make life's end both normal and familiar. This approach provided explanations for death itself. Explanations that helped individuals and communities confront the mysteries and fears about death with greater ease and confidence. These rituals were visible, widely present, and deeply enmeshed throughout the everyday life of the traditional community.

While each of us comes into this world alone and leaves it alone, dying is not just an individual, personal experience of a human being. Dying takes place within a specific historical and cultural context. It is that context that influences how death is viewed and how it is experienced. In this way, the forms of death are not universal and unchanging;

they are variable and reflective of the ways of life in the broader culture. In this regard, it may be said that the ways of death are reflective of the ways of life, and in turn, the ways of life shape the forms that dying and death assume.[22]

> The role of death in the traditional context was quite different than it is now.

It is a long distance from the traditional deathbed, where the dying person is surrounded by community and comforted by rituals, to the ICU where a dying person is surrounded by sophisticated machines and taken care of by highly trained, paid professionals. As we will see, hospice and palliative care have emerged in response to the indignities brought about by high-tech dying. As they developed their specialized skills in caring for the dying, they sought to restore a more-dignified approach to the ending of life; one most interestingly that resembles the support and comfort found in traditional death practices. In assessing this evolution, it is critical to note that hospice and palliative care services take place in a context wherein the simplicities and comforts of traditional patterns of dying have ceded to the fears and aversions of death. In fact, it is precisely the fears of indignity that have given rise to the supportive care movement. For this reason, it is useful to explore the evolution of traditional attitudes toward death in Western society; how they have given way to recent patterns of avoidance and worrisome indignities; and how in this context, palliative and hospice care are seeking to recapture the practices that once surrounded the traditional ways of dying.

One overarching distinction between the traditional and modern patterns of death resides in how visible a place suffering, dying, death, and grieving hold within the social life of the community. In traditional contexts, dying was visible throughout much of cultural life, whereas as society progressed through the Industrial Revolution and on to modernity and post-modernism, it has become less visible. The visibility of death in the traditional pattern led to dying and death's becoming a familiar presence in the life of the community: a familiarity that "normalized" death's presence and promoted an attitude of acceptance. To the contrary, in the modern context, death is far less visible in daily life, which in turn renders it less familiar. This "unfamiliarity" undermines death's once-held sense of being a normal and an accepted part of life (Figure 1.3).[23]

In the early Middle Ages, for example, the dying person was typically surrounded by members of the family and community. Death and dying were communal experiences and in a sense the deathbed was public. The focus of attention was on the dying person, and rituals known as the *ars moriendi*, the "art of dying," shaped interactions around the deathbed. The prevailing expectation was that a person should not be alone while dying. Goodbyes were to be exchanged, prayers said, and the community was expected to remain in mindful presence and support throughout the dying process until the moment of death. In this framework, dying was not an isolated, private experience. On the contrary, it was connected to the fabric of the community. As the historian Philippe Aries describes it:

> . . . death is celebrated by a ceremony that is always more or less solemn and whose purpose is to express the individual's solidarity with his family and community. . . .

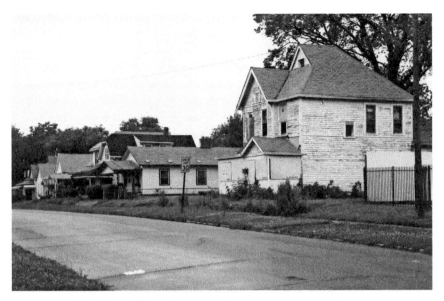

FIGURE 1.3 The landscape of "The Other America."

> This community gathered around the bed . . . later, in its rites of mourning, it expressed its anxiety caused by the passage of death. The community was weakened by the loss of one of its members. It expressed the danger it felt; it had to recover its strength and unity by means of ceremonies the last of which always had the quality of a holiday, even a joyous one.[24]

In this framework, death was not an isolated personal drama as it is in the 21st century. Instead, it was an event embraced by the community, which created elaborate rituals to support its members through the ordeal of dying. Traditionally it was the *ars moriendi* that established normative expectations for regular, ongoing presence of community members at the deathbed. As they kept their vigil—and this included the presence of children—death became something that was seen, known, and familiar. It is this familiarity that helped generate a sense of calm and acceptance. It bestowed a sense of peace upon the dying person—dare we say, even "tamed" death in a way that is very difficult to imagine today.[25]

Clearly, the role of death in the traditional context was quite different than it is now. Death literally was a regular and noticeable part of social life. People went to great lengths to remind themselves of the unavoidability of death. Ancient cemeteries, for example, were located in the courtyards of churches in the center of the town. These cemeteries were composed of mass graves that would contain hundreds and hundreds of bodies. The bodies were piled on top of one another, in communal fashion, so to speak. It was not unusual for one or more of the mass graves to be open, with the sights and smells of death present.

When graves were full, they would be covered with dirt, and others dug nearby. As this process continued, sooner or later, the digging of a new grave would unearth the skeletal remains of those previously buried. These remains would be exhumed in order to make room in the pit for the burial of new bodies. These bones upon removal were stored in the charnel houses or ossuaries that surrounded the cemeteries. But the charnel house, or "house of bones," as it has been also called, was more than an improvised storage area for the unearthed bones. It was designed as an exhibit to be seen. Reflective of an open relationship between life and death, the bones and skeletal remains were arranged in artistic display, and the charnel house became a sort of museum of the dead that people would visit. Some are still open and available to visit in cities throughout Europe today.

It is intriguing that, unlike modern cemeteries, which tend to be more private and secluded places, the traditional cemetery, even with the presence of the charnel houses and open graves, was a focal point of the social life of the community. It was where people gathered and carried on with their religious and earthly affairs. As Aries described it, the cemetery was the noisiest and busiest place in the community. It was where people gathered, socialized, conducted business, and even recreated. In short, the cemetery was the public square and ancient version of the modern shopping mall.[26]

One would have to believe, even notwithstanding the objection of public health concerns, that open graves and utilizing the cemetery as a focal point of social activity would be unappealing and even offensive to modern sensibilities. The contrast between then and now is striking. Once omnipresent, death has become banished from everyday experience. This disengagement creates a distance between life and death that ultimately renders dying both unfamiliar and unknown. The unity of living and dying in the more traditional setting created an openness and visibility that led to death's not being a matter of overly dramatic consequence. It was more widely accepted as a natural and inevitable part of living. People knew how to die and did so in the manner in which they had witnessed many others before them do. The community also knew what was required of it in the face of death. Acting in a manner that was commonly practiced, they gathered around the deathbed and participated in the *ars moriendi*. As a result, isolation in dying was not a social norm. Nor was social discomfort or uncertainty of how to be present in the midst of the dying process.

This relationship of proximity between the living and the dead lasted for millennia. While there would be fluctuations in form, the open relationship between living, dying, and death was a persistent one throughout the ages and was characterized by:

- Familiarity and acceptance;
- Communal presence and support;
- Deeply established religious rituals;
- Ceremonies and rituals that provided meaning;
- Practices that comforted grieving survivors in its aftermath.

To return to Becker's discussion, these long-lasting practices served as a "hero system" of sorts: they eased the suffering of death and imbued it with deep spiritual and cultural significance. Put simply, they helped humanity to cope. Thus, the *ars moriendi* offered a "taming" of death's terror and crafted an important, meaningful, and visible place for death and dying in the life of the community for a very long time.

It has been said that from a single acorn the mighty oak tree shall grow. With that as a guiding image, it is useful to note that the seeds of our modern aversion to death and dying were planted centuries ago, primarily around the time of the scientific/industrial revolution in Europe.

Specifically, the advance of science along with the abdication of community to the rising tide of individualism profoundly impacted social life and the way it was organized. It did so in ways that would ultimately redefine the relationship between human beings and mortality, and the ways in which dying, death, and grief would come to be experienced. Broadly speaking, these two changes were seminal in establishing the foundation upon which modern societies have been built, sowing the seeds for what might be termed the *modern pattern* of death. This introduced a new way of responding to death which is characterized by:

- A sense of personalized high-drama that impacts individuals (not communities);
- A specter of cultural and social denial;
- Feelings of anxiety and anticipatory fear;
- Waging of high-tech battles to fend off impending death.

As the Industrial Revolution swept across Western societies, the authority of religion was challenged by values and activities that established a different view and set of explanations for the world and human existence. This evolving paradigm was grounded in science and technological development, which became strong sources of cultural authority.

> He immediately begins to ponder how to employ his knowledge. And he proceeds without ever stopping to pause and consider if this is something he should be doing at all.

The change, so profound and impactful, has been the focus of intense sociological and historical study. The meaning of the sweeping changes, particularly as relevant for our purposes, may have been best captured, not in the landmark historical texts that have been written about it however, but rather by myth and storytelling. The subtitle of Mary Shelley's classic work *Frankenstein* which is; *or, The Modern Prometheus,* is of note. It offered a forewarning about the dangers that lie within science, specifically of the potential for harm that exists when technology and science progress without humanism. It illuminated the consequences of scientific and technological advances unaccompanied by wisdom. In particular, Shelley was focused on an ethical and moral issue about the development of science, namely, the need for balancing technological capacity with the wisdom on how, when, and whether these advancements should be even utilized. This is a warning not just about the general reliance on technology in the broader culture, but one that is specifically applicable to the use of technology in high-tech hospital settings near the end of life.

Prometheus was the Greek god who stole fire from Mount Olympus, against the will of Zeus. He gave fire to humanity and is credited in Greek mythology as being the creator of humans and all humanity. Shelley's intent, in selecting her subtitle, was to offer an alert about the dark side of science and technology and their potential for creating "monsters." She provided a prophetic warning about potential dystopian consequences that can occur when technological development outpaces morality and humanism.

Consistent with the open relationship between life and death that persisted at the time, her gothic tale is filled with images of cemeteries with mass, open graves and charnels. So, despite being at the threshold of major change in society, death was still widely present and visible in the towns, villages, and cities. But something subtle was happening and a new attitude was slowly forming, one in which denial of death and the urge to conquer it was entering into social consciousness. Her novel captures this attitude in its nascent form and presents a chilling and full-blown analysis of its potential consequences. Specifically, it warns that the development of technology and its "unethical" application could have troubling consequences. In particular, she was referring to the growth and use of new technologies untempered by ethical judgement on whether and how to use them, and the absence of the courage it takes to not utilize them in certain situations.

It was within this context of social evolution toward denial that Victor Frankenstein's explicit and stated goal was to defeat death:

> I entered with the greatest diligence into the search of the philosopher's stone and the elixir of life; but the latter soon obtained my undivided attention. Wealth was an inferior object; but what glory would attend the discovery if I could banish disease from the human frame and render man invulnerable to any but a violent death![27]

Broader cultural values at the time were starting to emphasize scientific exploration and discovery. In this context, gross physical anatomy was seen as a means to unlocking the secrets to life. Once exclusively explained through the authority of religious doctrines, answers to the mysteries of life were now being sought through the scientific method. It is especially fascinating to note that dissections during this time were being held in public amphitheaters in local communities and even in private homes of the affluent. Science was being established as the new paradigm that could best explain life and death, and anatomy was part of its toolkit. Frankenstein's activities were reflective of this zeitgeist:

> To examine the causes of life, we must first have recourse to death. I have become acquainted with the science of anatomy, but this was not sufficient; I must also observe the natural decay and corruption of the human body.[28]

Consequently, he immersed himself in the sights, textures, and smells of death, not in the ways that folks in traditional communities would have been exposed to them in the cemeteries and charnels, but rather with a single-minded purpose of scientific study:

> [I was] forced to spend days and nights in vaults and charnel-houses. . . . I saw how the fine form of man was degraded and wasted; I beheld the corruption of death succeed to the blooming cheek of life; I saw how the worm inherited the wonders of the eye and brain.[29]

Frankenstein had embarked on a quest to discover the means to create life:

> After days and nights of incredible labor and fatigue I succeeded in discovering the cause of generation and life; nay, more I became myself capable of bestowing animation upon lifeless matter.[30]

Shelley's admonition comes into sharp focus at this point in the story. Knowledge is one thing, but acting on that knowledge is entirely another matter. When Victor Frankenstein discovered the secrets to the creation of life, he immediately begins to ponder how to employ his knowledge. And he proceeded *without ever stopping to pause and consider if this was something he should be doing at all.* As the expression goes, be careful what one wishes for. Very quickly, the beauty and promise of his dream and newfound capability devolved into a horrible reality:

> I startled from my sleep with horror. . . . I beheld the wretch—the miserable monster whom I had created. He held up the curtain of the bed; and his eyes, if eyes they may be called, were fixed on me. . . . Oh! No mortal could support the horror of that countenance. A mummy again endued with animation could not be so hideous as that wretch. I had gazed upon him while unfinished; he was ugly then, but when those muscles and joints were rendered capable of motion, it became a thing such as even Dante could not have conceived.[31]

The ultimate message that Shelley puts forth revolves around the consequences of overstepping the core nature and bounds of our humanness in the pursuit of becoming "greater and more god-like." It points to the danger of acquiring knowledge and technological capacity that are not restrained by understanding and moral judgment about:

- Whether the knowledge or capability *should* be used;
- What purpose and in what manner and with what limitations they should be utilized.

These are questions that Frankenstein failed to consider. The result of his efforts was an achievement that was frightening and it filled him with regret. He despaired with "breathless horror and disgust [filling his] heart" over what he had done.

The best of science and technology lies in their great-hearted humanism. Danger, however, lies in their potential to be used in ways that, either intentionally or unintentionally, are destructive. It is not difficult to see that scientific discovery and technological advancements have contributed to improved health, well-being, safety, comfort, enjoyment, and longevity of people's lives in the industrialized world. But that is not the whole story. They have also had deleterious consequences.

Shakespeare once wrote: "Ignorance is the curse of God, / Knowledge is the wing wherewith we fly to heaven."[32] Shelly counsels, however, that real knowledge must go beyond know-how and technological capability. She warns that if science and technological expertise are not balanced with wisdom, they can and do lead to malefic consequences. An obvious example lies in the destructive capabilities of modern weaponry and how it can be mobilized to advance the cause of evil, such as we saw during the holocaust. A less obvious example would be a person lying in an ICU with extremely poor prognosis, body withering, and the person within the body suffering, all while being artificially maintained by mechanical life support. This is a terrible image that is made possible by the advancements of medical technology, and one that occurs too frequently in hospitals all across the country.

The indignities that surround dying in the ICU are pervasive and the suffering that is involved is often extreme. This is where Shelley's insights become suggestive of the need for developing approaches to patient care that are more merciful, kind, and person-centered, rather than death-prolonging. In this regard, I posit that there is a moral obligation to be more discerning about the type of care that is delivered to patients near the end of life. In particular, the focus should be on providing care that is truly beneficial and in the best interests of the patient. By extension this involves avoiding doing something just because something can be done. This approach requires that we become more thoughtful and "choose wisely" about what treatments should be offered at life's end. In order to do so we must be willing to ask and answer some hard questions when providing aggressive, life-prolonging treatments:

- What are we doing and why are we doing it?
- Should we be doing it?
- Is aggressive treatment consistent with our duty to serve patients in ways that are beneficent and non-maleficent?
- Are we enhancing life or protracting death?
- Is what we are doing beneficial?

The failure to actively incorporate these considerations into the daily practice of medicine will only result in failure to provide the best care possible.

> These are, in many ways, miraculous times in medicine. The medical center has become the place where hearts are kept beating, cancers combatted, seriously-ill newborns and neonates saved, joints replaced, and organs transplanted. The capacity to extend life is unprecedented, but it is the very utilization of that capacity that has also exacerbated discomfort, suffering, and social isolation—particularly near the end of life.

These are, in many ways, miraculous times in medicine. The medical center has become the place where hearts are kept beating, cancers combatted, seriously ill newborns and neonates saved, joints replaced, and organs transplanted. The capacity to extend life is unprecedented, but it is the very utilization of that capacity that has also exacerbated discomfort, suffering, and social isolation—particularly near the end of life.

The point to be made is that the seeds of rationality, science, and technology that were planted during the Industrial Revolution have profoundly changed the end-of-life experience. They have led to what might be called the medicalization of dying. The implications of this transformation were brought to our attention nearly one-half century ago by Elizabeth Kubler-Ross. As she observes:

> One of the most-important facts is that dying nowadays is more gruesome in many ways, namely, more lonely, mechanical, and dehumanized. . . . Dying becomes lonely and impersonal because the patient is often taken out of his familiar environment [. . .]
>
> [The dying person] may cry for rest, peace, and dignity, but he will get infusions, transfusions, a heart machine, or tracheostomy if necessary. He may want one single person to stop for one single minute so he can ask one single question—but he will get a dozen people around the clock, all busily preoccupied with heart rate, pulse, electrocardiogram, or pulmonary functions, his secretions or excretions, but not with him as a human being. . . . Is the reason for this increasingly mechanical, depersonalized approach our own defensiveness? Is this approach our way to cope with and repress the anxieties that a terminally or critically-ill patient evokes in us? Is our concentration on equipment, on blood pressure our desperate attempt to deny the impending death which is so frightening and discomforting to us that we displace all our knowledge onto machines, since they are less close to us than the suffering face of another human being which would remind us once more of our lack of omnipotence, our own limits and failures, and last but not least perhaps our own mortality?[33]

The situation that she describes stands in dramatic contrast to the peace, serenity, and meaningfulness that were typical of the traditional deathbed. It is reflective of a new model of dying wherein:

- Avoidance replaces acceptance;
- Anxiety replaces peacefulness;
- Technology is used to fight against death, sometimes at "all costs;"
- Traditional rituals and the *ars moriendi* disappear;
- The disappearance of community presence at the deathbed leads to isolation and loneliness; and
- The place of death is largely transferred from home to the hospital or nursing home.

Underlying the modern pattern of dying is an attitude steeped in uneasiness and uncertainty. Dying and death, once visible and easily recognizable, have become distanced and disconnected from the mainstream activity, and something to be fought against.

Consider, for example, even the very language by which we converse—or don't converse—about mortality. *Dying–death–dead:* the words are very easy to pronounce. Clearly, they are not tongue twisters of any sort. However, despite simplicity in pronouncing them, there is not ease in actually saying them. In fact, the words have largely become "unmentionable;" a taboo of sorts. So, an array of euphemisms is drawn upon to talk about *dying, death,* and *dead.* This enables us to enable refer these facts of life without actually having to use the words directly. Such expressions as "passed away, has gone to heaven, is with God now, is finally at peace, looks like he is asleep," all refer to the ending of life but in a way that is softer than the stark reality conveyed by "those three words." The utterance of *Ms. Smith has passed away* is easier to say and hear than *Ms. Smith is dead.* The latter is stark and direct, whereas the former offers a cushion, a softening of the harshness of death.

As discussed, throughout the patterns of traditional death, humans went to great lengths to remind themselves that death is a part of life. The cemeteries, bustling with social activity amid the presence of mass, open graves, were only one part of the visibility. The reminders of mortality ranged from its representations in art, literature, and poetry throughout the ages, to elaborate forms of personal expression found, for example, in the elaborate tombs of the Victorians and the public expressions of mourning that included wearing of jewelry and clothing that were designed intentionally to give visibility to a person's grieving. It is fair to say that, in the context of these traditional folkways, death was represented in ways that were communal, familiar, and openly accessible. The drift of modern culture, however, has been toward removal of death from public conspicuousness, and the medicalization of dying is part of that removal. As Aries notes:

> The dying man's bedroom has passed from the home to the hospital. For technical medical reasons, this transfer has been accepted by families, and popularized and facilitated by their complicity. The hospital is the only place where death is sure of escaping a visibility—or what remains of it—that is hereafter regarded as unsuitable and morbid. The hospital has become the place of the solitary death.[34]

A new relationship between humans and death is emerging: it is one where social and religious rituals and their attached meanings give way to a sense of fear, repulsion, and aversion. In this framework:

> Death no longer inspires fear solely because of its absolute negativity; it also turns the stomach like any nauseating spectacle. It becomes improper, like the biological acts of man, the secretions of the human body. It is indecent to let someone die in public. It is no longer acceptable for strangers to come into a room that smells of urine, sweat, and gangrene, and where the sheets are soiled. Access to this room must be forbidden, except to a few intimates capable of overcoming their disgust, or to those indispensable persons who provide certain services. A new image of death is forming: the ugly and hidden death, hidden because it is ugly and dirty.[35]

What is happening in the new model is that the ways in which society defends itself from the threats posed by death are changing significantly and in ways consistent with broader social trends where:

1. Community has abdicated to a model of individualism in which the life of the personal self takes on tremendous importance;
2. Technology has become a "go-to" answer in order to fix problems that challenge human welfare, including the problems of disease, dying, and death.

Thus, as communal values begin to disappear in an age of individualism, the community itself becomes less involved in the death of one of its members. This decline in solidarity and connectivity means that a dying person and a small contingent of loved ones are left facing mortality pretty much on their own. (Facebook, Twitter, and Instagram, or even specifically designed sites such as Care Bridge are not optimal means of sharing suffering and providing authentic support in the torment of loss and grief. They may bring a broad range of people together but only transiently and momentarily.) The isolation that surrounds dying and grieving can exacerbate uncertainty and anxiety, as people feel less secure in their capacity and understanding of how to get through these difficult experiences. Isolation not only increases unfamiliarity, but diminishes the ability to cope. In the framework of isolation and lack of confidence, one response is to turn to medical professionals and give over control of the dying process to them. This transfers the dying process from a community-based experience to one that takes place in a medical setting. In turn, reliance on medical technology becomes a way for Americans, often fearful of death, to cope with it.

> We tend not to pause and ask: What are we doing and why are we doing it?

Ironically, in the 21st century, where a decreasing sense of privacy has been created by social media and its ability to intrude into lives virtually everywhere, dying and death have become increasingly privatized. For example, a widow is no longer obvious by the way she dresses, and her rituals of mourning have become largely hidden. This is not to suggest that she is not grieving. Rather, it is to note that her emotional displays find little acceptance in the public arena and are constrained to far more private and isolated settings such as her home, therapist's office, or support group. The dying person similarly is no longer the focus of attention of a broad-based, supportive community. Instead, he or she is most likely to be sequestered in a hospital or other institutional setting. As a result, the deathbed is no longer communal. It has become isolated and separated.

In this regard, the contemporary model of death is shaped by a sense of privacy and individualism. Ironically, however, the drama that surrounds dying plays out in "public settings," not in the privacy of the home for the most part. This makes no sense upon first glace. But on deeper consideration, it is reflective of a widespread incapacity to effectively cope with the threat of death on one's own, without professional intervention and expertise. So a newly molded form of privacy in dying has been created in that, by placing death within the confines of public institutions, it is secluded away from ordinary life. This situation is very different from the traditional attitude in which death was tamed by the rituals of the *ars moriendi*, and wherein the dying person was comforted by the fellowship of a caring community. In this new model, dying is handed over to healthcare professionals and technology mobilized to fight against it.

Something profound yet subtle appears to be happening. Dying itself is becoming a source of shame; something to be hidden and avoided.[36] No longer being able to find protection from the threat of death in the traditional practices, modern society calls upon the profession of medicine to "eliminate" death, control its symptoms, or delay its inevitability. Death has become uniquely unsettling and "savage" in this framework, and high-tech medical invention has evolved as a means of defending against it.

As described, the meaning of a person's individual self has taken on enormous significance as society has modernized; the worth of a singular individual becoming extremely important. In the traditional context, the value of an individual's life was subsumed by the importance of church, clan, guild, and community.[37] In this pre-modern environment, the welfare of the community was far more consequential than the well-being of any of its individual members. In this new social order, the individual is emancipated from traditional moorings, including the overarching influence of communal expectations, and the value of the individual becomes a ruling precept.

While there has been a slow and evolving drift toward individualism throughout the 20th century, the past five decades have brought it to unprecedented levels. These years have been filled with practices and urgings designed to prompt people into maximizing their own potential, and holding people personally accountable for their own happiness. From Oprah Winfrey to self-help gurus and on to social media, the notion of the enhancement of the individual has taken strong hold in American culture. This movement corresponds with developing inclinations toward self-focus (some would argue "self-obsession"), self-creation, self-reinvention, and the pursuit of self-satisfaction. There can be humanistic values at play here as society evolves toward greater respect and valuing of the moral worth of individuals. This evolution does bespeak a respect for life and personhood. Yet, at the same time, there is also a diminishment of shared concerns among people in the society as well as a decline in solidarity, fellowship, and community attachments.

In this overall framework, several things are happening. The first is a redefining of death from a communal experience into one that is individualized. As a result, dying becomes a lonely experience and the dying person is isolated in ways that would have been inconceivable during the earlier eras. In addition, the meaning of death, once grounded in communal experience and practices, now becomes focused on the individual. In part, the modern fear of dying/death is derived directly from how central individualism has become. In a period where much of living revolves around self-seeking and self-enhancement, and wherein the value of the individual person is strongly endorsed, it is difficult to contemplate the ending of the life of the individual self. A common question of this age is, "What's in it for me?" The obvious answer with respect to dying and death would be, "Not much. Just suffering and the ending of yourself and your life." Such endings in the traditional model were normal, familiar, expected, and eased by a sense of shared meanings and purpose. In the modern context, however, such endings are often devoid of shared, communal meanings and supportive rituals. For this reason, dying and death become especially difficult, and it is not unusual for individuals to rant and rage against the ending of their own lives or the lives of their loved ones. It is difficult to imagine relinquishing oneself; dying; not being.

The second thing that is relevant is the emergence of a societal attitude of denial wherein the unpleasantness and sufferings that surround dying are avoided as much as possible. Denial generates a shroud of secrecy, hiding dying and death from everyday visibility. When the silence is broken from time to time, as it must be, it is often done with a protective veil of detachment or perhaps even indifference, so to protect against the stark discomfort that is elicited. For example, while the emotions may be raw for the immediate members of a grieving family at a wake or funeral, for most of the attendees the simmering uneasiness of being present in the presence of a dead body, and its reminder of the universality of death, becomes masked by a veneer of pleasantries and superficialities surrounding most of the conversations and interactions. Vacations are talked about, or sports, or what is happening with the family, or a new car or home purchase, and so forth. It is almost as if neither individuals nor the group at large in attendance can squarely face the visibility of death in front of them.

The third major part of the transformation is that death is now given over to the medical specialists whose charge is to battle against it, utilizing their professional skill and technological capability. As the process of dying becomes medicalized it has also become drawn out. And, as dying becomes protracted, it often results in a distressing portrait: a person who is withered by disease, physically and existentially suffering, languishing in deterioration while holding on to physical life, existing someplace between life and death, and being maintained in that state by artificial, mechanical means. In the vein of Frankenstein, there is something monstrous about this picture.

As concerning as this situation is, some good news has come from it. The recognition of the harm and increased suffering associated with this type of death has given rise to the hospice and palliative care movements. Their ultimate mission is to tackle the inhumanity that can result from high-tech dying and replace it with practices designed to ease suffering, maximize comfort, and promote dignity.

Although these movements have developed within the healthcare community, they also reflect broader social concerns. Their development embodies, in part, a growing awareness that overreliance on aggressive interventions near the end of life can create intense indignity and suffering. Ironically, despite this being an age of time of death avoidance, many people are aware of stories of people suffering greatly while dying. Many have personally observed such sufferings throughout the death of a loved one. Others have heard about it from neighbors, friends, or co-workers. Thus, although we remain largely in an age of denial, images of dying undignified are beginning to break through the taboos and galvanize another sensibility: the fear of death not just because it is the ending of one's life but because what happens during the process can be pretty terrible. This social concern about the indignities associated with medicalized dying is notable. In some sense it reflects a yearning for past practices, in particular for recapturing the customs of earlier eras that "tamed" the experience of dying, promoting comfort, peace, tranquility, and meaning.

The first hospice was created in the United Kingdom by Cicely Saunders, who by training was a nurse, physician, and medical social worker. It is no wonder that, given this rich, multidisciplinary background, she sought to improve patients' experience at the end of life by transforming care through an interdisciplinary approach. But equally, it is no wonder that she sought to remedy the problem with a largely clinical approach, as opposed to a community-based initiative, for example. As she sought a new model of caring for the dying, she focused her attention specifically on pain and symptom relief, along with holistic care of patients that addressed not only physical but also existential, spiritual, and psychosocial suffering. Thus was born the concept of specialized care for

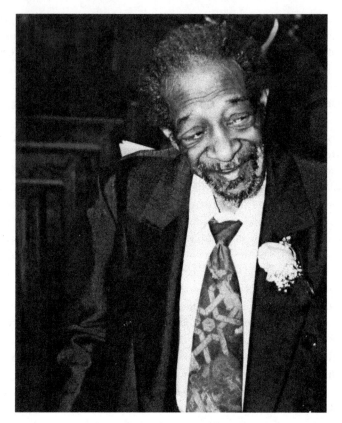

FIGURE 1.4 A smile graces the face of Reverend Bryant as he attends his beloved church for the final time before dying.

the dying *within* the system of medicine and healthcare, even if that system did extend into the home.

It is useful to note that, while the goals of hospice and palliative care are synonymous with the practices of the traditional patterns of dying, they are organized by a clinical and professional model. That is to say, they are based on a model whereby professional services are provided to patients (and sometimes families), and those services are paid for by private and government insurance. Whereas, during the traditional eras, relief during the process of dying was explicitly connected to communal, social, and religious folkways. Care of the dying was personal and communal, not a reimbursable professional service (Figure 1.4).

Thus, as hospice and palliative care evolved and developed within a clinical model, there has been emphasis on not only patient care but teaching and research as well. While hospice and palliative care emerged to provide more humane care for people dying of terminal illness, the movement also grew in ways that were inevitably influenced by organizational, political and economic factors. This growth included achievements such as:

- The Joint Commission (JHACO) initiating hospice accreditation;
- Congress establishing the Medicare Hospice Benefit;

- Private insurance companies offering a hospice care benefit;
- Hospice becoming legitimized as a part of the continuum of medical care;
- Major grant makers pouring significant money into funding for research into best practices to transform end-of-life experience in America;
- Major universities and teaching hospitals establishing end-of-life care institutes;
- Reflecting this growing cultural acceptance, the US Postal Service issued a Hospice Care commemorative stamp;
- Professional societies dedicated to advancing the fields of hospice and palliative care were established;
- Center to Advance Palliative Care (CAPC) was established;
- Research demonstrated the cost savings of hospice and palliative care;
- Advanced directives became commonplace in institutional settings such as hospitals and nursing homes.

To put it simply, there has been tremendous effort dedicated to creating better and more humane ways of caring for seriously-ill persons since Kubler-Ross described the dehumanization of dying in 1969 and America's first hospice program was established in Connecticut in 1974. These changes have had unquestionable positive benefits for many, including increasing the number of people who die at home and not in hospitals, reducing the number of invasive procedures that people get while in intensive care, reducing the number of hospital stays, and reducing the costs of care near the end of life. In short, there can be little doubt that hospice and palliative care are associated with improved quality of life,[38] which, for our purposes, maybe even more aptly described as improved *quality of dying.*

That said, despite 40 years of commitment and dedicated work by accomplished professionals, the state of dying in America still remains rather bleak. The groundbreaking project popularly known as SUPPORT (Study to Understand Prognoses and Preferences for Outcomes and Risks of Treatment) was the first major study to explore what the experience of hospitalized dying was like (Phase l) and seek to ease the indignities that surround the experience of dying in America by providing a greater voice for patients in decision-making (Phase II).

Overall, this study's findings revealed that care received at the end of life was often at odds with care desired by terminally ill patients; a divergence explained best by a tension between patient preferences for dignity and the locomotive of high-tech interventions that drives much of care delivered. It is fair to conclude from SUPPORT that:

- The culture of high-tech medicine is often at odds with patient needs for dignity, kindness, and mercy;
- Far too many patients suffer in pain;
- Communication between patients and physicians is less than optimal, especially around difficult issues;
- The high cost of medicalized dying, especially in the ICU, is cause for alarm.

In some ways, the study's results shook the medical world, and the authors in their summary of the findings expressed deep concern: "We are left with a troubling situation. The picture we describe of the care of the terminally ill or dying persons is not attractive."[39]

In many ways, the flurry of activity to improve the experience of dying in American society during the past 30 years was precipitated by SUPPORT findings and the widespread attention it generated, including more than 24,000 citations in the professional literature. So, it is fair to ask how much have things changed in the three decades since its release.

On one hand, as noted, there has been remarkable growth in the fields of palliative and hospice care. In some important ways, palliative medicine has become a common presence in many hospitals. Hospice utilization has increased significantly. And there has been a proliferation of conversation about end-of-life matters through professional societies, journals, books, and conferences. While there has been a lot of focused attention on the "failure" of Phase II, which was the planned intervention to improve the experience of dying in American hospitals, the remarkable success of SUPPORT resides in how it galvanized professional concern and activity around improving end-of-life care. In this regard, it is fair to say that a lasting and invaluable legacy has been created because of the researchers' efforts.

In September 2014, nearly 30 years after SUPPORT prompted some professional soul-searching and helped promote the growth of the palliative and hospice care movement, the Institute of Medicine published a report entitled *Dying in America*.[40] It clearly articulated that there is still "the pressing need to improve end-of-life care" in America today. So, despite the dedication of professionals all across the country to improving the experience, peace and meaning in dying can and do remain elusive. In specific, the report noted opportunities for improvement in the following areas:

- Delivery of person-centered, family-oriented care;
- Clinician–patient communication and advance-care planning;
- Professional education and development;
- Policies and payment systems to support high-quality care;
- Public education and engagement at three levels:
  - The societal level, to build support for public and institutional policies that ensure high-quality, sustainable care;
  - The community and family levels, to raise awareness and elevate expectations about care options, the needs of caregivers, and the hallmarks of high-quality care; and
  - The individual level, to motivate and facilitate advance-care planning and meaningful conversations with family members and caregivers.

A conclusion that can be drawn from the recommendation on public engagement is that there exists an urgent need to design and tailor programs in each of these areas that are attuned to the specific needs of people in community settings, including those of marginalized populations.

Overall, however, despite these efforts there remains in hospitals and medical centers throughout the nation a high-tech and high-pressure environment to aggressively treat at the end of life. Simultaneously, there are suboptimal conversations about and consideration of the consequences of aggressive and unbeneficial care. *We tend not to pause and ask: What are we doing and why are we doing it?* This lack of pause and deliberation can be due to the teaching and research mission of academic medical centers. It can also be related to the professional socialization of physicians that trains them to take technology-oriented actions to "fix" problems. This curative approach is embedded in medical training. Additional complexity is brought into play by physicians who feel that unless they offer every treatment to prolong life, they may be made vulnerable to lawsuits. Frankly, this concern is real and can lead physicians into the practice of "defensive medicine." In addition, families may insist on aggressive care because they are not prepared to deal with the death of their loved one. These pressures to treat, while driven by unrealistic expectations, can be difficult to address or resist. Additionally, in-depth conversations with patients and families about dying are both time-consuming and stressful for providers. Physicians are generally underprepared by their training to engage these conversations with skill and comfort, and it may just be easier to order a battery of tests and perform procedures to assure the family that "everything has been done." To be fair, this lack of preparation places physicians in a very difficult position and pressures them toward decision-making that is aggressive rather than supportive, and not always in the best interests of patients.

All in all, there remains a discomfort within the society and in hospitals about directly dealing with the issues that surround dying. Direct conversations are postponed or avoided entirely. Sometimes it seems that the silence around dying is deafening. It extends throughout the ranks of professional caregivers who are busy with clinically focused tasks, as well as to patients and families who are struggling to come to terms with things.

Despite the growing worries throughout society about the indignities associated with high-tech dying, Americans still place faith in the curative possibilities of that care. The practice of hospitalizing people throughout the trajectory of advanced illness, including near the end of life is common. When a medical episode takes place in the home, the default response is to call 911. The result is that when 911 is called, people often find themselves admitted to the hospital through the emergency department. From this point of entry, they are then swept along into a process of care that is highly specialized and technologically sophisticated. This care can be invasive and have a traumatic impact, resulting in distress, suffering, and agitation. In this pattern, the focus is not on generating peace and quality of life, for the most part. Rather, it is on physician expertise and technical capability to fight the medical problems that brought the patient into the hospital in the first place. The result is that, despite general wishes to the contrary, people are far more likely to die in the hospital than at home. Because that is where they go when sick. And to be honest, it is all of us—patients, families, and healthcare professionals—who are complicit in this happening.

It is useful to think about what a peaceful death might entail, how it differs from medicalized dying, and how in the hospital setting it can be elusive to achieve. In thinking about this, Daniel Callahan[40] expresses what would give peace at the ending of life. While his is but one version of a peaceful death, it is helpful to compare and contrast it with the qualities of high-tech death. He declares that a peaceful ending of one's life might include:

- Some meaning in the death;
- Respect and sympathy along with spiritual and personal dignity;
- The death mattering to others;

- Not being abandoned;
- Not being an undue burden on others;
- Dying in a society that does not dread death;
- A process that is not drawn out;
- The body and spirit are not overwhelmed by pain and suffering.

Hospice and palliative care services seek to help patients and families achieve peace in dying. However, there remains a bold overuse of technology and a timid underuse of hospice and palliative care near the end of life.[41] A major consequence is that patients lie dying in prolonged suffering, while they are being actively and aggressively treated in ways that are unbeneficial. They are often sustained by mechanical life support wherein the benefit of treatment is outweighed by the burden it imposes. The ramification is that suffering and harm are exacerbated without any reasonable expectation of benefit.

This reliance on technology to postpone and combat death cannot be separated from the deep uneasiness that we have in facing mortality in 21st century America. The reality is that families, patients, and physicians often deal with dying in a state of uncertainty and chaos; a process that undermines peace and acceptance in deference to technological interventions. It is not pressing too far to state that this very situation is playing itself out, in frustrating, complex and confusing ways, at this precise moment, in hospitals and medical centers throughout the country.

DYING AT THE MARGINS

As underutilized as hospice and palliative care generally are, their underuse is especially acute with respect to marginalized populations. As there are inequities that subvert the health and wellness of those challenged by economic and racial barriers throughout life, there are also clearly established disparities in end-of-life care. These include sub-optimal relationships between providers and patients. Most providers come from very different backgrounds than their inner-city patients. So it is very difficult for them to "walk in their shoes." The social and economic divide that separates providers from patients is reflective of divisions that persist throughout the broader culture. According to the Institute of Medicine:

> Racial and ethnic disparities in healthcare occur in the context of broader historic and contemporary social and economic inequality and evidence of persistent racial and ethnic discrimination in many sectors of American life.[42]

For this reason, it is fair to say that the unevenness of care and unique sufferings that run through the stories in *Dancing with Broken Bones* are not isolated experiences. To the contrary, they are reflective of injustices that exist broadly and systemically throughout American life and that specifically affect racial and economic minorities.

It is worth highlighting two major factors that play into race-based inequities that surround end-of-life care in the inner city. The first is the **unconscious stereotypes** that healthcare providers have toward racial minorities; stereotypes that impact provider–patient relationships. These biases are reflective of attitudes and prejudices that many

Americans have and that embody a lack of cultural sensitivity, or as I prefer to term it—"cultural humility." These stereotypes are deeply rooted in American folklore and are based on pejorative caricatures that portrayed African Americans as "bungling buffoons." These historical images include archetypes such as Mammy, Golliwog, Sambo, and Jezebel. They accentuate physical characteristics such as "toothy-white smile," "over-sized red lips," and being shabbily dressed. More modern imagery casts blacks variously as drug dealers, drug abusers, street drunks, welfare queens, unintelligent, irresponsible, lazy, criminal, and angry. They are further degraded by their association with fried chicken, watermelon, and rap music. The stereotypes demean their humanity and suggest an "unworthiness."

These stereotypes often find their way, unconsciously, into the worldview of doctors, nurses, and others who work in healthcare. In turn, once again unconsciously, they can impact not only attitudes but decision-making by providers, thereby resulting in the possibility of a different kind of care being delivered. An example is how racial and class biases play into generating stereotypes of patients as "drug-seekers," which can lead to undertreatment of pain for people living in poverty and for racial minorities as well. This situation is only likely to worsen given the opioid-addiction crisis that is capturing the attention of healthcare institutions. As physicians and hospitals are increasingly under pressure to restrict the amount of opioids they prescribe, it is fair to imagine that unconscious stereotypes will play a role in how the poor and racial minorities are treated for severe pain.

> The canons of "good medicine" make it morally mandatory to learn about the cultural milieu of our patients.

Unconscious stereotypes are not the result of the predispositions of morally-insensitive professionals. Instead, they are normative responses in a society in which prejudice remains active. They are part of a general perception that denigrates the poor and racial minorities and which separates them from the rest of us. We all make decisions about what feels safe, likeable, and familiar in everyday life. We tend, in the vein of confirmation bias, to make decisions and judgments that reaffirm existing beliefs and, in doing so, these beliefs impact the way we perceive ourselves and others, and influence the way we interact with those who are different. I have little doubt that the physician who spoke about the irresponsibility of the poor, in response to my conference presentation, was commenting not out of malevolence but from a place that was safe, familiar, and comfortable to him and his view of the world. In his mind he meant no harm or prejudice, I imagine. Yet, I would have to think that when patients who typified the characteristics of the people portrayed in *Dancing with Broken Bones* entered his professional practice, he would relate to them in a fashion consistent with his pre-formed conceptions. He would do so not with conscious intent, but rather with the security of unawareness about his judgements. For this reason, I believe there would be no escaping the impact that his hidden, personal biases would have on his relations with these patients. I also have little doubt that patients and their loved ones, drawing on their "street savvy and heightened sensitivity" to prejudice, would recognize or "sense" his perceptions and that would sow the seeds of disconnect and their distrust of him.

The point to be made is that physicians, and all who work in healthcare, are human beings. They are exposed to and influenced by prevailing folkways of society. It is only natural that they embody the imperfections that come with being human and are likewise impacted by pejorative perceptions of the poor and racial minorities that prevail in the larger society. It should not be surprising, therefore, that physicians' attitudes about race and poverty, even if deeply unconscious, affect the patient–doctor relationship in ways that contribute to stereotyped judgments and disparities in care.

This issue connects directly to a second major factor that influences end-of-life care for marginalized populations; namely, **mistrust.** This mistrust is not so much an intentional rejection by patients of individual providers who are perceived as being untrustworthy. It is instead a suspicion of the system itself. Lack of trust in the medical establishment is related to its history of mistreatment of African Americans, which is most notably evidenced by the US Public Health Service study of syphilis in black males. The study exploited blacks for scientific purposes, actually ensuring their suffering and death. Known as the Tuskeegee study, it was originally intended to follow the course of syphilis in this population as it naturally occurred within the body. While motivated by beneficent intentions, perhaps, it instead devolved into something sinister. The fact is that when penicillin was discovered, which was after the study began, it was not made available to those men who were enrolled in it. For decades the deceit and deprivation of care continued, inevitably leading to horrible outcomes. This narrative of exploitation has been passed down from generation to generation in African-American culture and serves as a bedrock of distrust in the medical establishment.

One result within the African-American population today is increased suspicion of any recommendations made by medical professionals that do not revolve around life-saving and life-prolonging efforts. Thus, understandably the cultural lens through which supportive or hospice care is viewed within the African-American community is more likely to create feelings of mistrust, both of the intentions of the hospital itself and of those who work in it.

The trials, tribulations, and humiliations of being poor and a racial minority in America play out every day. When one is stigmatized by racial and economic disenfranchisement, it is hard to trust the intentions of those who are a part of mainstream institutions. And this includes physicians. The poor and racial minorities are people who have been victimized, ridiculed, and exploited throughout their lives by those in power. For this reason, the mistrust of the medical establishment is a result of the experiences people have outside the hospital throughout their lives which predispose them to mistrust.

It is difficult for most empowered people, including healthcare providers, to empathize with and understand their suspicions, because we do not walk the same journey in life. To be sure, the intentions of doctors, nurses, and other clinical caregivers are overwhelmingly altruistic and benevolent. That is why they do what they do. Thus, it can be difficult for these honorable men and women to understand why they are the object of derision and distrust, when all they are trying to do is be helpful. So when patients, families, and loved ones present with anger and preformed, disrespectful attitudes, it is hard for providers to understand why this is happening. In this framework, it is not unusual for patients and families to be judged as difficult and unlikable.

The sufferings that are associated with poverty and racism run deep and inter-generationally. The newest generation is raised with stories about the harm and injury that its elders have endured, and they learn suspicion and mistrust as a survival skill. For this reason, pervasive mistrust among the poor and racial minorities should not surprise us.

It should not be shocking, then, that marginalized populations will be less recep-tive to hospice and palliative care, as these are models of care that, in their view, would deprive them of "life-saving" services. They are less likely to believe that hospice or sup-portive care could actually be beneficial to them and their loved ones. One could imagine patients and families, when presented with options for less-aggressive care near the end of life, thinking something like, "We have been enduring deprivation all of our lives. Now you are recommending we discontinue treatment, opt not to be resuscitated, don't call 911 . . . you have to be kidding. Not happening!"

For this reason, while hospice and palliative care are becoming somewhat more of a norm of practice in the United States, there is much in the experience of economic and racial disenfranchisement among vulnerable populations that makes them suspicious and less receptive to their aims. The National Hospice and Palliative Care Organization reports that of the patients who utilize hospice, about 80% are white, while a mere 8% are African American.

Those facing racial and economic disengagement throughout their lives have experi-enced discrimination, negative stereotyping, neglect, abuse, disrespect, and disregard in varying combinations. It should therefore not be surprising that vulnerable populations will approach end-of-life experience and decision-making with great caution. Victimized by structural racism, poverty, and discrimination, they are wary of mainstream institutions and how they represent the interests of a status quo that has been unhelpful to them throughout life. Given that palliative and hospice care discussions are initiated by health-care professionals, patients and families may be skeptical. They may be afraid that doctors are seeking to terminate their lives earlier because of their social status. They may feel that doctors and nurses are serving the economic interests of the hospital and therefore are recommending discontinuation of curative treatment. For these reasons, it may very well be that in order to optimally serve marginalized populations near the end of life, the next generation of palliative and hospice care will need to establish strong collaborations with community partners who can legitimize their value and ease suspicions about them.

I suspect that, the degree to which palliative and hospice care remain primarily seen as a part of the medical establishment, marginalized populations will continue to be leery of them. They utilize skills and practices that are an established part of medical care and medical institutions. The goals of hospice and palliative care are laudable and deeply hu-mane, yet, as long as they function in connection with mainstream institutions, racially and economically vulnerable populations will be more likely to remain skeptical and dubious about their value.

A CONCLUDING REFLECTION

The voices of patients and loved ones in *Dancing with Broken Bones,* around which the re-mainder of this book will specifically revolve, declare that dying among the inner-city poor is far more than a clinical and medical issue. They illuminate not only the deep personal significance of dying, but also the cultural and social factors that shape patient and family experiences. In some fashion, these factors must be addressed in ways that extend beyond clinical care if we are to become more successful in meeting the needs of the dying poor.

If we listen attentively to their voices, they suggest that their end-of-life experience was shaped by factors that persist in the everyday social, cultural, and economic fabric of their lives, and were characterized by:

- Indignities in care that were clearly associated with their disempowered socioeconomic status;
- Anger and a general sense of mistrust that were a product of having lived at the margins and all of the personal harm that marginalization entails;
- Complicated and sometimes unreliable systems of support;
- A disconnect between the world of patients and families, and the providers who cared for them;
- Some stereotyping among providers about who they were as people and some perceived judgments about their behaviors;
- A feeling that they were not fully or meaningfully understood;
- Daily struggles being created by economic and social hardships few of us can imagine and that sometimes resulted in poor choices and unhealthy lifestyle behaviors, for which they were judged.

On the other hand, their voices also revealed personal and social factors that enabled them to survive and get along both in life and while dying. These included:

- The development of adaptive coping skills and "street-smart" ways that helped them to deal with the rigors of living in inner-city poverty and navigate the overwhelming bureaucracy of the healthcare system;
- A spirit of resilience and hardiness that was cultivated by confronting the daily grind of living poor;
- An unwavering faith that God would see them "home" and thus the corresponding belief that the sufferings of earthly life would be relieved upon their death;
- The uplift provided by sources of social support, even if unevenly and chaotically present;
- A deep spirit of appreciation whenever they felt well cared for and respected as persons;
- A sense of gratitude when they felt that their caregivers were actually interested in them and in their stories. They also trusted that those would hear their stories would not judge them harshly;
- A dignity and self-respect that was remarkable and which stood in stark contrast to their sufferings and dismal life circumstances.

In listening to their stories and attending to the lessons contained within them, the need to develop and systematize practices uniquely tailored to serving their needs becomes apparent and suggests that we must:

- Improve our understanding of the human impact of economic and racial disenfranchisement on individuals, families, and communities if we are to effectively improve end-of-life experience for the inner-city poor;
- Enhance cultural humility among healthcare providers, including creating initiatives that challenge all of us to deepen awareness of our unconscious biases and how those biases influence not only our view of others but also how we relate to them;
- Advance the skills of providers in caring for the unique needs of marginalized populations;
- Develop community-based initiatives that are grounded in culturally-sensitive understandings and grassroots collaborations;
- Create learning experiences for healthcare professionals around the skills and qualities that are required to provide optimal care for vulnerable populations.

A transformation in practices of care for vulnerable populations can be best accomplished if we accept the proposition that, as a wealthy and democratic society, we do have a unique obligation to care for those who live at the margins. In order to do so we must approach the task with cultural humility and in ways that are particularized to addressing their unique vulnerabilities and needs.

All human beings will become ill, will suffer, and will die at some point. The degree to which we can enhance the dignity of all persons in life and while dying is a reflection of the integrity and humanity of our culture and society. While "that physician" is most likely correct in noting that the poor will always be with us, we don't have to accept that to be poor means that one is destined to "die poorly."

In fact, we can choose another path in providing care for those who live at the margins. One which recognizes that we have a moral obligation to improve the quality of their lives. I will conclude by noting the words of Edmund Pellegrino, which state that we do have this moral obligation specific to African-American experience. But I would emphasize that his words also have great relevance for understanding and caring for all marginalized populations:

> . . . . There is a special obligation to African Americans. Their numbers are significant, and their assimilation into the American life has been slow. Their forebears were not willing immigrants, but slaves. There are also the special of the black health experience—the prevalence of poverty, the higher incidence of certain diseases, the alarming infant mortality, the limited access to healthcare, and the paucity of black healthcare professionals.[43]

Pellegrino goes on to add that the canons of "good medicine" make it morally mandatory to learn about the cultural milieu of our patients. Developing practices in palliative and supportive care in ways that are better informed by cultural humility and competence would be to advance the state of the art toward a "next generation" of capability in serving the underserved.

The reflections of the contributors to this volume that you are about to read seek to achieve precisely that. Not only are these professionals true luminaries in palliative and hospice care. Through their participation in this book, they are advancing the cause of

Pellgrino's vision of "good medicine." By their "dialogues" with patients from *Dancing with Broken Bones* (now all deceased), they illuminate a deeper understanding of the role that hospice and palliative care can play in serving the most vulnerable. My hope is that these conversations will promote awareness and enhance practices in caring for the most vulnerable among us, thereby making them "strangers among us" no more.

Emily Dickinson once wrote:

> Death is a dialogue between
> The spirit and the dust.
> —"Death Is a Dialogue," 1890

It can be said that what follows in the remainder of this book is a dialogue between those who live, die, and provide care at the margins.

REFERENCES

1. Harrington M. *The other America: poverty in the United States.* New York: Macmillan; 1962.
2. Powers M, Faden R. *Social justice: the moral foundations of public health and health policy.* New York: Oxford University Press; 2008:90–91.
3. Ahmed SW, Lenkau JP, Neabigh N, Mann B. Barriers to healthcare access in non-elderly urban poor American population. *Health Soc Care Commun.* 2001;9(6):445–453.
4. Rittner B, Kirk AB. Healthcare and public transportation use by poor and frail elderly people. *Social Work.* 1995;40(3):365–373.
5. Levy BS, Seidel VW (eds.). *Social injustice and public health.* New York: Oxford University Press; 2006:5.
6. Tavernese S, Gebeloff R. Smoking proves hard to shake among the poor. *New York Times.* March 24, 2014, A17.
7. Drewnowski D, Specter SE. Poverty and obesity: the role of energy density and energy costs. *Am J Clin Nutr.* 2004;79:6–16.
8. Shuval K, Leonard T, Murdoch JO, Coughy M, Kohl HW. Sedentary behaviors and obesity in a low-income minority population. *J Phys Activity Health.* 2013; (1):132–135.
9. Coleman-Jensen A, Rabbitt M, Gregory C, Singh A. Household food security in the United States. *United States Department of Agriculture. Economic Research Report No. 173.* 2014.
10. National Center for Health Statistics. Health, United States, Special Feature on Ethnic and Health Disparities, 2015. Tables 712, 773, 783, 785.
11. DeNavas W, Proctor BD. Income and poverty in the United States: 2014. Washington, DC: US Census Bureau; 2015.
12. Buffet W. United States Senate Committee on Finance. October 14, 2007.
13. Domhoff W. Who rules America? New York: McGraw-Hill Press; 2006.
14. Fry R, Taylor P. A rise in wealth for the wealthy. Pew Research Center: Social and Demographic Trends. April 23, 2013.
15. Lowry A. The wealth gap in America is growing, too. *New York Times,* Economix Blog, April 2, 2014.
16. Health Disparities. NIH Fact Sheet. 2013.
17. Becker E. *The denial of death.* New York: The Free Press; 1973:ix.
18. Becker E. *Escape from evil.* New York: The Free Press; 1975:11–12.

19. Becker E. *Escape from evil*. New York: The Free Press; 1975:124–125.

20. Nisbet R. Death. In Nisbet R. *Prejudices: a philosophical dictionary*. Cambridge, MA: Harvard University Press; 1982:87.

21. Field M., Cassel C (eds.). A profile of death and dying in America. Approaching death: improving care at the end of life. *Natl Acad Sci*. 1977: 33.

22. Moller DW. *Confronting death: on values, institutions, and human mortality*. New York: Oxford University Press; 1996.

23. Aries P. *Western attitudes toward death: from the Middle Ages to the present*. Baltimore, MD: Johns Hopkins University Press; 1974.

24. Aries P. *The hour of our death*. New York: Oxford University Press; 1981:605.

25. Aries P. *The hour of our death*. New York: Oxford University Press; 1981:28.

26. Aries P. *The hour of our death*. New York: Oxford University Press; 1981:64, 69, 70.

27. Shelley M. *Frankenstein; or, the modern Prometheus*. New York: Airmont Books; 1963:44.

28. Shelley M. *Frankenstein; or, the modern Prometheus*. New York: Airmont Books; 1963:529, 55.

29. Shelley M. *Frankenstein; or, the modern Prometheus*. New York: Airmont Books; 1963:55.

30. Shelley M. *Frankenstein; or, the modern Prometheus*. New York: Airmont Books; 1963:55.

31. Shelley M. *Frankenstein; or, the modern Prometheus*. New York: Airmont Books; 1963:61–62.

32. Shakespeare, Henry the 6th Part 2, scene 7.

33. Kubler-Ross E. *On death and dying*. New York: Macmillan Press; 1969:8–9.

34. Aries P. *The hour of our death*. New York: Oxford University Press; 1981:371.

35. Aries P. *The hour of our death*. New York: Oxford University Press; 1981:569.

36. Moller DW. *Life's end: technocratic dying in an age of spiritual yearning*. New York: Baywood Press; 2000.

37. Nisbet R. *The quest for community*. New York: Oxford University Press; 1974.

38. Rubin R. Improving quality of life at the end of life. *JAMA*. 2016;20(316):2110–2112.

39. Connors W and The SUPPORT Principal Investigators. A controlled trial to improve care for seriously ill hospitalized patients. The Study to Understand Prognoses and Preferences for Outcomes and Risks of Treatment (SUPPORT). *JAMA*. 1996;275(16).

40. Callahan, D. Pursuing a peaceful death. The Hastings Center Report. 1993;23(40): 33–38.

41. National Hospice and Palliative Care Organization. *Facts and Figures, Hospice Care in America*; 2015.

42. Unequal Treatment: Confronting Racial and Ethnic Disparities in Healthcare. Washington, DC: The National Academies Press; 2003:6.

43. Segundy MG. *Trials, tribulations, and celebrations: African American perspectives on health, illness, aging, and loss*. Yarmouth, ME: Intercultural Press; 1992:xxl.

2

COWBOY

FROM SOUTHERN PLANTATION TO URBAN HOMELESSNESS: A PORTRAIT OF AN AMERICAN LIFE

David Wendell Moller

His name is Milton, actually, but he prefers to be called "Cowboy" these days. The month is September, and Linda and I are on our way to visit him at home. However, this will be no ordinary visit, for Cowboy lives under a bridge in a Midwestern city. He is a striking, light-skinned 73-year-old man of biracial descent. At first sight, he looks thin but vibrant. His marvelously-bright eyes seem betrayed by an unclean appearance, and his weathered face reveals a life of long-term suffering and hardship. Greeting us with enthusiasm, he scurries inside and returns with gifts. He presents Linda with a bunch of freshly picked flowers. "I'm not going to tell you where I got them," he says to her mischievously. For me, he has a can of Pepsi wrapped in foil and accompanied with a straw. "You take this and drink it, it's good, you know," he instructs. I also notice that he is clean-shaven and sporting a nice-smelling cologne. I came to learn later on that this was far more for Linda's benefit than for mine and was a part of his pattern of relentlessly flirting with her.

Immediately I sense that, although he lives in an unusual way, Cowboy is a unique and special man. He is engaging, articulate, and gracious. Despite these appealing qualities, however, he is rendered "socially invisible," having been disregarded, perhaps even disdained, by the thousands of people who literally travel over and past his home every day. Daily he faces the challenges imposed by poverty, homelessness, mental instability, and recently diagnosed lung cancer. Yet he remains fiercely independent, retaining great capacity for joy, love, and an appreciation of life. Most people ignore, fear, or disrespect him because, in a culture of affluence and materialism, he embodies economic failure and its moral shame. In this way, people tend to avert their eyes when they encounter Cowboy and others like him, the result of which renders them "invisible." Homeless people live on the margins and in the shadows of acceptability and make us uncomfortable. We typically prefer not to give much thought to them as we scurry past. Nevertheless within each of them is a story which can reveal great insights into the human condition. Cowboy's story contains important lessons about societal responsibility, empathetic connection, the nature of suffering, the resilience and creativity of the human spirit, and the possibilities for transcendence. It demonstrates that the injuries of slavery and segregation are not a vestige of times past. They afflict people still today. And, as we shall see, it also declares the amazing work of palliative care "done right"—that is to say, care that is delivered with cultural competence and single-minded dedication to the service of vulnerable populations.

Cowboy has lived under the bridge for years. The site once housed a colony of homeless men, but they were all chased away by the police. Cowboy was allowed to stay because of his respectful demeanor and the fact that he was judged not to be a threat or a nuisance. As I got to know him I learned how adept he was at human relations and steering interactions with others so they would work in his favor. He loves his home and speaks affectionately about it, calling it "the cave." He is keen on giving us a tour of the premises.

"This is the lounge area," he begins, referring to the first section we come upon after passing through the plastic tarp that serves as the front door. Two bar stools are placed against the back wall, both covered with a film of soot. Remarkably, in this dirty and dingy place that Cowboy calls home, an ironic sense of order and neatness is evident. All his personal items, from medicines, razors, and shave cream, to soaps, deodorant, and toiletries, are impeccably organized. He knows where his every possession is and takes pride in telling us that he is always fixing things up. "I'm an organizer and fixer," he says with a wry laugh, "always have been."

Continuing with the tour, he takes us deeper into the cave, apologizing for the lack of light. "My gas lantern is broken but it'll be fixed soon. So when you come back, things will be nicer." This area is beyond a dead tree that we have to climb around or under and contains all kinds of paraphernalia one might expect a "homeless" person to have: shopping cart, charcoal grill in which wood is burned for heat or to boil water for coffee, and boxes of clothes. (Again, as indicated in the Preface, I must note that I place "homeless" in quotes because if Cowboy were to hear himself described as such, he would say, "That's B.S. What are you talking about? The cave is my home!") Burning torches, filled with a mixture of diesel fuel and gasoline, provided a bit of lighting in the tunnel. Smoke from the burning fires fills the air, bringing irritation and tears to my eyes, and I cannot help but think it is no wonder he is dying from lung cancer.

Venturing deeper still into the furthest and darkest recesses of the cave, we come to the bedroom. Here is a twin-size box spring and mattress that has sheets, two blankets, and pillows. I take note of how neatly the bed is made. There are more boxes of clothes against the wall. Next to the bed is a table where he keeps things he might want during the night. Immediately behind his bed is "the toilet." This is a cardboard box that he fills with dirt, "You know, like cat's litter," he unashamedly explains. "I empty it every day, but usually I go to the bathroom out in the neighborhood." Somehow, I feel impressed with Cowboy's serenity in living with poverty (Figure 2.1).

I later discovered poverty has been the only life he has ever known. Cowboy grew up in the Deep South, picking cotton on a plantation. "We were beyond poverty," he lamented. "Our 'boss man' would lend us enough money to get through the month, but it always ran out in the third or fourth week. We were always in debt to him and could never get out of it." In a very strange way, the foundation for self-sufficiency that would enable him to live productively as an urban, homeless person was laid in the impoverishment of his youth. As his family literally struggled to eat and survive, Milton learned the arts of hustling and entrepreneurship. He raised some chickens that provided eggs and meat, along with a small monthly income. "And I'm not going to tell you how I got it all

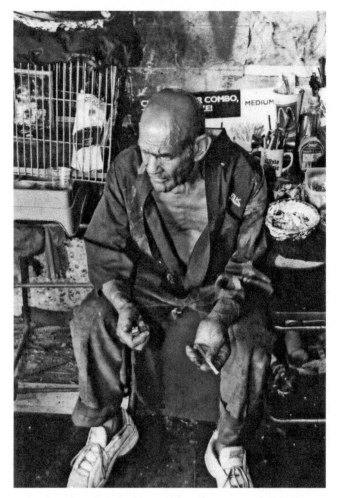

FIGURE 2.1 Cowboy explains that it is not appropriate to label him "homeless," because the cave is his home.

started," he would tease. He did odd jobs for affluent families and earned enough money to eat well throughout the month. "They would go hungry, but not me," he often said with a trace of bitterness in his voice, referring to his own family. His memories of those days in Mississippi are mixed. He takes enormous pride in having survived, especially in his ability to find ways of exceeding the standard of living to which others in his family and community succumbed. Even so, the circumstances of economic deprivation created enormous hardship that not only became his constant companion but also defined the boundaries of his life.

> "They would go hungry, but not me," he often said with a trace of bitterness in his voice, referring to his own family.

In addition to the injuries inflicted by severe poverty that prevailed for families living in the tenant-farmer sharecropping system, prejudice and racism also shaped his youthful experiences. Born out of wedlock, he was conceived by a mother of African-American heritage, while his father was Greek. Even before his birth, his mother was sharply ridiculed by her family and community. She suffered this rejection less for having become pregnant outside of marriage at the age of 14 than because her baby's father was of a different race. As a result of his conception and birth, life was made difficult for Milton's mother, and she deeply resented him. She abused him physically and verbally. He was another mouth to feed, and his presence in her community was a constant source of insult and derision for her.

> He speaks with rage and fury every time he mentions his mother. Her words "I wish I had flushed you down the toilet" remain a hurtful mantra that he has never been able to reconcile.

For 13 years she passed on this iniquity to her son. He angrily explains that those times were filled with physical and verbal harm: how boiling water was poured over him, the scars being visible decades later; that his mother and cousins would beat him regularly; that he was repeatedly called the most vicious names by his family and neighbors; and that he was told on more than one occasion that "everybody would be better off if you were dead." Cowboy's boyhood experiences torment him to this day. He speaks with rage and fury every time he mentions his mother. Her words "I wish I had flushed you down the toilet" remain a hurtful mantra that he has never been able to reconcile. The heart of the matter had to do with race. Compared to his family and others in his community, Cowboy was light-skinned and therefore he was despised because of the significance that carried in the culture and experience of blacks in the deep South during slavery and segregation.

Just as regrettable, Cowboy has passed the legacy of harm on to his own children. He has three by different women. One child is a Christian pastor. Another graduated from Ohio State University and went on to Harvard to study theology with Harvey Cox. But he was unable to complete his journey out of the margins and was drawn back to the streets where he began selling bootleg goods out of the back of his van. He subsequently converted to Islam and became a sheik, living in severe poverty. The third child, his only daughter, is in middle-level management for a national pharmaceutical company. The children want absolutely nothing to do with their father, and Cowboy despises them. "They just don't accept my lifestyle," he says with resentment. Both Linda and I have sought his permission to contact them so they may say goodbye to their dying father and attend his funeral. He becomes irate every time the matter is brought up, and we have been instructed never to mention it again. I cannot help but contemplate how the injustice of poverty and the wickedness of racism, which Milton suffered as a boy, have influenced not only his view of the world but his capacity to relate to it. I often wonder what his life would have been like had not the severity of poverty and evil of prejudice overwhelmed his body and soul during his formative years.

When he was 13, his mother, wanting to be entirely rid of her burden, sent him north to Indianapolis to live with a grandmother. Although he yearned for an education in his new environment, he was told he was "too stupid to learn" and that he should accept who he was. In response, he turned to the streets and received an education of a different sort. He joined the army during the Korean war era at the age of 18 and served for two years in Texas. After being honorably discharged, he worked at many jobs in Chicago and Indianapolis, including driving taxis, bartending, and shining shoes. He always took great delight in "dressing fine and enjoying life." With money in his pocket, he "dressed to impress," especially the ladies, referring to this manner of self-presentation as "cash and flash-flash and cash." He loved and still is passionate about music, which he describes as "my true mistress." Nonetheless, throughout his life he was always haunted by a sense of exile, never feeling comfortable with himself regardless of his surroundings. His abusive upbringing, coupled with his failed marriages, inadequate fathering of his children, and other failed relationships throughout life, has created pain and mistrust, both of which have increasingly become manifest in mental disquiet wherein he is prone to excitability and angry expressions. He does not have a formal diagnosis. However, the best informal medical opinion is that he is manic and perhaps mildly schizophrenic.

> "She's my best friend and I have to take care of her," he quipped about his nine-month-old puppy, Cowgirl.

Recently, Cowboy had been having enormous difficulty breathing, and his legs had swollen to elephant-like dimensions. He rode his bicycle to the local public hospital and was found wandering the hallways. He was immediately taken to the emergency department, where he was evaluated and subsequently admitted to the hospital. Tests revealed that he had lung cancer. After being stabilized and regaining some strength, he would sneak out in the afternoons. The staff assumed he was just running back to the streets for illicit purposes, but these afternoon disappearances had a different meaning. He was returning to the cave each day to feed his dog. "She's my best friend and I have to take care of her," he quipped about his nine-month-old puppy, Cowgirl (Figure 2.2).

Since his diagnosis, Cowboy's life has increasingly become connected to the public hospital system. He began chemotherapy, has met the palliative care team, has spoken to medical students, and has been to the ER four times. Each trip to the ER resulted in admission to the progressive intensive care unit (PICU). His experience as a patient in a safety-net hospital has been both positive and negative. He loves visits by medical students, who have taken an interest in this man from "the other side of the tracks." He thinks the world of his oncologist, although he has met her only once. He loves Linda, the palliative care social worker, and cannot wait for "Dr. G.," the medical director, to visit. It is also instructive that, unlike many inner-city poor who have no choice but to rely on a county hospital for their healthcare, Cowboy, as a veteran, had the option to go the Veterans Administration (VA) hospital. But he opted to seek care at this safety-net hospital because he felt it best served his needs. On the other hand, he has been the recipient of some abusive and impatient treatment by some nurses in the ER, who have

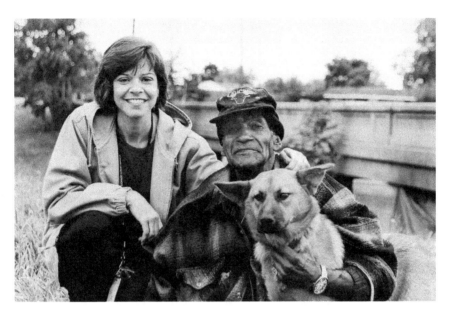

FIGURE 2.2 Cowboy with his beloved Cowgirl and dedicated social worker, Linda.

been frustrated by his return visits. (As it turns out, he had not been fully compliant in taking the antibiotics to treat his pneumonia. Part of the reason was that his eyeglasses were broken and he could not read the discharge instructions or the instructions on his pill bottles.)

He was confused and disorderly during a recent PICU admission, and the nurses exacerbated the situation by huddling outside his door, trying to figure out how to deal with him. He overheard the muddled tones of their conversation and became paranoid because they were talking about him. He started snarling at them, and they decided it was necessary for him to be restrained, Fortunately, at this time, Linda was stopping by for a visit. She was able to tell the nurses about Cowboy's history and needs. Although his history is indeed complex, his needs are rather simple. He needs to know that he matters and will not be mistreated because of how he lives. He needs reassurance that he will not be abandoned, and he requires recognition and respect for his uniqueness as a person. After talking to the nurses, Linda went into his room. Sitting on his bed, she took his hand and spoke with a comforting tone. Within a matter of minutes, the transformation was phenomenal. His ranting and raving were replaced by calm and gratitude. Having witnessed such a dramatic change in behavior, the nurses learned how better to interact with Cowboy, and their relationship with him has improved significantly. Part of this transformation was related to their becoming aware of Cowboy's life story. As his narrative was revealed they were able to deliver care that was informed by cultural humility and compassionate understanding of who he was as a person outside the hospital.

Cowboy was discharged from this hospital admission early in November. He is currently living in a room at the local YMCA. The rent has been paid for two weeks by a Catholic layperson who runs a metropolitan-wide street ministry for marginalized populations in the inner city. Cowboy goes each day to the cave to check on Cowgirl. His faith in God is a source of strength during this difficult time.

> I noticed out of the corner of my eye a Bible neatly placed on a table. Observing me looking at the Bible, he went on to say, "I don't read it so much anymore, and the ministers, they have rejected me a long time ago."

"I'm surprised you ask me about God," he admonished when I questioned him about his beliefs. "God makes all this possible. Yup, He does," he said with conviction. I noticed out of the corner of my eye a Bible neatly placed on a table. Observing me looking at the Bible, he went on to say, "I don't read it so much anymore, and the ministers, they have rejected me a long time ago." I find it interesting that his faith is as private as it is deep. His belief in God is strong, but his disconnection from a faith community and its supportive rituals seem intractably solidified by his lifestyle and its rejection by local faith communities. The cave is located within 500 feet of a church whose clergy and members have no involvement whatsoever with Cowboy. The result of this separation is that he is facing the end of life with regrettable spiritual isolation (Figure 2.3).

I do not know what the future holds for him at this point in his story. He could die this week or live for six months. It is also unclear where he will live after his two weeks at the YMCA are over. Winter is coming, he is sick, and something will have to be worked out for him, and hopefully for Cowgirl as well.

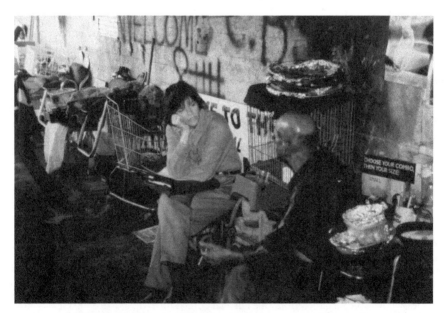

FIGURE 2.3 Everyday racism, as expressed and experienced in American life, reverberates through Cowboy's life story.

The overall purpose of this book is to revisit the portrait presented in *Dancing with Bones* of what is like to live and die in urban poverty, advancing understanding of the unique needs that beleaguer patients and their loved ones, and stimulate a dialogue about best practices in caring for populations who are vulnerable specifically in the intersection of serious illness with racial and economic disparities. So, the beginning of Cowboy's story is in essence the beginning of this effort.

The reflections of Terry Altilio on Cowboy's story, which appear in the next chapter, get us moving toward that end. They initiate that dialogue and set forth a prescription for improving care for marginalized populations near the end of life.

3

NOTES FROM THE TRENCHES
A CONVERSATION WITH COWBOY
AND HIS TEAM

Terry Altilio

A Special Observation

Just as the inhumanity of humanity is revealed throughout much of Cowboy's life, as poverty and racism created indelible harm to him from boyhood and onward, so are opportunities revealed to create moments of compassion when clinicians make efforts to connect with empathy and respect.

Take-Home Lesson

Any belief in the notion of American exceptionalism is seriously challenged by the circumstances that surrounded Cowboy's life as a child and adult. From birth, clearly he was *not created equal*. Nor was he afforded any semblance of equality of opportunity to achieve and be successful. From the beginning, poverty and racism served as barriers to wellness and kept him imprisoned within an "outlier" status in society. He experienced the hatred that flows from bigotry and prejudice. He struggled with injustice and economic disparity; which for him were tethered to the legacy of slavery and the exploitations of tenant farming that are a part of American history. As a result, his life was exceptionally difficult, and in many ways, he became fractured both emotionally and socially. As he lived at the margins, he found within himself strategies for coping and survival that allowed him to live with purpose and meaning. He was creative and resourceful. Despite the tribulations and hardships that weighed him down, he found joy in life. He lived on "his own terms" so to speak, "doing it his way." And it was within his relationship with a best friend, his dog, Cowgirl, that he found comfort and an ability to love for she did not judge him severely as he had been judged throughout his life by so many.

—David Wendell Moller

Note: This commentary reflects thoughts and wonderings that evolved after reading Cowboy's journey with illness, reported through the eyes of those who joined with him as he negotiated this passage. In some ways it is written as a missive to him.

INTRODUCTION

Amid a climate of hopefulness and caution, Linda and David are received as guests in your home and given gifts; flowers for the woman ("I'm not going to tell you where I got them") and a soda for the man. In this one act you have given gifts and simultaneously volunteered that you hold back parts of yourself, vulnerabilities that if exposed might put you at risk. Mischief, engagement, ambivalence, and mistrust are reflected in words and acts; characteristics that may infuse most relationships, yet, based on your early life, may be most pronounced with women. In the course of this visit, you share some essential values and aspects of who you have come to be. Your revelations will help build both relationships and a beginning plan of care that may sustain and protect you through an illness that will force interaction with a healthcare system, with the potential, while often unintended, to recreate the rejection and despair of your early years. So, there is a lot at stake and the risks for you are high. This same system, however, and those individuals who work in it can also craft an experience for you, in your dying, that affirms your right to be who you are by caring for you with empathy.

The fact that Linda and David have been allowed to visit your home bespeaks a number of tentative hypotheses, some hopeful and some cautionary:

- *Hopefulness*
  - You have chosen to allow "institutional others" into your "cave" and begun to share the narrative of your life on your terms and in your space;
  - These same clinicians and their palliative care team can provide some coherence over time and across settings to assist as you manage a progressing disease, treatments, and a fractured healthcare system;
  - There is the prospect that the healthcare system and those who work in it may provide an experience that legitimizes your personal struggles and acknowledges what you have created in your life;
  - People of good intentions may craft an environment that hints of a trust that will allow you to risk being cared for in spite of the racism, cruelty, and disinterest that you have come to know;
  - Some of the same people who may have "walked over" or "driven over" you while you were at home under the bridge may feel redeemed as they provide care in the safety and structure of an institutional setting;
  - Lastly, the skills that have helped you to survive may serve to engage those in the healthcare system who remain available for engagement.

- *Caution*
  - The sparkle in your eyes may mask a range of fears, beliefs, suspicions, and emotions that have the potential to ignite under the stress of illness, its debilitating symptoms, and your evolving dependence;
  - Seeking medical care forces an entrée into a system that has the power to validate schemas of defectiveness, shame, rejection, and mistrust that pervaded your early life;[1,2]

- There will be a range of responses from staff—some may feel empathy and shared responsibility for the dehumanizing effects of racism and poverty; others may wish to flee, blame, or punish;
- The palliative care clinicians working to serve you through this illness may not always be there, nor always be able to influence the hospital environment to support and respect your unique self;
- Dependence on others will be a risk. The charm, respect, and resourcefulness that enhance your relationships may be more difficult to garner as illness evolves; anger and rage may surface at times when you need others the most;
- The order and control that you have created in your "cave" and the alliance with police authorities contribute to your sense of safety. Transferring this "formula for safety" to a healthcare system may be complicated both by illness and by the reality that the "boss man" is represented by multiple and ever-changing staff.

SETTING A CONTEXT: WHAT HAVE WE LEARNED THAT MAY TEACH US HOW TO BEST SERVE YOU?

You have survived where others have not. You learned at a very early age that survival depended on you, and you alone. You learned that sharing with others or trusting them often strengthened the harmful capacities of those who would damage you or prefer to see you dead. As a biracial child in the South and a biracial adult in the United States it was as if you were victim of both whites and blacks; finding comfort or acceptance from neither. Many of those in similar circumstances who lived around you were also desperate to survive. Internalized rage fueled by destitution and racism may have prompted the cruelty, physical and emotional, that you experienced. Yet your skills as a hustler and entrepreneur have served to help you survive, but they never taught you how to love. You were able to engage in relationships with the three different women who bore your children. But beyond the biological act of fathering, the experience of parenting and sustained giving relationships was not possible for you. It was never learned or received in your own childhood. Reflective of your early life, the needs of others, including those of your own children, may have been perceived as threatening to your very survival and the lifestyle that you worked so hard to create. While this lifestyle may have been mediated by loneliness and aloneness that served to protect you, it was also celebrated by pleasures that included women, music, and being publicly acknowledged by awards such as "Best Dressed Black Man" in Chicago. It gave you identity and helped you to survive living in circumstances that are hard for most to fathom.

While poverty and probable mental illness have derailed aspects of your "cash and flash" identity, you have created a sense of order, a secure, private, and protected space where you live at the behest of the "boss man" represented in your current life by the police. They have privileged you and allowed you to live in a place where others have been forced out. Your charm and respectfulness to those in power allowed you to remain, and you have established a home. Cowgirl has entered and stayed in your life, providing a singular and chosen relationship of mutual nurture and dependence.

SOME WONDERINGS AND WORRIES

Hospitals and people who work in them have a respect for order and control similar to yours. While they may respect independence in their own lives, independence in a health-care setting sometimes disrupts the order perceived to be necessary to meet the needs of patients and staff. There are rules and uniforms; forms that ask for data such as address, next of kin, and insurance; forms that may cause distress if they symbolically reflect what has been so missing in your life. They will ask about social and family supports; Cowgirl, while a cherished relationship, may not be viewed as sufficient support. Although she may very well be able to seek help should an emergency evolve, Cowgirl will not be able to help with decision-making should there come a time when you cannot guide us. It will be important to consider sharing your ideas and values about what makes your life meaningful. The beginning of your life was controlled by others; the end can be lived in a way that is coherent with who you have become.

> You have survived where others have not.

The diagnosis of lung cancer will most likely force a relationship with the healthcare system and oncology clinicians over time. Relationships of long duration have not been your strong suit! If the disease progresses quickly, the challenges of sustained relationship will be replaced by an intimate connection to a system and staff you have not been able to test for reliability and safety. Regardless, your identity as "Cowboy," one who lives in the "cave" under a bridge, nurtures and cares for Cowgirl, is the father of three, a lover of music, "flash and cash" is likely to broaden as you become a patient, a cancer patient, a homeless cancer patient, and one who has alienated your family. The lack of family to advocate for you creates an additional vulnerability. It may make you more susceptible to the power of the healthcare team who may assert their own values in caring for you and remain unchallenged in doing so because of the absence of family or friends. Healthcare systems, at their worst, foster identity theft: people often lose much of themselves as they become a "patient." In the best of circumstances, identity is not shattered but evolves as a person is helped to bring coherence to their experience with illness, symptoms, the healthcare system itself, and eventually death. While many will celebrate you as a survivor with resilience and strengths, others may confer an identity of victim—unclean, disheveled, homeless, and indigent without necessary resources to support a treatment plan for cancer. Your identity as "survivor" may take on different meaning as you anticipate the end of life and consider the legacy you might leave beyond your lived experience. Clinicians may label you as "noncompliant" or perhaps use a gentler version of the term, "non-adherent." While both words may cause you to feel judged or infantilized, well-intended clinicians will be reflecting their judgment that your social environment and skills will not support safety and allow you to manage the treatments or medications necessary to treat your diseases. These worries may be used to justify clinicians' decisions to withhold certain treatments that would be suggested for others, impacting your quality of life and perhaps your survival and validating the reinforcing nature of destitution.

These worries are not unfounded. Lung cancer at a relatively young age may, at one and the same time, be a consequence of destitution and the precipitant that drives you to move from living in your beloved "cave" to a different environment. Treatments may require a range of medications, interventions such as catheters or intravenous lines, and perhaps oxygen, should you become short of breath. This disease and its treatments may force conversations that are not intended to disrespect the life you have created in your "cave," but rather to anticipate possibilities and protect you from medical crises that cannot be handled at home. Such protection is not meant to diminish you, and it may seem peculiarly ironic that the protection that you needed as a child is now being offered at the age of 73 (Figure 3.1).

While exploring and anticipating possibilities, it is helpful to ponder how early abuse and victimization may add to the vulnerability implicit in illness and the role of patient. Interacting, asking for help, and depending on others is unavoidable. The structure and schedule are often set by others. Privacy is essentially gone. Dogs are generally unable to visit. Sometimes we cause "hurt" in the course of treating serious illness. We give injections; chemotherapy that may cause side effects and pain. This dynamic can mimic early trauma. Will you flee, attack, or attribute cruelty to those who are intending to help? This "hurt," often unavoidable, is not intended to harm. On their better days, clinicians will do their best to create predictability and a structure that minimizes re-traumatization, respects your history, and accomplishes the medical tasks. It is possible that simple interventions delivered with calm and respect for your unique narrative will not compound the impact of trauma and destitution as you receive medical care. Toward this same end, perhaps we can arrange a visit with Cowgirl, help you to plan for her so she is cared for as you come to the end of life.

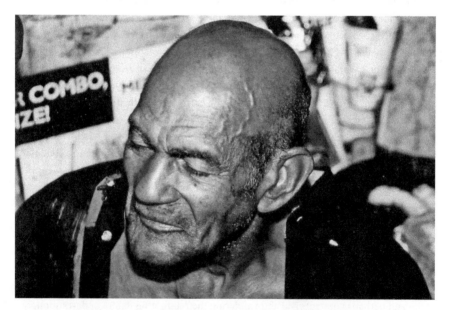

FIGURE 3.1 The story of Cowboy illustrates the need for cultural curiosity to discover the dynamics that evolve at the intersection of person, illness, and institution in order to provide the best care possible for people who live their lives at the fringes.

One last worry—many people who are living with life-threatening illness are asked to appoint an "agent," generally a trusted person who can assist with medical decision-making. These conversations will invite reflection on your aloneness and fractured relationships with your children and their mothers. Clinicians will ask about resuscitation, artificial hydration, and nutrition and may offer their best medical opinion, share the benefits and risks of these interventions, and suggest that, in the setting of progressing lung cancer, you forego these interventions. It will be hard to imagine that the world that has been so depriving would have your best interests at heart. The emotions and thoughts that surround these considerations are often complex. Making decisions based on the values that bring meaning to your life may be clouded by the experience of deprivation and a wish for reparation. Consider that resuscitation or artificial nutrition could never compensate for the cruelty and destitution that have been part of your life. The act of resuscitation in its aggressiveness toward your body may seem a congruous ending to your life; you may want to fight for continued survival. It is possible also to choose to allow your life to end in a peaceful and calm manner in a setting of familiarity and comfort. These are important discussions to be held with those you may come to count on.

THE TEAM: "WE WILL LOVE HIM UNTIL HE DIES"

Palliative care teams have a collective and individual focus; shared and individual expertise. The challenge of "We will love him until he dies" may place shifting and unique demands on each discipline. Cowboy's narrative presents a tapestry of opportunity for psychosocial-spiritual intervention—housing, fractured family relationships, spiritual and social isolation, psychiatric vulnerability—to name a few.

The environmental aspects that revolve around housing, Cowgirl, medications, and safety are intertwined, infused with complex meaning, emotion, and practical challenges. The ongoing adjustments in these aspects of a palliative plan of care rest essentially within the relationship with a social worker who, as a woman, may be a recipient of ambivalent and powerful emotions. This aspect of care becomes a magnet for the judgments of healthcare professionals about Cowboy's cave—judgment juxtaposed with the value that Cowboy places on his home and possessions and the social worker's effort to respect his autonomy and self-determination. Our perception of safety and an adequate setting for a sick and aging man may differ significantly from that of Cowboy, whose home is infused with complex meaning and memories. This discrepancy in perspective is reflected in his words, "You can't worry about these things more than I do."

Securing adequate housing will be challenging due to the nature of the man and his illnesses, both medical and psychiatric, and it can become a focal point for those who may question Cowboy's capacity to make good decisions. The complexity of this aspect of care is reflected in the effort of the social worker to secure, over time, four housing arrangements, overcoming multiple obstacles only to then be judged by medical students for allowing herself to be exploited and manipulated. Medical students in their role as learners were gifted by Cowboy's teaching, an activity that reflected his resilience and ability to overcome. Teaching others validated and enhanced his self-esteem at the same time that it represented a victory over those who had diminished his ability to learn. Teaching provided an avenue to express his beliefs and views about race and poverty to a young generation who were not his troubled and disappointed children. They simply received and became a part of a legacy provided to the next generation in a relatively conflict-free manner.

> Can a father rest when he has come to experience a caring—an acceptance that is so diametrically opposed to what he created with his children?

Creating a successful plan for housing would not be conflict-free. Cowboy would leave most of his possessions and Cowgirl. He would be asked to follow rules stifling his independence and containing his creative efforts to create a living space that reflected his unique identity. Painting the walls in the YMCA red might be a glaring representation of both protest as well as a need for expression of self. Expecting to become sicker and more symptomatic, his survival skills, resilience, and lack of concern for consequences allowed him to take risks and make choices that were potentially life-threatening. For example, after an expected eviction from a residence that could not manage his emerging incontinence, he disappeared into the street for two weeks. Perhaps in Cowboy's lived version of a life review, he returned to touch and grieve aspects of his life where he felt respect and an established identity. It is possible that because of the accepting and mutually respectful relationship he had with the palliative care team, he felt the freedom to "disappear" and "reappear," trusting that he would be cared for. Perhaps he considered abandoning the others before they abandoned him. Yet, Cowboy returned, allowed himself to be cared for, paid his debts, and let God enter his life.

The team's mantra to "love him until he dies" has different meanings in his life, dependent on role and relationship. Beyond the team, Cowboy's relationships with his family are troubled and infused with anger, resentment, and themes of abandonment. His ability to create meaningful and valued relationships with medical students and healthcare staff as he comes to the end of his life is one aspect of a legacy that complements or counters what his children have known of their father. They may be confused and need help to understand how Cowboy has come to give to and accept from healthcare providers when he was so unable to give to them. The death of their father means the death of his physical self and whatever hopes they might have had for more time and reconciliation. "Loving him until he dies," while possible for staff, was not possible for his children and was not expected, nor forced by the staff caring for Cowboy and his family. Yet through the process of their father's illness and death, his relationships with his care team, and the celebrity he came to attract, they may come to know each other and aspects of Cowboy that may help them, over time, to create lives that integrate a more complex legacy that goes beyond his inability to nurture them.

SUMMARY

The clinicians who assisted Cowboy through this last chapter of his life attributed the outcome to the "redemptive power of love" and "mindful presence." There are many other notable aspects of Cowboy's narrative.: Unconditional acceptance, searches for housing, attention to symptoms, trust building, and partnership formation. As he struggled in illness these were components of the care provided to him and which comforted him throughout his end-of-life experience. Beyond the core palliative care team, there were also community contributions, ranging from the police who protected the cave to the landlady who was asked to face her son's dishonesty and her fear of Cowboy dying in her home who then went on to become a part of the rescue of Cowgirl.

Cowboy's journey leaves one with many questions and wonderings. Do medical treatments that are offered, withdrawn, and accepted have attributed meanings that go beyond the treatments themselves and become symbols of caring—remedies for past deprivations? Can a father rest when he has come to experience a caring and acceptance that is so diametrically opposed to what he created with his children? Is it possible that this caring is so excruciatingly absent from his relationship with his sons and daughter as to cause an unrest that may never be soothed? Is this perhaps a most poignant lesson from Cowboy's final legacy?

REFERENCES

1. Parsonnett L, Lethborg C. Addressing suffering in palliative care: Two psychotherapeutic models. In Altilio T, Otis-Green S. *Oxford textbook of palliative social work.* New York: Oxford University Press; 2011:191–200.
2. Young JE, Klosko JS, Weishaar M. *Schema therapy: A practitioner's guide.* New York: Guilford Publications; 2003.

4

EXPLORING THE EXPERIENCES
OF MR. J. W. GREEN
INJUSTICE, POVERTY, MISTREATMENT, AND
EVIL SURROUNDING SERIOUS ILLNESS AND
DEATH IN POOR AFRICAN-AMERICAN PEOPLE

Richard Payne

Everybody wants to go to heaven, but nobody wants to die. It's not so much the act of dying itself, but the things that are surrounding death: injustice, poverty, mistreatment and evil. . . . There's a sense that we won't be stopped by those things—our "somehow theology." Somehow, some way, we will get through this.
—Rev. Frank Jackson

J. W.—A Snapshot Reflection: A Story of Racism and Injustice

The experience of being black and poor in America cannot be separated from our societal history of institutionalized racism in the form of slavery, segregation, and blocked opportunity. J. W. Green was a product of that history.

J. W.'s ancestors were slaves on a Southern plantation. The son of tenant-farmer sharecroppers, he was raised in Mississippi. The sharecropping experience has faded from American consciousness, and many people know little about it. For those who were part of the streaming exodus from the Deep South to urban ghettos in the 1950s and 1960s, however, the imprint of this form of rural poverty—which evolved directly from the institution of slavery—was an inescapable part of the socioeconomic identity that shaped who and what they were to become in urban life.

Tenant farmers and sharecroppers living on the plantation were technically free, but the burden of poverty was inescapable and imprisoning. After the Civil War ended the slaves were emancipated, but they lacked skills and opportunities to build economically independent lives. Consequently, they entered into what was essentially a new system of servitude. As tenant farmers, they would be provided a parcel of land to grow crops, along with basic necessities—primitive housing, food, clothing, seeds, and farming equipment. When the crops were finally harvested, the owner of the plantation would take his share (50% typically). He would also deduct from the proceeds the costs of food, shelter, and so forth that he had provided to the tenants. Sharecropping remained a regular part of Southern life until the middle of the 20th century. It created debt cycles and a sense of despair and hopelessness that trapped many in an economic and race-based system of exploitation. In short, black people in the South may have been formally free during this era, but many remained subservient, poor, and lacking in opportunity to improve their lives.

This was the economic, cultural, and personal reality that J. W. experienced for the first two decades of his life. His family lived in constant debt to their "boss man," as the plantation owner was called. Daily life was filled with hardships and the struggle to survive in the grip of sharecropper poverty. His family history, where his ancestors were unable to move up the economic ladder, taught him that there was virtually no escape from this life of subsistence. Ironically, however, his memories of these years were not entirely resentful. He spoke about how rich his family life was—not in the sense of material wealth, but in the love of each other, the simplicity of their lives, and their deep and abiding faith in God. He took great comfort in this richness, and it would influence him for the rest of his life.

Despite this solace, he realized that he was doomed to destitution and a life in "plantation poverty" unless he made a move. So J. W., as did many of his generation, said goodbye to his Southern roots and migrated to a Northern/Midwestern city. The promise and hope was for a better life, one where the strain of racism and economic hardship would be eased by a spectrum of new possibilities. Life was indeed very different up north for J. W., but not in ways he had hoped for. Racism, while differently expressed in Northern cities, still existed. Because of his race and his lack of education and skills, his employment opportunities were limited, and he had left behind the support of family and community, which grounded and comforted him back in Mississippi. In the chaos and stymied opportunity of his new world, J. W. began to learn the fine art of street survival. He eked out a living by hustling, stealing, and running the neighborhoods scouting for opportunities to make money and engage in mischief. Drinking and womanizing became dominant activities and offered some escape from the demands of ghetto life. In many ways, if the truth be told, J. W. lived his life as a "poster boy" for the irresponsible black man in the inner city, an image that was created and popularized in the broader society with little understanding of the damage that these people had endured in their lives. He had multiple wives and children and never fulfilled his responsibilities as a husband or father. As he submitted to the pull of the streets, drug dealers, prostitutes, and numbers runners became influential in shaping who he was. Unlike many American children who are born into privileged lives and have futures that are far more hopeful, J. W. was never able to overcome the impact of poverty and racism that shaped and limited his opportunities in life—both on the Southern plantation and in the urban-ghetto streets. Thus, the "ways of the street" became the defining pathway to his ways of life and ultimately shaped the way in which he would die.

Six decades after his birth in Mississippi, J. W. became a patient in the urban public hospital system, having been diagnosed with advanced prostate cancer. His illness narrative is one of disempowerment, neglect, and fear. He was disempowered in his role as a patient to the degree that he did not understand his prognosis or even treatment regimen. He also endured numerous indignities in care that most would find unacceptable. As his disease spread into his spine and he was on the verge of becoming quadriplegic, he was admitted to the county nursing home. Once there, inattention and neglect led to the development of horrific bed sores that persisted until he died. He endured this indignity without ever voicing a complaint to the staff but, nonetheless, held the distinct belief that the deficiencies in his care were a consequence of his being poor. He often talked about how in life he was one of the "have-nots," and he distinctly believed that the less-than-optimal care he received in the nursing home was directly a result of his being poor.

Perhaps most distressing of all for J. W. was the fear of abandonment and loneliness. He had deserted his children and wives a long time ago, and perhaps turnabout is fair play. None of his seven children and five former wives was interested in his suffering or impending death, and they wanted nothing to do with him. The result was that he worried intensely about being alone in dying. However, in the midst of the chaos, a nephew stepped up to the plate and promised that he would support him throughout his illness—and that is exactly what his nephew, Frank, did. Each day, for the final four months of his uncle's life, Frank would be found "mindfully present" at J. W.'s bedside in the nursing home.

Another striking aspect of J. W.'s end-of-life experience was his faith-based acceptance of dying. Despite pain and discomfort, J. W. was never angry or bitter. To the contrary, he looked forward to the future with great optimism, believing that God would take him "home." J. W. viewed his disease as a necessary part of that journey and faced its tribulations with the firm belief that at the end of his life there would be great reward. Somehow, all these decades later and in spite of his personal imperfections and the burdens created by poverty and racism, the faith that helped sustain him as a boy on the Southern plantation guided and comforted him as he was dying in the nursing home. The result was that he died spiritually rich, at peace with God and himself.

A Special Observation

J. W.'s struggle in life and illness was directly linked to being a poor, black man in American society.

Take-Home Lesson

The vicissitudes of race and poverty shaped J. W.'s upbringing in the Deep South as well as his adjustment to urban living as an adult. His lack of education, employment opportunity, and personal empowerment led to a "life on the streets." His personal journey as an adult, tied explicitly to the legacy of race and class in his life, led to irresponsible behaviors toward his wives and children. In turn, he was abandoned by them during his illness and encountered the anxieties that surround loneliness in dying. A lack of education and empowerment resulted in misunderstandings about his disease and its corresponding treatment, compromising his ability to advocate for himself with his caregivers. Stoic faith saw him through a life and death in poverty.

—David Wendell Moller

INTRODUCTION

As chronicled by David Moller in his book *Dancing with Broken Bones*, J. W. Green was a poor African-American man who migrated from rural Mississippi to the Midwest in early adulthood, and died at 60 years old from metastatic prostate cancer.[1] He lived a life on the streets, disconnected in many ways from his family responsibilities as a father and husband. His disease was diagnosed at an advanced stage, and, as the cancer invaded and compressed his spinal cord, he was rendered quadriplegic. In the hospital, the quality of his care was compromised by the poor communication between him and his medical team of caregivers. He also received substandard care in the nursing home when he was no longer able to live independently, developing painful, infected bedsores in the last months of his life as a result. During the pain and suffering and the assault on his dignity, Mr. Green remained relatively tolerant of his caregivers' behaviors and mistakes and made few complaints during the last phase of his life (Figure 4.1). He had a great fear

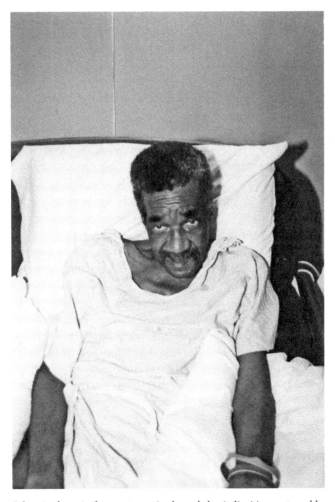

FIGURE 4.1 Suboptimal care in the county nursing home led to indignities most would never tolerate.

of isolation and abandonment—ironically, despite his own abandonment of his wives and children as a younger man. The attention and compassionate presence of a nephew who protected him from his angry, vengeful sons at the end of his life quieted this fear. Because of his strong faith in God, Mr. Green was able to accept the circumstances of his dying and achieve some measure of peace.

Mr. Green's case raises so many important issues that will be briefly summarized here and detailed further in subsequent sections. First, it is critical to recognize that his life story is inextricable from the fact that he was born a poor African-American male who "immigrated" (this word is used deliberately) from the South to the North in search of a better life. In some ways his "immigration" was beneficial to him, but, alas, he could not escape a fate that was largely determined by his economically deprived childhood and young adult environment.

His death from prostate cancer, and the inadequate care he received prior to death are all too common for African Americans. A landmark Institute of Medicine (IOM) Report, *Unequal Treatment: Confronting Racial and Ethnic Disparities in Health Care*, published more than a decade ago, concluded that:

> a consistent body of research demonstrates significant variation in the rates of medical procedures by race, even when insurance status, income, age, and severity of conditions are comparable. This research indicates that U.S. racial and ethnic minorities are less likely to receive even routine medical procedures and experience a lower quality of health services.[2]

These disparities in care are reflected in worse health outcomes for African Americans, and contribute to excessive mortality associated with cancer and other chronic diseases. As Mr. Green experienced, even nursing home care is beset with inequalities arising from segregated facilities and affects those with limited available resources.

David Williams, a sociologist, epidemiologist, and public health researcher, has documented that there are many ways in which racism and perceived discrimination may affect health and influence mortality.[3] Some of these factors are illustrated in Figure 4.2. The net effect of these negative practices in healthcare settings engendered by poverty and associated health disparities is the nearly 1 million "excess deaths" in African Americans over the course of a decade.[4]

Mr. Green's life and death typified very important characteristics of African-American life: in particular, the importance of care by a dominant family member—even care by a so-called fictive (non–biologically related) kin—and the critical role of faith and religion in everyday life. Religious and cultural beliefs of persons like Mr. Green, and his social and cultural expressions of same, may impact health caregiver perceptions and treatment of serious illness and end-of-life care. These will be discussed in the section on the importance of religion in African-American life and the section on dignity.

RACIALLY-BASED DISPARITIES IN HEALTHCARE

Of all the forms of inequality, injustice in health care is the most shocking and inhumane.
—Dr. Martin Luther King, Jr.

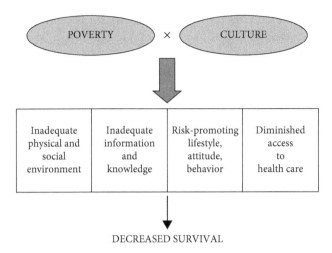

FIGURE 4.2 Medical neglect syndrome. This figure diagrams the factors that are associated with decreased survival in poor and medically-underserved communities. Recent social and environmental factors that support health and longevity have been shown to have biological correlates that may ultimately provide a mechanistic understanding of the ways in which psychological stress associated with poverty, racial discrimination, and other social ills influence excessive mortality.

This famous quote is attributed to Martin Luther King by Dr. Quentin Young, Chair of the Medical Committee for Human Rights in Chicago, who heard a speech given by Dr. King to their group in 1966. Dr. Young noted that King actually said that health inequalities are "inhuman," which, in my view, is an even stronger criticism than to call them "inhumane." Yet, as the 2003 IOM report documented, racially based disparities are prevalent in all areas of healthcare. More recent studies than the IOM report have documented the persistence of racially based health disparities, and as Williams has stressed,

> The residential concentration of African Americans is high and distinctive, and the related inequities in neighborhood environments, socioeconomic circumstances and medical care are important factors in initiating and maintaining racial disparities in health. . . . Health and health disparities are embedded in larger historical, geographic, sociocultural, economic, and political contexts. Changes in a broad range of public policies are likely to be central to effectively addressing racial disparities.[5]

Inequalities in healthcare can have lethal outcomes, whether they occur in the hospital, the cancer clinic, or the nursing home. Mr. Green received very poor care in the nursing home, suffering bed sores from inadequate turning, care, and attention. This should not be surprising, as highly segregated, understaffed, and poorly resourced nursing homes are common in African-American communities. Nursing homes, like residential housing in many areas, are highly segregated. African Americans make up less than 15% of the US population, and live in all parts of the country. Yet 60% of African Americans reside in fewer than 10% of the nursing homes because nursing home demographics closely reflect the housing patterns in their neighborhoods. A recent study documented the poor care that African Americans receive in many nursing homes in their communities.[6] African Americans like Mr. Green, the study found, were substantially more likely than whites to reside in nursing homes with major deficiencies on inspection reports, staffing shortages, and financial difficulties. Ironically, nursing homes in the South were less segregated than nursing homes in the Midwest, with Indianapolis, where Mr. Green lived, ranking among the highest in segregated nursing homes providing poor-quality care.

Medicaid, the federal and state program funding care for the poor, is also the major funder of nursing home care in the United States. Long-term nursing home care for the poor, or those who progress to poverty when their financial resources are depleted, is funded by Medicaid. Although it is good that there is a source of funding for nursing home care, it is also true that Medicaid pays nursing homes substantially less than private payers do. African-American nursing home residents like Mr. Green are almost twice as likely to live in places that were terminated from Medicare and Medicaid participation because of poor quality. One obvious policy recommendation is to close the gap between amounts paid to nursing home by Medicaid and private payers, and to insist on implementing quality measures that promote better care. Among these measures should include higher minimum staffing levels that would allow more attention to the physical care of residents like Mr. Green who require frequent turning and high personal touch care.

In particular, Mr. Green's story is typical of the plight of so many poor people—white and non-white—who have cancer. Many years ago, cancer surgeon and pioneer Dr. Harold Freeman, one of two African-American presidents of the American Cancer Society, initiated a program to address the greater lethality of cancer in poor Americans.[7] His pioneering work was a response to data showing that for men and women, the five-year survival for all cancers combined is 10 percentage points lower among persons who are poor.

Furthermore, Mr. Green's burden of living in poverty carries additive risks and liabilities associated with race-related inequalities of cancer care and related outcomes.[8] African-American men have a 60% higher incidence (rate of new cases per 100,000 population) of prostate cancer, and two to three times higher death rate than white men with prostate cancer.[9] We have no information as to whether Mr. Green had prostate cancer screening at age 45 as is currently recommended by the American Cancer Society (ACS) "for men at high risk of developing prostate cancer. This high risk group includes African Americans and men who have a first-degree relative (father, brother or son) diagnosed with prostate cancer at an early age (younger than age 65)."[10]

There is controversy about screening for prostate cancer. Recent guidelines from the US Preventative Task Force (USPTF) recommend less aggressive screening of all men for prostate cancer.[11] However, others have argued that African-American men are at such a greater risk than other men for developing the disease and dying from it that the 2012 USPTF guidelines should not apply to them. Supporting this argument are studies that suggest that prostate cancer behaves biologically more aggressively in African-American men than in whites.[12] This controversy is largely irrelevant to Mr. Green, and, indeed, most individuals like him, who are unaware of the guideline recommendations, and, even if they were, would have substantial hurdles in getting to medical facilities to receive even the reduced level of recommended screening. It is highly doubtful that Mr. Green had any prostate cancer screening at any time, much less at age 45, but such screening could detect early prostate cancer, which is curable.

There are a myriad of reasons for higher rates of cancer and worse outcomes from cancer in poor and African-American people. These factors involve the interplay among economic, social, and cultural—and perhaps even biological variables. These elements influence all aspects of cancer care, including prevention, early detection and diagnosis, treatment adequacy, patient compliance, post-treatment quality of life and support, and, ultimately, survival. Poverty has a particularly pernicious influence on health outcomes from all disease, especially cancer.

In describing Mr. Green's life at one point, David Moller offered this commentary:

> However, in getting to know J. W. during his time of serious illness, I saw a different side of him and was able to understand how many of his actions were *traceable to the terrible hardness of his life*. Although the impact of extreme poverty that was his "birthright" can never be precisely defined or measured, there is no doubt that it held sway over his view of the world and his actions in it. . . . [emphasis added].[1]

There is/may be a pernicious social disempowerment at play here where persistence of excess mortality among the African-American population is a desirable outcome.

Mr. Green's life was indeed "hard," chiseled by the mix of poverty and the structural racism that enabled so much of it, ultimately leading to a shortened lifespan for him. As diagrammed in Figure 4.1, poverty and the effects and life stressors that are associated with institutionalized poverty can become embedded in one's culture and daily lifestyle. For example, an inadequate physical and social environment often leads to unhealthy diets, overconsumption of alcohol, the use of tobacco products, and chronic disease (asthma, chronic obstructive pulmonary disease [COPD], etc.) Inadequate health information and health illiteracy associated with resource-poor environments all have powerfully negative effects on health. For example, it is doubtful that Mr. Green had any adequate knowledge about choices in cancer screening, particularly for African-American men who are at higher risk for developing prostate cancer and dying from it. Clearly Mr. Green lived a risk-promoting life style on the streets of Indianapolis, involving himself in prostitution, and perhaps illicit drug use (which closely follows prostitution and street life). He had limited access to routine, preventative healthcare based on his lack of health insurance, and probably fell victim to the variable quality of healthcare often associated with public insurance programs such as Medicaid. Importantly, there is an emerging body of evidence in molecular biology, genetics, and epigenetics that demonstrate that social and environmental factors associated with poverty and *biological processes* can adversely affect health.

There is/may be a pernicious social disempowerment at play here where persistence of excess mortality among the African-American population is a desirable outcome. An analysis of 73 million US deaths from the years 1970 to 2004 estimated that approximately 1 million black votes were not cast in the presidential election in 2004 by people in the age range of 40–60 years of age because of deaths in this age group. Although these additional black voters would have been likely to overwhelmingly vote for the Democratic candidate, Senator John Kerry, it would not have been enough to change the result of the election. However, the effects of excessive mortality on black "disenfranchisement" are, in fact, magnified by the additional loss of African-American voters related to felony convictions and disenfranchisement laws that predominantly affect the poor and communities of color. This is another fact of life placement and choice that is connected to poverty, poor education, and a lack of economic opportunity. In fact, the authors of the study concluded: "Systematic disenfranchisement by population group yields an electorate that is unrepresentative of the full interests of the citizenry and affects the chance that elected officials have mandates to eliminate health inequality."[13] We do not know Mr. Green's voting habits or his political preferences. It is likely, however, that he, like many poor African Americans, did not regularly vote or otherwise participate in the political process. The life trajectory of the Mr. Greens of America must change so they are functioning and contributing members who participate to effect health policy changes that will be of benefit to their communities and thus the overall health of our populace.

> Socioeconomic status is a major factor determining life expectancy in the United States for males and females of all races and ethnicities.

We don't have much information about Mr. Green's perceptions of racism and discrimination, but surely he experienced it. If we take the most-commonly accepted definition of racism, by which we mean people and organizations who "categorize population groups into 'races' and use this ranking to preferentially allocate more societal goods and resources to groups regarded as superior,"[14] it would be beyond belief to assume that Mr. Green did not experience racism personally as he lived poor in the rural South and then in the urban Midwest. My primary argument in this chapter is it is impossible to understand Mr. Green's illness experiences, and his reactions to them, without a sense of the institutionalized systems of racism that give rise to persistent poverty and the manifestations of health inequalities in our society. A critical aspect of this argument is that racist practices and policies become deeply entrenched in the culture of society and its institutions, so that discrimination can persist in a succession of healthcare settings such as professional medical societies, hospitals, clinics, and nursing homes—*even as levels of individual racial prejudice and discriminatory practices decline.*

There is now a large body of evidence documenting the idea that the life stresses associated with being targets of discrimination—actual and perceived—can have profoundly negative effects on health.[15] The negative effects of life stressors associated with racism can be as far-ranging as effects on cardiovascular reactivity and blood pressure control to cancer susceptibility.[16]

Important recent data also suggest that racism and life stresses may influence biological responses related to aging and disease susceptibility, thereby affecting mortality. For example, women who have "triple-negative breast cancer," a type of breast cancer in which the tumor cells lack estrogen, progesterone, and HER2-receptor hormone proteins, have a worse prognosis for survival than women who have forms of breast cancer in which one or more of these receptors are present on their cancer cells. A higher percentage of African-American women have triple-negative breast cancer compared to white women, for reasons unknown, and this partly explains the higher overall death rates of black women compared to white women with breast cancer. However, it is also known that when African-American women and white women with triple-negative breast cancers are compared, African-American women *still* die at higher rates than white women. Recently, a biopsychosocial model of breast cancer has been proposed in which social determinants of health, such as eating habits, level of exercise, and obesity rates, among other factors, may be correlated with elaboration of biological mediators that influence the aggressiveness of the cancer biology in women with triple-negative breast cancer.[17] It is theorized that these social "determinants" of health may influence biological responses through the stimulation of hormones such as cortisol and others that may then mediate or moderate other biological pathways and mechanisms.

Another example of this correlation comes from studies by the 2009 Nobel Laureate in Medicine or Physiology, Elizabeth Blackburn. She elucidated the biology of telomeres. Telomeres are repetitive sequences of DNA at the ends of chromosomes. The function of telomeres is to protect the DNA against degradation. This is a function that is fundamental to the regulation and aging of cells. In 2014, she and colleagues published a study in which they found a correlation between perceived racism and psychological stress and the shortening of telomeres in African Americans, as measured in white blood cell samples taken from the participants in the study. Telomere shortening has also been observed in other situations of psychological stress—for example, associated with caregiving—and has been associated with other chronic diseases such as arthritis, diabetes, and Alzheimer's disease. It is quite intriguing to speculate that there may be a mechanistic link (not yet proven) between psychological stress related to negative experiences associated with perceived or actual racism and the increased prevalence of some diseases and premature aging and death seen in the African-American population. In fact, Blackburn and colleagues concluded in their paper that "Results suggest that multiple levels of racism, including interpersonal experiences of racial discrimination, and the internalization of negative racial bias, operate jointly to accelerate biological aging of African-American men."[18] Correlation does not equal causation, but nonetheless the findings are worthy of further study.

It is now known that environmental factors can influence the ways in which genes are turned on and off; in other words, the ways in which they are expressed and regulated. *Epigenetics* is the name of the field of study about the linkage between environmental factors and gene regulation. Epigenetics involves the study of heritable changes in the phenotype (the observable physical traits or biochemical characteristics of an organism based on a combination of the organism's genes and environmental factors) that do *not* involve changes or mutations in the underlying DNA sequence. We now appreciate that social determinants of health—decisions such as your diet, how much you exercise, and conceivably the amount of psychological stress you feel based on social factors such as discrimination and racism—can eventually cause chemical modifications in the gene that will have the effect of turning those genes "on" or "off" over time. These are potential mechanisms by which social and environmental factors may influence genetic expression. Additionally, we now know that some epigenetic changes can be inherited.[19] Experiments in non-human animal species such as bees and mice have even shown that *social* information can change the way brain signals are encoded, which then changes gene expression in a way that can be inherited![20] If this biology is applicable to humans, it gives new meaning to perspectives on the persistence of negative social behaviors (e.g., intergenerational racist beliefs, negative behaviors, and attitudes), as well as positive social behaviors (e.g., intergenerational academic achievement), and their impact on health. Thus it is possible to speculate that environmental factors and stressors (e.g., perceived discrimination related to racism) can produce profound changes in fundamental biological processes like gene expression, and this may provide a basis for understanding the negative health effects associated with racially based health inequalities that sometimes persist (and even seem to be passed down) from generation to generation.

It is important to realize that these effects can happen in both directions. That is, improvement in socioeconomic status and the associated benefits realized with higher educational status, wealth accumulation, and changes in health-related behaviors, may have a positive effect in increasing life expectancy. For example, there is a persistent mortality gap of about 5.4 years between black and white populations in the United States. Despite a ten-year increase in life expectancy for black males in the United States between 1975 and 2011, their life expectancy is only 72.2 years, compared to 78.2 years for white males, and 81.2 years for white females. However, despite progress in some areas, something interesting and tragic has been happening in the past two decades in the United States—I might add, coincident with the rise of increasing income inequality.

Socioeconomic status is a major factor determining life expectancy in the United States for males and females of all races and ethnicities. For example, a recent report from the Social Security Administration reported that, after age 65, the top half of male earners had five-year advantage in life expectancy over the bottom half of earners. The situation is even worse for people like Mr. Green.

In 2006, for the first time, whites with a high school education or less experienced death rates that *exceeded* those of blacks. While this phenomenon can be explained in part by the improving life expectancy of African Americans, alas, it appears to be primarily driven by negative health behaviors producing excess mortality in white people between the ages of 45 and 54 with relatively low levels of education. A *New York Times* article of findings by 2015 Nobel Laureate (Economics) Angus Deaton and his wife, Anne Chase, concluded that "rising annual death rates among this group are being driven, not by the big killers like heart disease and diabetes, but by an epidemic of suicides and afflictions stemming from substance abuse: alcoholic liver disease and overdoses of heroin and prescription opioids."[21] These are the kinds of risky behaviors that lead to premature mortality in poor African Americans like Mr. Green as well, but they have become less common in more highly educated and higher income African Americans in the past three decades, leading to an overall improving health status of higher socioeconomically situated blacks.

THE GREAT MIGRATION: IMPACT OF PERSISTENT POVERTY ON HEALTH INEQUALITIES AND EXCESSIVE MORTALITY

We were poor. Dirt poor.
The rich people don't even know how a poor person lives. . . .
—J. W. Green

Mr. Green was part of the Great Migration, that period in the early 20th century, chronicled in the Pulitzer Prize–winning work of Isabel Wilkerson, *The Warmth of Other Suns*,[22] in which millions of African Americans moved from the Deep South to the Northeast and Midwest, looking for social and economic opportunity. For many, the move out of the South opened opportunities for educational and economic advancement that were unimaginable prior to what Wilkerson also called the great "immigration."

My family's history is part of this Great Migration. Like Mr. Green, my parents left rural Georgia shortly after the Great Depression for the hope of greater economic opportunity in the Northeast. They were also leaving the racial terrorism of the Jim Crow South. Although my father had little formal education, he (and other members of our extended family) was able to secure employment in New Jersey sufficient to support a large family. My parents lived to a reasonably old age, both dying in their eighth decade. They lived to see many of their children graduate from college and build professional careers, and to see many of their grandchildren grow into young adulthood—all within two generations of their migration from South to North. They were a success of the Great Migration. This success allowed the growth and development of a thriving black middle class, with each generation doing better in economic and educational achievement and in overall health and longevity.

> The emotional, spiritual, social, and indeed at times even physical support provided by the black church to African Americans, especially poor African Americans like Mr. Green, cannot be underestimated.

Mr. Green's path during the Great Migration was not as successful as my parents'. Of note, a recent analysis of economic and health outcomes resulting from the Great Migration actually showed that there was a subgroup of African Americans like Mr. Green who did not benefit economically, and, paradoxically, experienced increased mortality compared to cohorts who stayed in the South.[23] The reasons for the variances in experience between Mr. Green and my father are surely complex and therefore incompletely understood. Seth Saunders and her colleagues formulated several hypotheses to explain the negative consequences of migration from South to North for people like Mr. Green. It is now evident that simply increasing wages in the absence of gaining material wealth (defined as capital accumulation and the associated benefits derived thereby) does not produce any advantage in health outcomes. Marginal increases in wages for people like Mr. Green came with increased costs of living, which predominantly advantaged the Northern businessman/landlord, but not the Southern migrants. Another explanation raised by economic and public health experts is that much of our lifetime health is determined during childhood and early adult development, and that wealth acquired later has limited ability to raise health and increase longevity. Of course, it is likely that there is an interaction between these possible mechanisms.

IMPORTANCE OF RELIGION IN AFRICAN-AMERICAN LIFE: IMPLICATIONS FOR CARE WITH SERIOUS AND TERMINAL ILLNESS

Sure God will take care of me after I die. Because you don't need no keep. . . . You don't have no pain. You are well taken care of after death.
—J. W. Green

Mr. Green's strong religious faith is not surprising to me. The Pew Research group regularly reports statistics on the religious life of Americans. Their 2014 study reported that between the years 2007 and 2014, there were 5 million fewer individuals in the United States who identified themselves as "mainline Protestants," that number declining from 41 to 36 million in that seven-year period. During that same period of time, the number of African-American Protestants increased slightly, from 15.7 million to 15.9 million. In fact, they noted that,

> of all the major racial and ethnic groups in the United States, black Americans are the most likely to report a formal religious affiliation. Even among those blacks who are unaffiliated, three-in-four belong to the "religious unaffiliated" category (that is, they say that religion is either somewhat or very important in their lives)— compared to one in three of the unaffiliated overall.[24]

The emotional, spiritual, social, and indeed at times even physical support provided by the black church to African Americans, especially poor African Americans like Mr. Green, cannot be underestimated. There is a rich tradition in African-American culture and religious life formed in response to the realities of living and surviving (and, in many instances, thriving) despite social, economic, and healthcare discrimination.

African-American religious tradition and their interpretation of biblical scriptures and theology has grown a nuanced, sometimes even dualistic perspective, on attitudes toward death. There is a tension. On one hand, traditional interpretations of biblical theology focus on the notion of accepting death as an inevitable part of the life cycle, and one that is required to experience the fullness of eternal life in heaven. As David Moller observed in describing Mr. Green's acceptance of his fate and death, "J. W. spoke of death almost as a friend."[1] Another view, however, asserts that there is an obligation to not accept the inevitability of death, especially premature death which is associated with the evils of poverty and racism. Resisting death, according to this perspective, becomes a form of resistance and is part of the struggle for social justice.

Palliative care physician and researcher Kimberly Johnson has studied African-American spiritual beliefs to understand what impact they have on medical decision-making and other practices influencing end-of-life care.[25] In a review of multiple surveys of African-American spiritual beliefs that might influence end-of-life care, she and colleagues found several consistent themes, including these:

- Only God has power to decide life and death;
- Spiritual beliefs are the most effective way to influence healing;
- There are religious prohibitions against limiting life-sustaining therapies;
- There is a strong belief in divine intervention and miracles;
- The doctor is God's instrument.

An overarching perspective concerning these views is that spiritual beliefs and practices are an important source of comfort, coping, guidance, and healing. Findings such as these are consistent with Mr. Green's religious beliefs and practices. Other studies have confirmed that, compared to other patients, African-American patients suffering from cancer are more likely to find solace within religion and spirituality.[26] Mr. Green is a shining example of the seemingly passive and accepting behaviors associated with these kinds of religious beliefs. His religious beliefs and spiritual practices were a source of strength and support that gave him a way to cope with the distress and suffering associated with coming to terms with his impending death.

Alternatively, there is a perspective on the interpretations of biblical theology and scriptures—perhaps best exemplified by the Rev. Martin Luther King's philosophy and leadership of the civil rights movement—that requires one to actively resist injustice and evil in the world. Consistent with this understanding of morality and ethics, this leads one to resist notions about getting "comfortable with death," especially death that might be hastened by social discrimination and unfair treatment.

This duality of perspectives on death and dying is beautifully expressed in African-American spirituals and other literature. For example, belief in transcendence is expressed in such works as James Weldon Johnson's funeral sermon "Go Down Death"[27] and Maya Angelou's famous poem "Still I Rise."[28] While the scars and harm of slavery and injustice may seem endless, storytelling, mythmaking, and singing offered hope for transcendence and a promise of survival. They were the safe places in a world of unimaginable cruelty where people found refuge and strength. Through them they could imagine a brighter future. One that would be filled with kindness and caring. Clearly, Mr. Green found strength in his faith and his personalized expressions of it.

Even the very title of Maya Angelou's poem, "Still I Rise" emphasizes the capacity of black folks throughout history to rise above suffering. It speaks not only to strength and resilience, but to resistance as well. Other canons of African-American literature also speak to strength and resilience. There is a particular literary and artistic genre that depicts domineering African-American matriarchs who support and hold families together at great costs, even at the expense of their own health. Their strategies for coping with prolonged exposure to stresses such as social discrimination often required expending high levels of effort, which results in accumulating physiological costs. Examples in literature and the performing arts include works such as Lorraine Hansberry's *A Raisin in the Sun*, James Baldwin's *Go Tell It on the Mountain*, or Toni Morrison's *Beloved*. As Trudier Harris put it in her 1995 paper titled *The Disease Called Strength*, these African-American matriarchs were "towers of strength," and "Historically African-American women have been viewed as 'balm of strength,' the ones who held a people together against assaults from outside as well as from within the known community."[29] Yet this virtue of strength can become "its own form of ill health," as Harris put it, with negative consequences of taciturnity, romantic loneliness, emotional isolation, and even a denial of their own femininity and/or sexuality. Ironically, they may come to alienate the very children they are trying to protect, as depicted in the play *A Raisin in the Sun*.

There is an African-American male equivalent to this matriarchal "disease of strength." It is called "John Henryism." This subject takes its title from African-American folk hero John Henry, who was famous for hammering holes into rock with his steel hammer to place explosives for construction of railroad tunnels. Legend has it that his strength and prowess were such that he once won a race against a steam-powered hammer, only to die afterward from stress-induced heart failure, with his hammer in hand. Public health specialist and sociologist Sherman James has advanced a "John Henryism" hypothesis to explain excessive deaths in African-American males. James defines "John Henryism" as

> a strong behavioral predisposition to cope actively with psychosocial environmental stressors that interacts with low socioeconomic status to influence the health of African-Americans. Hypertension, a leading cause of disability and premature death among African-Americans, will be the focal health problem, although much of what I will say has implications for understanding other "stress-related" health problems that affect African Americans disproportionately.[30]

I think, in his own way, Mr. Green's womanizing and street life were, for him, a way of living as well as he could despite his poverty, poor education, and general lack of any real economic opportunity within mainstream society.

In the book written by Julius Lester, the John Henry character famously says, "dying ain't important. Everybody does that. What matters is how well you do the living."[31] While not offering this as an excuse for his behaviors, I think, in his own way, Mr. Green's womanizing and street life were, for him, a way of living as well as he could despite his poverty, poor education, and general lack of any real economic opportunity within mainstream society. Mr. Green strives hard to succeed, but his life is ultimately shortened by the crushing influences of poverty and associated maladaptive health behaviors that ultimately result in his premature death.

DIGNITY PRESERVATION: THE ROLE OF CULTURE AND RELIGION IN AFRICAN-AMERICAN LIFE

I come here tonight to plead with you. Believe in yourself and believe that you are somebody. . . . I want to get the language so right that everyone here will cry out: "Yes, I'm black, I'm proud of it. I'm black and I'm beautiful!"
—Dr. Martin Luther King, Jr.

At one point, David Moller said of Mr. Green, "J. W. was waging two battles. The obvious one was his fight against cancer. Less obvious, but of equal compelling importance, was his struggle to preserve independence and dignity."[1] And Mr. Green himself said (like the mythical John Henry):

> I don't think about dying, nothing like that. I'm going to die anyway. I might as well make the best of my life while I got it. The only thing that I've thought about is that I don't want to be a burden on my people.

Mr. Green's desire to not be a "burden" expresses in an indirect way a sense of preserving his dignity as a "somebody." The Rev. Martin Luther King, in his encouragement to black people to believe that they are "somebody," is an expression of the notion that the dignity of an individual life should result simply from the fact that they are a human being. As explained by physician and philosopher Danial Sulmasy, this notion of dignity being intrinsic to being a human being, formed in the image of God, has roots in religious and theological writings dating back to Thomas Aquinas in the Middle Ages, and has been a major teaching of the Catholic Church over many centuries.[32] This is the notion of an intrinsic human dignity that is possessed by each person, by virtue of their "humaneness," or in Martin Luther King's word, their "somebodyness."

Notice that King did not say "believe in yourself so that you can *become* somebody." He said "believe in yourself because you *are* somebody." This is a subtle difference in language with profound importance. Intrinsic human dignity flows from the essence of being human, as opposed to concepts of "innate" dignity in which we attribute to others some sense of worth based on their capacity to make moral decisions and to exercise free will. Often when we speak of "dignity," we are referring to some attribute of the individual. Of course, the fear of the concept of attributed human dignity is that it is based on some notion of a personal or societal judgment of worth; these judgments are almost always made by the powerful and privileged upon the weak, the poor, and the vulnerable—people like Mr. Green.

With this important caveat concerning the concept of attributed human dignity, it is worthwhile to note the important work of psychiatrist and researcher Harvey Chochinov, who has done empirical studies of ways to provide end-of-life care that are dignity-conserving.[33] This type of empirical research must make judgments about attributes of care and physical and emotional states of patients that one would find desirable and consistent with preserving dignity. It is important to note that these decisions are made by directly asking patients what they cherish, and this is good. Empirically derived and validated constructs that operationally define dignity, such as the importance of maintaining one's independence, the desire not to be a burden to others, and a sense of maintaining hopefulness, are extremely important in constructing ways to provide quality end-of-life care. Nonetheless, these self-attributed notions of personal and human dignity are, by their very nature, subjective and change according to the mores, customs, and cultural norms of the time. Improving care to vulnerable and different patient populations will require a multilayered approach that more effectively "hears" what vulnerable sick people—and their families—need to maintain a sense of integrity and wholeness.

Chochinov's research addresses a concern voiced by bioethicist Ruth Macklin, who famously opined that dignity is a "useless" concept.[34] Her argument is that in modern bioethics, the term "dignity" is often evoked as a synonym for the moral principles of autonomy and respect for persons. She goes on to say, "In the absence of criteria that enable us to know just when dignity is violated, the concept remains hopelessly vague." It seems that Chochinov's research, and more recent refinements, attempt to do just that.[35]

Mr. Green experienced many personal indignities in his care at the end of his life, yet he maintained personal "dignity" and integrity because he did not waver in his sense that, despite being poor and black, he was "somebody"—especially in the eyes of God.

ONE PERSON, THREE IDENTITIES

EVERY MAN is in certain respects;
a. like all other men,
b. like some other men,
c. like no other man.
—Henry A. Murray and Clyde Kluckhohn

This quote from Murray and Kluckhohn's famous book on personality formation is wonderfully applicable to medicine and the challenges of providing comprehensive healthcare.[36] This observation applies to all of us, and could be particularly helpful in informing caregivers how to approach our fellow humans suffering from illness. For example, Mr. Green shares a common humanity (like all others), a common cultural heritage with other African Americans (like some others), and is unique in his individual preferences and personality (like no others).

LIKE ALL OTHERS

I just want to know. I want to know just about what they know.
—J. W. Green

J. W. was a poor black man, raised in poverty in rural Mississippi, who spent his adult life as a street hustler in Indianapolis. Yet, he had needs and wants concerning his end-of-life care that every human being shares, regardless of race, ethnicity, and station in life. Two critical common needs are the desire for honest communication, and the desire not be abandoned while dying. Mr. Green's desire to not be abandoned was fulfilled by the loving presence of his nephew, Frank. Unfortunately, his desire to have open and honest communication with his doctors was not fulfilled.

> Mr. Green experienced many personal indignities in his care at the end of his life, yet he maintained personal "dignity" and integrity because he did not waver in his sense that despite being poor and black, he was "somebody"—especially in the eyes of God.

Like almost all other areas of medicine and healthcare, the type and quality of communication between doctor and patient is influenced by race. A recent study evaluated communication behaviors of doctors when dealing with black and white patients.[37] In this study, the researchers demonstrated that in relaying factual information to patients, there was little difference between black and white patients. However, in critical nonverbal, so-called rapport building modes of communication, such as the spatial difference between doctor and patient when talking, and the assumption of an inviting "open" body posture versus a distancing "closed" body posture, they found significantly fewer positive cues with black patients compared to with whites. Although this may seem paradoxical, I suspect that it is precisely these more positive, rapport-building, nonverbal modes of communication behaviors that Mr. Green was hoping for in his providers—and not just the simple exchange of facts when Mr. Green says that he just wants to "know what they know." Indeed every patient wishes for these elements of empathic, human–human conversations with their doctors.

LIKE SOME OTHERS

I don't think about dying, nothing like that. I am going to die anyway. . . . The only thing I've thought about is that I don't want to be a burden on my people.
—J. W. Green

Mr. Green's statement about not wanting to be a burden to his family is, of course, shared widely by many people. However, bioethicist Gilbert Meilaender offers an unexpected perspective on "being a burden"[38]:

> None of us wishes to imagine his children arguing together about who really knows best how he should be treated (or not treated). We hate to think that our children's last thoughts of us would be interwoven with anger at each other, guilt for their uncertainty about how best to care for us, or even (perhaps) a secret wish that we'd get on with the dying and relieve them of this burden. . . .
>
> But still, there is here a serious point to be considered. *Is this not in large measure what it means to belong to a family: to burden each other—and to find, almost miraculously, that others are willing, even happy, to carry such burdens?* Families would not have the significance they do for us if they did not, in fact, give us a claim upon each other. At least in this sphere of life we do not come together as autonomous individuals freely contracting with each other. We simply find ourselves thrown together and asked to share the burdens of life while learning to care for each other [emphasis added].

This sense of willingly taking on the "burden" of caring for family is shared across many cultures and religious groups, to be sure, but is particularly strong in traditional African-American culture. We see this exemplified by Frank, who took on the "burden" of being present with his "Unc," Mr. Green, even when his sons abandoned him. This notion of "familial" obligations to take on the burdens of caring for the weak and vulnerable—especially when sick, flow from Christian tenets as expressed in parables of the Good Samaritan and in other teachings by Christ, in particular, His call to care for "the least of these."

LIKE NO OTHERS

I got so many girlfriends . . . I take care of them and they take care of me. They say, "we'll be with you as long as you treat us nice and we'll treat you nice."
—J. W. Green

Mr. Green's life on the street certainly defined him as an individual. The fact that he shared this aspect of his life so openly with David Moller supports how important this aspect of his life was to him. David Moller's sensitive and generally non-judgmental portrayal of this part of Mr. Green's narrative models how providers can discuss the deepest personal aspects of a person's life in an attempt to understand their individual preferences and motivations that drive health behaviors (Figure 4.3).

THE WAY FORWARD: REFLECTIONS ON HOW WE CAN IMPROVE CARE FOR MR. GREEN AND POOR PEOPLE OF COLOR

We have much to learn from exploring Mr. Green's life and experiences as a poor African-American man facing the end of his life. First and foremost, he teaches us that everyone comes to this phase of life with strengths to cull from their cultural and spiritual beliefs. Mr. Green came to his death having achieved a kind of peace with his dying that many

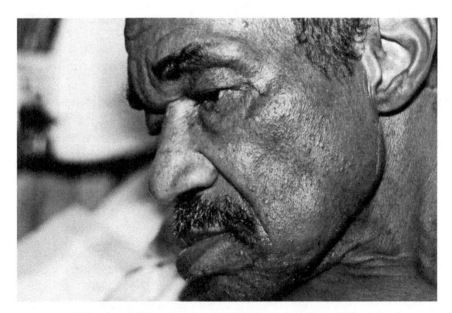

FIGURE 4.3 J. W. smiles mischievously as he reminisces about some of his misbehavior on the streets.

middle class and wealthy people wish they could attain. This peace was buttressed by his strong religious beliefs and the loving support from an extended family member that are intimately coupled to the cultural norms of African-American life. This fact requires that doctors and other healthcare providers explore the cultural beliefs and value systems of our patients. For many, if not most, African Americans, this also requires an exploration of religious and spiritual beliefs.

Mr. Green also teaches us that dignified dying does not require the unfettered exercise of personal autonomy, although a deep and abiding respect for the self-worth of the individual is necessary. Respecting preferences for family involvement in decisions is needed, as is a sense that "family" can extend beyond the immediate biological relatives, and it may even include a community that can provide emotional and spiritual support.

> Mr. Green came to his death having achieved a kind of peace with his dying that many middle class and wealthy people wish they could attain.

Mr. Green's death at the relatively young age of 60 from a disease that is essentially curable when diagnosed early must also force us to confront the realities of persistent racially and economically-based health disparities that all too often lead to excessive mortality in poor communities of color. As discussed, declining life expectancy increasingly occurs in poor and lower middle-class white communities as well. What is required in addressing the problem is to confront institutionally-based assumptions, policies, and in some instances, frank racism, that drive these inequalities. It requires acknowledgment of the existence of prejudicial policies and practices and willingness to change them through enforcement of evidence-based clinical guidelines and health policies that could improve healthcare overall and outcomes in particular.

Systemic, stigmatized treatment of patients resulting from preconceived cultural biases toward race, gender, socioeconomic/educational status (SEES), and lifestyle choices leads to poor care and neglect of their needs. These biases may cause health caregivers to miscommunicate, misdiagnose, mistreat and mismanage certain population segments of our society—especially black and brown people, and people who are impoverished. Ironically, the health caregiver can be of the same race or gender as the patient and still practice what I shall term the *medical neglect syndrome* (MNS).

Patients like Mr. Green have experienced poor healthcare and MNS over a lifetime. His living and dying would have been immeasurably improved if he had had access to more material resources. Discussions concerning the elimination of poverty are certainly beyond the scope of this chapter. However, it is worth noting that poverty, disease susceptibility, and lifestyle choices are directly related to the poor management of the illness of our most vulnerable. Consider the life of Mr. Green and the probable healthcare he experienced whenever his life/illness interacted with our healthcare system. Throughout his life, and as it ended, we did not provide him with optimal or even adequate care. We honor his life, and the life of our collective humanity, when we commit our emotional, intellectual, and physical capabilities to address suffering in all forms (but especially when it is driven by the persistence of poverty in the wealthiest nation on earth) of our fellow human brothers and sisters (Figure 4.4).

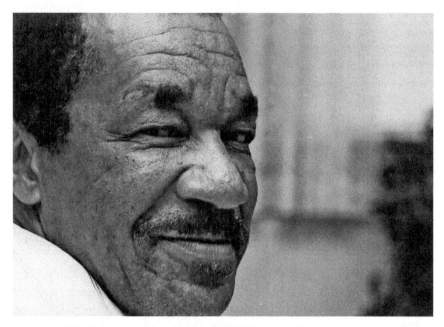

FIGURE 4.4 "It's all about the money; they have it and I don't," J. W. laments.

REFERENCES

1. Moller DW. *Dancing with broken bones: race, class, and spirit-filled dying in the inner city.* New York: Oxford University Press; 2012.
2. Smedly BD, Stith AY, Nelson AY. *Unequal treatment: confronting racial and ethnic disparities in health care.* Washington, DC: National Academy of Medicine Press; 2003.
3. Williams DR. Discrimination and racial disparities in health: evidence and needed research. *Behav Med.* 2009;32:20–47.
4. Levine RS, Foster JE, Fullilow RE, et al. Black–white inequalities in mortality and life expectancy, 1933–1999: Implications for Health People 2010. *Public Health Rep.* 116: 476–483.
5. Williams, DR, Jackson PM. Social sources of racial disparities in health. *Health Aff.* 2005;24(7):325–334.
6. Burton D, Feng Z, Fennell M, Zinn J, Mor V. Separate and unequal: racial segregation and disparities in quality across US nursing homes. *Health Aff.* Sept/Oct 2007;26(5):1448–1458.
7. Freeman, H. Cancer in the socioeconomically disadvantaged. *CA Cancer J Clin.* 1989;39(5):266–288.
8. Ward E, Jemel A, Cokkindies V, et al. Cancer disparities by race/ethnicity and socioeconomic status. *CA Cancer J Clin.* 2004;54:78–93.
9. Horner MJ, Ries LAG, Krapcho M, et al. (eds). *SEER Cancer Statistics Review, 1975–2006, National Cancer Institute.* Bethesda, MD: National Cancer Institute; 2009. http://seer.cancer.gov/csr/1975_2006/, based on November 2008 SEER data submission, posted to the SEER web site, 2009. (Accessed March 25, 2016.)
10. American Cancer Society Recommendations for Prostate Cancer Early Detection. https://www.cancer.org/cancer/prostate-cancer/early-detection/acs-recommendations.html, Last revised, April, 2016. (Accessed March 20, 2017).

11. Moyer VA, on behalf of the US Preventive Services Task Force. Screening for prostate cancer: US Preventive Services Task Force recommendation statement. *Ann Intern Med.* 2012;157:120–134.

12. Powell IJ, Bock CH, Ruterbush JJ, Sakr W. Evidence supports a faster growth rate and/ or earlier transformation to clinically significant prostate cancer in black than in white American men, and influences racial progression and mortality disparity. *J Urol.* 2010;183(5):1792–1796.

13. Rodriquez JM, Geronimus AT, Bound J, Doring D. Black lives matters: differential mortality and racial composition of the US electorate, 1970–2004. *Soc Sci Med.* 2015;136–137:193–199.

14. Bonilla-Silva, E. Rethinking racism: toward a structural interpretation. *Am Sociol Rev.* 1996;62:465–480.

15. Clark R, Anderson NB, Clark VR, Williams DR. Racism as a stressor for African Americans: a biopsychosocial model. *Am Psychologist.* 1999;54(10):805–816.

16. Williams DR, Mohammed SA. Discrimination and racial disparities in health: evidence and needed research. *J Behav Med.* 2009;32:20–47.

17. Dietz EC, Sistrunk C, Miranda-Carboni, O'Reagon R, Seewaldt VL. Triple-negative breast cancer in African American women: disparities versus biology. *Nat Rev Cancer.* 2015;15:248–254.

18. Chase DH, Nuru-Jeter AM, Adler N, et al. Discrimination, racial bias and telomere in African American men. *Am J Prev Med.* 2014;46(2):103–111.

19. Jirtle RL, Skinner MK. Environmental epigenomics and disease susceptibility. *Nat Rev Genet.* 2007;8:253–262.

20. Robinson GE, Fernald RD, Clayton DF. Review: genes and social behavior. *Science.* 2008;322(5903):896–900.

21. Case A, Deaton A. Rising morbidity and mortality in midlife among white non-Hispanic Americans in the 21st century. *PNAS.* 2015;112 (49):15078–15083.

22. Wilkerson I. *The warmth of other suns: the epic story of America's Great Migration.* New York: Random House; 2010.

23. Black D, Sanders SG, Taylor EJ, Taylor LJ. The impact of the Great Migration on mortality of African Americans: evidence from the Deep South. *American Economic Review.* 2015;105(2):477–503.

24. Pew Research Center, May 12, 2015. America's changing religious landscape. http://www. pewforum.org/2015/05/12/americas-changing-religious-landscape/#. (Accessed March 22, 2016.)

25. Johnson KS, Elbert-Avila KI, Tulsky JA. The influence of spiritual beliefs and practices on the treatment preferences of African Americans: a review of the literature. *J Am Geriatr Soc.* 2005;53(4):711–719.

26. Dessio W, Wade DW, Chao M, Kronenberg F, Cushman LE, Kalmuss D. Religion, spirituality, and healthcare choices of African American women: results of a national survey. *Ethnicity Dis.* 2004;14:189–197.

27. Johnson JW. *God's trombones.* New York: Viking Press; 1927.

28. Angelou M. *And still I rise.* New York: Random House; 1978.

29. Harris T. The disease called strength. *Lit Med.* 1995;14:109–126.

30. James S. "John Henryism" and the health of African Americans. *Culture Med Psychiatry.* 1994;18:163–182.

31. Lester J. *John Henry.* New York: Dial Books; 1994.

32. Sulmasy D. Dignity, vulnerability and the personhood of the patient. In: *The rebirth of the clinic—an introduction to spirituality in health care.* Washington, DC: Georgetown University Press; 2006:24–43.

33. Chochinov HM. Dignity-conserving care—a new model for palliative care. *JAMA.* 2002;287(17):2253–2260.

34. Macklin R. Dignity is a useless concept. *BMJ.* 2003;327:1419–1420.

35. Chochinov HM, Krisjanson HL, Hack TF, Hassard T, McClement S, Harlos M. Dignity in the terminally ill: revisited. *J Palliat Med.* 2006;9 (3):666–672.

36. Murray HA, Kluckhohn C. *Personality in nature, society, and culture.* 2nd ed. New York: Alfred A. Knopf; 1953.

37. Elliott AM, Alexander SC, Mescher CA, Mohan D, Barnota AE. Differences in physicians' verbal and nonverbal communication with black and white patients at the end of life. *J Pain Sympt Manag.* 2016;51(1):1–8.

38. Meilaender G. I want to burden my loved ones. *First Things.* October 1991.

5

THE WHITES

EXPRESSING UNIMAGINABLE INDIGNITIES

Christian T. Sinclair

Snapshot Reflection: A Story of Undying Love and Horrific Neglect

"I hope she goes first," Ken whispered about his wife, Virble. He understood that after 43 years of marriage they were both coming to the end of their lives. Out of love, he wanted her to be spared the grief of his death and the burden of confronting her own death without him. His wish was not to be granted, however, as he would be the first to die. But before that was to take place, they would both endure neglectful treatment and indignity in the county nursing home that was incompatible with any sense of compassionate care or respect.

The first time I met Mr. White, he was wandering dazed and confused throughout the hallway of County Hospital, a place where the uninsured and poor go to receive care. He had been turned away from his appointment in the oncology clinic because he had no insurance and did not have the $25 copayment that was required. Our initial meeting was to get acquainted and solicit his participation in the *Dancing with Broken Bones* project, but his rejection from the oncology clinic forced us to shift gears. With a volunteer accompanying him, he was brought down to Social Services, where he could begin the process of obtaining "safety-net" insurance in the hospital's Advantage Program, which would make him eligible to receive care as an indigent person.

The next time we met, I visited him at his home. It was a boxy, red, small house with empty lots on each side. A chain link fence surrounded it. He and his beloved wife were most gracious and welcoming. They sat and talked about their life together, describing its difficulties without shame. Mr. White talked about his nearly three decades of bone-crunching work in a fish market—how the work was dirty, demanding, and frigid during winter months. The work, like all of his jobs, provided neither a pension nor health-insurance benefits. Even still, he worked relentlessly to support his family. There would always be enough money to pay for basic clothing, the rent, and utilities, to gas up the broken-down car he drove, and to splurge for a bit of beer over the weekend. Each week he would step on this "work-survival treadmill" anew, repeating it over and over again for the four decades of his marriage to Virble. The White's lived a deplorable version of the movie *Ground-Hog Day*, with their struggles being recreated anew on a daily basis. He worked hard, provided for the children, and loved his wife dearly. But despite the work ethic he possessed, there was scant opportunity for him to get ahead in life. He worked at menial jobs that provided no opportunity for advancement. Throughout the hardships of their lives together, he remained faithful to his belief in God and never strayed from his dedication to his family.

Illness throughout the family brought Virble and Ken's sufferings to a new level of difficulty. Their son Dean suffered a heart attack and died. Another son, Danny, suffered a debilitating stroke. Ken was 10 years younger than Virble and was her primary caretaker. He had also suffered a stroke but continued to take care of Virble at their home. But when he was diagnosed with esophageal cancer, it all became too much, and they needed to look for options and develop a plan.

The first thing to do was to see what the doctors in the oncology clinic had to offer. Now that he had become a hospital "Advantage-insured" patient and had some healthcare coverage, he could be seen. The news he received in the clinic was not good, however: tests revealed that the disease had spread extensively, and the only thing the oncologist could offer was to enroll him in a research protocol. The idea of experimental chemotherapy did not sit well with Mr. White. He stated to the doctor that if the cancer was terminal, that was God's will and he was ready to accept it. Therefore, he would not give his consent to treatment. The doctor became impatient with the conversation and, rather than discussing hospice and palliative care options, abruptly told Mr. White that he would see him back in the oncology clinic in two months. Mr. White's view of the conversation was not only that the doctor was impatient, but that he was also "rude." "Tell me he wasn't rude," he challenged when he relayed his take on the encounter with the oncology fellow.

In addition to the abruptness that Mr. White experienced, he was also let down in a clinical sense. In his hurry and reliance on a technical/medical world view, in which the goal was to extend life through aggressive treatment, the physician missed a great opportunity to honor the patient's wishes and help him to make a smooth transition from a curative to a comfort-care approach, to one where dignity and quality of life would be of foremost concern. It would have been preferable and patient-centered to state something like, "Well, you know, Mr. White, while I do disagree with your decision, I respect your right to make it. Since you have decided against treatment for your cancer, let me talk to you about another option. Have you ever heard of hospice?" That conversation never took place, and Mr. White left with a slip of paper in hand that instructed him to return to the oncology clinic in two months, with no follow-up plan during that interval. He departed that day feeling displeased and disgusted with the whole interaction.

The second "decision" facing Kenny and Virble was essentially predetermined given the progression of his disease and the frailty of his wife. Inevitably, they decided upon moving to the county nursing home, the place where many of the inner-city poor without options go to die. From the onset, things did not go well. The first weekend they had settled in, Virble soiled her sheets, and the nursing attendants took over an hour and a half to get her cleaned and back into a freshly laundered bed. This negligence in care persisted over the course of four months, subjecting both of them to regular indignities of "excremental assault," as I termed it, in which the overburdened and/or indifferent staff of the nursing home inadequately tended to their toileting needs. Virble whispered to me one day, a sense of hurt palpable in her voice, "Those nurses don't have to get so rough with Kenny when he wets the bed. He can't help it, you know." Their room regularly smelled of urine and feces, and they lived in this humiliating situation for four months. Being poor and disempowered, with no other choice available, in their own way they each submitted to living in this deplorable condition with a mixture of depression, internalized anger, and sadness in witnessing what was happening to their beloved life partner.

A Special Observation

The shabby care they received in the nursing home degraded and humiliated them, depriving them of even basic human dignity.

Take-Home Lesson

To understand the Whites, it is critical to appreciate how the daily struggle of living in poverty shaped their spirit of independence and capacity for hardiness. They toiled hard throughout their lives to survive and raise their family, doing so with enormous dignity. As they faced their respective illness experiences, it was important for them to have their wishes honored and their dignity preserved. However, poor communication and inadequate patient-centered understanding in the oncology clinic led to decisions that did not serve Mr. White well. And inattentive care and lack of compassion exacerbated their suffering, creating indefensible indignities for both of them while they endured life in the nursing home.

—David Wendell Moller

INTRODUCTION

In healthcare, poverty is a major risk factor for morbidity and mortality. Unfortunately, in most situations, the risk poverty imposes is often hidden and undervalued compared to an elevated creatinine or abnormal electrocardiogram (EKG). In the ER and hospital, patients are frequently changed out of their everyday clothes into a hospital gown, thereby removing many of the informal indicators of their socioeconomic status. Even when there are some nonverbal clues about poverty or financial distress, the topic is often overlooked. With Mr. and Mrs. White, we hear through their voices how the healthcare system looked right past them and missed seeing the whole person. In knowing the larger story about Ken and Virble White, we can readily see where our approach to patient care fails and hopefully make the changes on a personal, system, and social level to prevent their sad tale from repeating and being experienced by other people who live at the margins.

In the story of Ken and Virble White, we come to understand how a life of skimming by week-to-week and paycheck-to-paycheck left them unable to get the care they deserved, especially after Mr. White's new cancer diagnosis. Ken and Virble had been married for 43 years when we met them in the story. Ken, the breadwinner, often did difficult and unpleasant work for little pay, while Virble focused on raising their four children. While Mr. White was regularly employed, they still struggled to make ends meet. He had no health insurance or pension, and the weekly financial demands prevented Ken and Virble from getting ahead and planning for the future. They lived in an unsafe part of the city that had a lack of public infrastructure and lacked the community cohesiveness that can sometimes buoy other families facing illness.

A quick summary of Ken and Virble's journey as we meet them in *Dancing With Broken Bones* follows.

Ken was diagnosed with esophageal cancer and had decided to forgo any chemotherapy, radiation, or surgery, a decision based on his Catholic faith and his interpretation that his cancer diagnosis was part of God's will. He framed this cancer diagnosis (along with his poverty and suffering) as part of a test of his faith. Ken did make a visit to the oncologist, and there he saw an oncology fellow whom Ken perceived as being quite disrespectful once it was clear Ken was not going to entertain any option of chemotherapy. The tone of the visit quickly changed when Ken expressed his desire to forgo treatment, and Ken focused on the incivility and rudeness of this physician long after the visit. Ken received an unhelpful follow-up appointment for two months later, without any plan or resources. A week later, he landed in the ER, and after a little bit more time and further functional decline, he and his wife moved into a nursing home together. Ken was also a caregiver for his wife, who could not do many of her own self-care activities in addition to being bed- and chair-bound because of her frailty and chronic lung disease.

In the nursing home, the Whites had the nursing home experience many people dread. Both of them were left to sit in their own soiled sheets for hours at a time, unable to help each other. Afraid to speak up and advocate for themselves, they continued to suffer these indignities. Once it became clear that Mr. White was closer to dying, Virble asked for help to get him a suit for his funeral. Ken received a donated suit from the palliative care team that had embraced Ken in a surreptitious chance encounter. Ken was buried without much ceremony, and Virble moved in with her daughter. Virble died about four months after Ken.

In my career as a hospice medical director and a palliative medicine physician, I have met many patients who remind me of various aspects of Ken and Virble White. This authentic story of a brief part of their life together highlights many parts of our healthcare and social services that undermine simple respect and dignity for people. Thankfully, there are ways in which many of the indignities the Whites faced can be overcome in a systematic fashion if we as individuals, we as organizations, and we as a society care enough to do something about it. Through their voices, there are three areas illustrating the challenges they faced and our opportunity for doing better: improving whole-patient assessment, equal access to palliative care, and caring for the family system through integrated health and social services. Once you read the story of Mr. and Mrs. White, the challenges that led to suboptimal care appear so obvious, yet from the viewpoint of the clinicians and healthcare system in the story, they did not have the benefit of seeing Ken's whole story, of having "walked in his shoes," if you will. If they did, it might have been more obvious what care and support Ken and Virble needed (Figure 5.1).

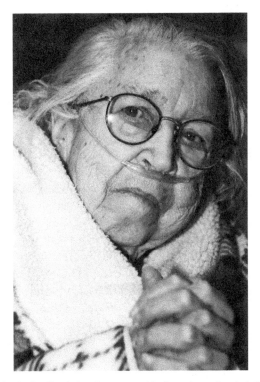

FIGURE 5.1 After the death of her beloved Kenny, Virble shares how, after their first date, she exclaimed to her momma, "He can park his shoes under my bed anytime." And so he did, for 43 years of a loving marriage.

PATIENT ASSESSMENT

There are many ways to view and assess a patient. To most clinicians, our healthcare culture has held up objective, quantifiable information as the gold standard. Patients become a collection of numbers and images, all collected in a digitized electronic health record, usually stripped void of any personal identifiers outside of date of birth, gender, and name. To our benefit, this infusion of objectivity and the application of the scientific method has been extremely helpful. Clearly, research into diagnostic and therapeutic advances have helped countless people. For that, we should be thankful. As with any tool, however, there is a balance in how it is wielded. As we increasingly concentrate on numbers and metrics, focus is shifted away from the humanity and dignity of being a person. Of course, there are many heartwarming stories of clinicians connecting with patients on a much deeper personal level, but in the business of healthcare, these experiences are more often the exception to the rule, since productivity, laboratories, procedures, and scans drive finances and therefore the clinical workflow.

The Whites had the nursing home experience many people dread.

Ken's retelling of his visit with the oncology fellow does not go into much detail about what occurred beyond the decision to forgo chemotherapy, and the rudeness of the oncology fellow:

> Tell me you think he wasn't rude. He went yeah, yeah, yeah, yeah. All I said was fine, fine. He then said we will go into chemotherapy and we will cut some of the cancer out. And I said not for one damn second. And he got up and left.

Based on these facts, it was likely that the visit was structured around the pathophysiology of Ken's cancer diagnosis instead of being focused on Ken, a person with a cancer diagnosis. In a busy clinic, it is easy to presume that there was a review of the medical records and an establishment of a chemotherapy regimen (and maybe an alternate regimen) before the visit started. The cancer diagnosis was probably reviewed in medical jargon that Ken may not have been able to understand. A 2008 study showed physicians were responsible for leading more than 64% of the time during a clinic visit, and if the patient was alone (as Ken was) or had a lower education level, then the physician was likely to talk more often. The study also reinforced that biomedical information was given a much higher prevalence than psychosocial issues.[1]

The exclusive focus on disease and a treatment plan probably contributed to the rudeness Ken felt when the oncology fellow appeared to change his tone once Ken shared his desire to forgo active treatment. Without the aggressive clinical treatment plan to structure all of their future visits, the oncologist may have felt that he had very little to offer. This led to a vague follow-up appointment without goals being clarified. If the majority of oncology visits are focused on disease and "the next chemo regimen," this fellow may have felt unprepared to offer up a different paradigm of plan. Without a plan, it may have been more difficult for the fellow and Ken to align on shared goals, and therefore the social structure of the visit (and any future visits) broke down, contributing to Ken's exacerbated suffering.

Even before the doctor visit, Ken was presented with obstacles to care. Not only was it difficult for him to get to the hospital, he was diverted from an appointment when he was told he needed to submit a $25 co-pay, a fee which he could not afford to pay. Ken's ability to qualify for a financial assistance program was not entered correctly in the computer and serves as a red flag that alerts us to the lack of whole-person support. Despite organizations' attempts to overcome financial burdens that may limit care, the complexity of being funneled through the system leads to inefficiencies and increased risk of diverting people from a proper care plan. Taking time to ask key questions of Ken about his financial distress and his financial responsibilities would have been helpful in uncovering barriers to effective treatment. Although Ken didn't highlight finances as being a reason to forgo chemotherapy, financial distress is a well-researched cause for suboptimal treatment for many people with cancer and other serious illnesses.[2] Universal screening for financial impacts of cancer care is beginning to be more widely utilized, but that is only the first step, as this is much more complicated than just the ability to pay for doctor's visits, lab tests, and medicines.

On an individual level, clinicians can all make a better effort to talk with patients about financial distress. One might begin to ask questions at the onset of care or at major changes in treatment plans about any financial distress experienced by patients. Many patients with cancer stop working during initial treatment, including absences of two to six months or even permanently.[3] Out-of-pocket medication expenses may cause patients to prioritize some medications over others or may lead to nonadherence, which creates even more complications. Understanding that medical costs are a major factor in bankruptcy, we must appreciate how ruinous a serious illness can be, not only for those patients who start near poverty, but also for people at other socioeconomic statuses.[4]

In addition to universal screening for financial distress, it would be helpful to know about Ken's roles and responsibilities in his personal life and how they may be impacted by cancer and any treatment decision he makes. One clue for any clinician was that Ken came alone to his visit. Most aspects of the social history in medicine are designed to elicit risk factors for certain illnesses. Asking about tobacco and drug use and sexual partners is the clinical way to narrow down a diagnosis and treatment plan, as all medical students are taught. Any other social aspects of a patient's life are merely part of the friendly banter before and after a visit, yet not important enough to document in the chart. Inquiring about family and friends who may be of support during a serious illness leads to many insights in a whole-patient assessment. Ken did not have anyone with him because his wife might be a hindrance because of her debility and his son also had difficulties because of his stroke. Family members or friends in attendance at healthcare visits can provide help with transportation, take notes, stay focused on the questions the patient needs answered, and in general be the voice of support during a potentially challenging experience. I often see patients in Ken's situation, where the patient or their significant other is the primary income generator and can't find someone to take off work to attend an appointment with them. This is in stark contrast to employed people with benefits that include access to the Family and Medical Leave Act (FMLA). FMLA includes time off to care for a spouse, son, daughter, or parent who has a serious health condition, in addition to caring for one's own serious health condition. Yet the qualifications for FMLA are not always met by people who live around the margins of the poverty line, in addition to its being a non-reimbursed leave entitlement. Not getting a paycheck could be catastrophic for families near poverty, so they may not make use of FMLA benefits even when they have full rights to do so. Poverty and the burden of serious illness throughout his family undermined Ken's ability to navigate through the system, leading to more suffering for all involved (Box 5.1).

Box 5.1 FMLA-Eligible Employees

Accessible at: https://www.dol.gov/whd/regs/compliance/whdfs28.pdf
Works for a covered employer:

- Has worked for the employer for at least 12 months;
- Has at least 1,250 hours of service for the employer during the 12-month period immediately preceding the leave*; and
- Works at a location where the employer has at least 50 employees within 75 miles.

An important part of Ken's story was his role as a caregiver, not just being a patient who needed care himself. Not only did Ken care for his wife, Virble, who was 10 years older and depended on him for basic care such as eating, toileting, and mobility, Ken also was a caregiver for his 40-year-old son Danny, who'd had a stroke when he was 39 and had to move in with his parents. Research demonstrates that caregiving is a major time and financial burden on families and on society by greatly increasing the risk of absenteeism, presenteeism (the need to go to work despite being sick and in poor health because of financial urgency), mental health issues, morbidity, and mortality compared to the general public.[5] Nearly 18 million Americans are family caregivers for someone age 65 and older who has a significant impairment. For those who have the financial means it is possible to hire private-duty assistance. But for the working poor like Ken and Virble, this would never be an option. The research is already clear about the magnitude of the problem with caregiver health, but the solutions are much more difficult. One could make an argument in Ken's case that he was already at increased risk for cancer, given that he was a caregiver in poverty with poor social supports, in addition to how it impacted his care after the diagnosis.

While not explicitly addressed in Ken and Virble's story, another key area for whole-patient assessment is health literacy. Far more than just reading comprehension, health literacy includes a variety of skills to obtain information and services, communicate needs, and understand the choices and consequences of medical decisions. Health literacy covers a breadth of important actions like the ability to decipher a complex set of medication prescriptions, and includes the ability to state what goals you are trying to achieve by pursuing a course of treatment. Even if Ken decided to pursue surgery and chemotherapy, there is a good chance that his health literacy might have undermined his chances of success. Bridging the literacy gap does not just happen. This is a difficult problem and "fixing" it is not easy. Attempts at resolution must be actively designed and come from the professionals and organizations who are charged with providing care to the marginalized. The experience of Ken and Virble is not isolated. Nearly 90 million American adults have difficulty understanding and acting upon health information.[6] As noted, solutions to this problem must come from clinicians and organizations that serve in healthcare leadership and from among leaders in public policy in the broader society. In order for this to happen in any meaningful way, however, societal commitment to improving the well-being of the poor and marginalized must be expanded.

While health-literacy research has shown us the breakdowns in care, clinical solutions have not been widely adopted, partially because the evidence of proven solutions is hard to apply broadly, and the financial incentives are not necessarily available to prompt investment of human and financial capital in such high-intensity projects. Occasionally, foundation grants may provide support for projects designed to improve health literacy among vulnerable populations. But overall, there remains absence of will to take on the problem. Ironically, if we did establish this as a national priority the likely result would extend beyond improving the lives of the poor to financial benefits that would accrue for the broader society. Inasmuch as lack of health literacy is associated with more hospitalizations, higher healthcare spending, and poor health status, there would potentially be far-ranging societal benefit to improving things. In fact, some have advocated for health literacy to become a vital sign to assess and improve the health of the nation.[7] That said, the problem is not an easy one to solve and would be very time-consuming and expensive in the short term. In a society interested in immediate results, enthusiasm for and investment in such long-term projects are difficult to generate.

There are numerous easy-to-use, health-literacy tools. But despite the correlation of illiteracy to poor health outcomes, they are not utilized frequently in clinical encounters. Nor are they pervasively utilized outside of the healthcare arena in local communities. While the issue of health literacy is critically important in all patients and may be a challenge even for those who do not live in poverty, the health of the poor is especially vulnerable because of it.

Back to the experience of Mr. White. It would have only taken four to eight minutes of conversation in the clinic to provide the foundation for better care. In those few minutes, four major barriers to optimal care could have been identified: financial distress, limited support network, lack of health literacy, and his being a patient with primary care-giver responsibilities. None of these hugely relevant factors, however, has anything to do with tumor type or genetic markers. But, in reality, they did have a major impact on his quality of life and his confrontation with mortality. Even though none of these factors were reasons voiced by Ken about why he ultimately chose not to pursue chemotherapy, they are a part of his story.

Ultimately, he placed the responsibility for his decision on his Catholic faith and his understanding that his suffering and illness was part of God's will:

> I've lived for 71 years with this, not with a terminally-ill part, but I've lived for 71 years. I am going to die. God is going to take me to a new life on His time for me to go, not before, and that's the way I feel about it. I've been hurt several times. Could have been dead a couple of times. I'm still here, so apparently God has some use for me yet. Until he doesn't, no cutting!

Clearly, Ken used his faith in God and his spiritual beliefs to help reinforce his decision not to pursue treatment. Without asking patients directly, it is unlikely that the role of spirituality and religion would ever come up in a medical encounter. In healthcare settings, religious preference resides on a demographics intake sheet, but it rarely makes its way into a physician's note or even decision-making unless a patient is vocal about an opposition to treatment. Understanding someone's faith and belief system and how it informs their healthcare decisions in light of a serious illness is an important screening tool that nurses and physicians must be competent and comfortable in using in order to serve the whole person.

In areas where values come into conflict, it is important to employ the expert guidance and counseling of chaplains. Healthcare chaplains have a unique role and the training to dive deeper into the complex topics of spirituality and health. People may find that spirituality and faith provide hope for cure in the face of an abysmal prognosis. Sometimes that serves as the basis for insisting on aggressive care, even when the medical indicators suggest that cure is not realistic. Or, for others, faith may offer strength and the feeling of being loved in times of sorrow and change and therefore provide a foundation of strength which allows an acceptance of death's approach. In any event, enhancing understanding of how faith impacts healthcare decisions for patients and families is an important function that chaplains can fulfill as members of the multidisciplinary care team.

In Ken's story, it would be beneficial for the oncology fellow to explore Ken's reasons for opposition to treatment. How a doctor approaches shared decision-making with a patient will vary if the reason for avoiding treatment is faith-based or if it based on other factors, such as fear of side effects for example. If the doctor understood the roots of Ken's decision-making he may have felt more comfortable with recommending a comfort-care approach and offering a referral to hospice. Using readily available tools like FICA (**F**aith, **I**mportance of it, membership in religious **C**ommunity, how do you want your needs **A**ddressed?) and HOPE (**H**ope, **O**rganized religion, **P**ersonal Practices in spirituality, **E**ffects these have on decision-making) can be very helpful for clinicians in exploring conflicts or understanding how a patient's faith and spirituality play out in their decision-making (Box 5.2). Serving patients requires spending time with them, listening with genuine inquiry, and discovering what matters most to them. Patients value their relationship with physicians who do this.

Even when there is no conflict to resolve, addressing faith and spirituality is still a core responsibility if care is to be delivered holistically. Studies not only show that patients commonly depend on spirituality and religion to cope with serious illnesses but also that they welcome interactions with their clinicians that explore how important they are in their lives.[8] For these reasons, understanding how a person copes and makes decisions can be indispensable in reducing the burdens of serious illness and relieving suffering. It is therefore an essential responsibility for physicians, especially when dealing with patients who are near the end of life

Meaningful assessment of the whole person extends beyond the task of filling out another checklist. The components highlighted here best serve as a conversation starter. They serve as a useful framework for clinicians to get to know their patients better. They emphasize the importance of thinking beyond the biomedical model and assert that factors such as social background, cultural beliefs, and personal values may impact the care of patients in even more significant ways than an elevated glucose or specific tumor marker might. Completing a whole-patient assessment may take more time but

---

Box 5.2 FICA and HOPE

HOPE

H: sources of Hope

O: Organized religion

P: Personal spirituality and practices

E: Effects on medical care and end-of-life issues

FICA

F: Faith and belief

I: Importance

C: Community

A: Address in care

is essential to optimal care, especially for those who live in the shadows of mainstream society.

The field of hospice and palliative care is steeped in the tradition of an interprofessional, multidisciplinary approach to patient care. It is precisely the team approach in healthcare that has been central to recognizing the need for whole-patient understandings. For this reason, it is routine in hospice and palliative care to explore the patient's social history beyond what is commonly taught and practiced. In medical school, students are taught to take social history by concentrating on behavioral risk factors such as tobacco use, alcohol use, and drug use, in addition to sexual activity. In a team approach, a patient is assessed and supported with a personalized care plan that includes psychosocial issues like financial distress and spirituality. The role of the social worker and case manager in helping identify and manage financial distress should not be overlooked. The emergence of nurse navigators who are advocates for patients is another area of promising impact.

> Ken used his faith in God and his spiritual beliefs to help reinforce his decision not to pursue treatment.

Understanding the particular aspects of Ken's life are important in creating a plan for providing optimal care for him. The same is true of all patients, but too often in medicine, we focus on the biological and physical. Labs and scans offer objective information about an illness, but they reveal little about how the patient is coping or what stresses are weighing on the person and the family. For many clinicians, there is comfort in focusing on the numbers. Doing so can give a sense of mastery over the disease. But it also leaves many big questions unanswered, especially those that revolve around how the illness is playing out in the patient's life. As pointed out earlier, physician documentation is organized around billing codes to secure reimbursement and as a result the physical facts of disease is what the electronic medical record emphasizes. In recent decades, there has been a minor revolt in medical training and practice, a movement which places a greater emphasis on patient centeredness and empathic care. This approach involves developing skills in effective communication, including the art of listening, so as to tease out a narrative that gives a fuller picture of the person than just the body sitting on the exam table. This is an important evolution in the care of patients but many pressures, financial and otherwise, threaten its universal dissemination.

In the clinic, it may be easy for nurses and physicians to quickly scan for possible signs of poverty or to stumble upon the fact the patient cares for his sick older brother at home, but these discoveries are often serendipitous, not a focused intent of the medical encounter. In addition, the love of data and a simplified "data-repository"—the electronic medical record—makes it harder for us to even see patients as individuals. But, as the story of Mr. and Mrs. White illustrates, when we lose sight of the array of factors that define people's lives outside of the medical arena their care becomes compromised—just as egregiously as it would be by the failure to order the proper diagnostic test or if they had been prescribed the wrong dose of a potentially-toxic medication.

Another critical discipline in holistic patient care is social work. The importance of social workers in providing assessment and support, from the unique perspective of their discipline, cannot be understated. A skilled social worker can make a large difference in crafting a treatment plan that is actually successful; that is to say, care tailored in a way to address a broader spectrum of issues and needs than pointed to by the biomedical approach. Under the Medicare Hospice Benefit, social workers have been established as essential members of the core team. This is because of their intrinsic value and unique skills in advancing holistic care of patients. Their role in navigating the difficult circumstances of people living at the margins is exemplified in the care that Cowboy received, which is being discussed elsewhere in this book. Unfortunately, however, throughout much of the healthcare system social workers are considered an afterthought, their purpose being narrowed to discharge planning designed to reduce length of stay and control costs. If we are going to change how the system cares for people like Mr. and Mrs. White, then we must make a commitment to broaden the presence of social work activity that is meaningfully focused on holistic patient care.

ACCESS TO PALLIATIVE CARE

Ken decided against disease-focused treatment for his cancer. Even if he was interested in aggressive treatment, the options would have been quite limited for his esophageal cancer. Regardless of his choice, Ken and many others like him are prime candidates for early referrals to palliative care services. Ken's plan of care was a follow-up appointment two months after the first oncology visit. Even if the oncology team didn't plan to give chemotherapy, there was still important anticipatory guidance to give Ken on future complications and challenges that he might face with progressive esophageal cancer. This was not done, nor was a plan for going forward made. He was kind of placed in a holding pattern where a wait-and-see attitude prevailed. But a lot can happen quickly during serious illness and the statement, "Come back in two months" had a ring of abandonment to it. The was no ongoing plan of support for Mr. White upon leaving the oncology clinic that day. He was being sent off to fend for himself, in a certain sense. Despite the good intentions of physicians to do the right thing, proactive planning for supportive care for patients like Ken takes a back seat to a willingness to aggressively treat disease. It may be, as his situation reveals, that supportive care sometimes can be taken to mean the absence of aggressive treatment, which sounds like, "keep doing what you are doing and wait until the next complication." Studies looking at best practices in supportive care show there is no standardized definition of it nor an established protocol of what must elements it must include. So even the notion itself of "supportive care" can become a misnomer at best and perhaps even a hollow lie causing more suffering at worst.[9] The bottom line is that we are far more advanced and proficient in our ability to offer sophisticated technolgies to combat disease than to provide the means to ease suffering and improve quality of life near life's end (Figure 5.2).

Palliative care services are varied across the United States. There is clustering in suburban/metropolitan areas and a high saturation of hospital-based palliative care teams that handle crises. There also exists a smaller but growing number of community-based and clinic-based palliative care options for more upstream access during an illness.[10] In general, access to palliative care is dependent on physician referrals, which can vary among individual providers. Therefore it is available in a non-standardized fashion. It is

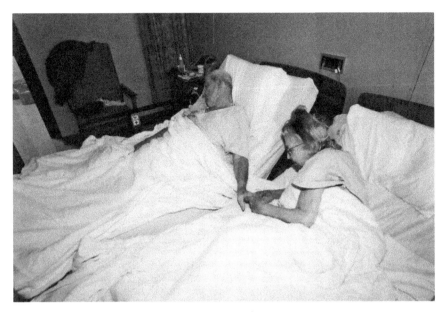

FIGURE 5.2 Having mutually endured the nursing home experience that many people dread, Virble says goodbye to her beloved husband.

not only dependent on geographical availability of services, utilization itself varies across populations. People of low socioeconomic status have less resources generally speaking. As a result of lower health literacy they often lack understanding of the value of palliative care. Their attitudes toward it may be reflective of a concern that, in some ways, palliative care may in fact have middle-class underpinnings. People who live at the margins tend to mistrust the mainstream. This generalized distrust and cultural estrangement may feed into an attitude of suspicion about the very nature of palliative care. Additionally, patients of low economic and social status often lack the empowerment to advocate for themselves in the medical encounter, as was clearly indicated in Mr. White's visit to the oncologist. Because of this, people with lower socioeconomic status are less likely to access palliative care.[11]

Personal finances, access to health insurance, and poverty play a large role in access to quality care near the end of life. Multiple studies demonstrate that areas with high poverty rates require more investment to achieve the same quality of care as is available in areas that are not in poverty. Some of these costs may be related to higher incidence of multiple comorbidities in lower socioeconomic levels, as witnessed by the multiple health issues faced by each member of the White family.

Ken also shared some mistrust of the healthcare system as a whole, which may have contributed to his lack of access to palliative care. There are marginalized groups in lower socioeconomic statuses that have a mistrust of healthcare in general and any perceived efforts to limit accessibility to "life-saving care" because of significant past wrongs that have been endured, like the historic cases of withheld treatment for minority groups for US medical research in the 20th century. From such a perspective, palliative care is likely to be seen as an unacceptable alternative to more aggressive curative treatment, even if there is no reasonable expectation for cure.

> We should be able as a wealthy country to find the ability to care for those who can least afford it.

To help counter the underutilization of palliative care services, clinicians and health-care systems can incorporate standardized screening and triggers for palliative care to help uncover need before a crisis occurs. But this increased demand needs to be paired with a ready and available palliative care workforce. In order to provide high-quality care, an expanded labor force is required, especially if community-based care is to be a part of the solution. This means the training of more professionals, which requires investment of both time and money. And if care is to extend beyond the walls of the hospital into the community, the inefficiencies of doing so will have to be addressed. For example, travel time to visit a patient in their own environment is a major cost factor to consider. In addition, there is the issue of the potential lack of sustainable reimbursable clinical services in home-based care outside of the regulated fields of hospice and home healthcare. Unfortunately, the American private and public reimbursement systems of fee-for-service does not cover the significant, interdisciplinary time investment that non-hospice, palliative care requires.

Some innovation is happening as part of a larger push for quality-based payment systems that may enhance capacity to deliver the right care at the right time. This may prompt development of strategies for providing more efficient care that also improves patient satisfaction and outcomes. This strategy is outlined in the Affordable Care Act (ACA) quality-improvement reform efforts that include programs like Medicare Access and CHIP Reauthorization Act (MACRA) and Merit-based Incentive Pay (MIPS), along with alternative payment models and accountable care organizations and some unique commercial-insurance programs. While it is good to see change is coming, it will take time before the reforms can impact the quality of care delivery across the system. And, despite the overall usefulness of these initiatives, there will still be people like Ken and Virble who will be left out and not be well served by these programs. Until then, we must continue to press for increased access to quality programs so palliative care can become a standard of care that is equitably available for all and not something that somebody happens to "luck into" like Ken White.

CARING FOR THE WHOLE FAMILY THROUGH INTEGRATED HEALTH AND SOCIAL SERVICES

Once it was clear that Ken was not planning to pursue chemotherapy, there should have been a whole different group called into action to help him make plans for his family, for moving to a nursing home, and to develop a plan for his eventual death. A palliative care team was involved, and it was clear they cared enough to donate a suit for him to wear to his funeral. Yet palliative care teams, if they visit the home at all, only visit a couple of times per week or make contact several times a week by phone. The need for social services and custodial care was probably much greater than for medical services at that time. A case manager or social worker could have helped plan the eventual transition to a nursing home better. They might be able to find creative ways to keep Ken and Virble in their own home with in-home caregivers through Medicaid programs. For people like Ken and Virble, social needs can outweigh the medical issues, but as a society we do not assign them adequate priority.

For a long time, the family tried to make things work in the home, as Ken and Virble sought to take care of each other despite their enormous challenges. The Whites are a prime example of America's reliance on family members to be caregivers. A study done by the American Academy of Family Physicians (AAFP) in 2009 showed that such care was equal to $450 billion in one year alone.[12] The human burden of caring placed on indigent families can be especially enormous, and the need to take time off from work, even if FMLA benefits are available, can be financially ruinous for a family.

Our fee-for-service reimbursement structure is in need of reform as well. Even at the end of life, there are counterproductive incentives to order additional tests, generate longer hospital stays, and refer for more clinic visits, even if in the big picture these are not medically beneficial or they do not fit with the goals of the patient or family. As noted earlier, the push toward improving quality outcomes will hopefully drive new plans with more aligned incentives and care strategies that are truly patient-centered as well as cost containing.[13]

SUMMARY

Ken and Virble White are part of our social fabric, the large group that is defined as the working poor. We know they are subject to worse health outcomes and have inadequate means to make the health system work in their favor, or even on par with the rest of the population. Elements of their story reveal the harm and injustice that people living in or near poverty suffer. In particular, the issues confronting the White's played out in chaos and confusion. Medical decisions being made based on religious faith without adequate understanding of the medical situation, inadequate patient–physician communication, low health literacy, and lack of access to social services did not contribute to a good outcome. Instead they led their story to a grim conclusion as they were subjected to unconscionable indignities in the nursing home facility. These facts of dying poor, however, are not exclusive to their story. They are present in different ways, in the experience of those who live and die near the margins throughout our society each and every day.

Listening to the story of people like the White's is invaluable to advancing the capacity to provide optimized care for vulnerable populations. When we begin to gain understandings of who we are caring for through mindful listening, cultural competence, and whole-patient assessment, we will better be able to care for people like Ken and Virble in a more compassionate way. It should not matter if a patient has insurance or can hire endless nurse aides: as a wealthy country we should be able to find the ability to care for those who can least afford it. In fact, it is precisely because we are so wealthy and committed to democratic ideals and the principles of Judeo-Christian heritage, that we have a moral obligation to do so.

REFERENCES

1. Dimoska A, Butow PN, Dent E, Arnold B, Brown RF, Tattersall MHN. An examination of the initial cancer consultation of medical and radiation oncologists using the Cancode interaction analysis system. *Br J Cancer.* 2008;98(9):1508–1514. http://doi.org/10.1038/sj.bjc.6604348

2. de Souza JA, Wong Y-N. Financial distress in cancer patients. *J Med Person.* 2013;11(2). http://doi.org/10.1007/s12682-013-0152-3

3. de Boer AGEM, Frings-Dresen MHW. Employment and the common cancers: return to work of cancer survivors. *Occup Med.* 2009;59(6):378–380. http://doi.org/10.1093/occmed/kqp087

4. Ramsey S, Blough D, Kirchhoff A, et al. Washington State cancer patients found to be at greater risk for bankruptcy than people without a cancer diagnosis. *Health Aff.* 2013;32(6):1143–1152. http://doi.org/10.1377/hlthaff.2012.1263

5. National Academy of Medicine; Committee on Family Caregiving for Older Adults. *Families caring for an aging America* (R. Schulz & J. Eden, eds.). Washington, DC: National Academies Press; 2016. Retrieved from https://www.nap.edu/catalog/23606

6. National Academies of Sciences, *Health literacy and palliative care* (J. Alper, ed.). Washington, DC: National Academies Press; 2016. http://doi.org/10.17226/21839

7. Weiss BD, Mays MZ, Martz W, et al. Quick assessment of literacy in primary care: the newest vital sign. *Ann Fam Med.* 2005;3(6):514–522. http://doi.org/10.1370/afm.405

8. Whitford HS, Olver IN, Peterson MJ. Spirituality as a core domain in the assessment of quality of life in oncology. *Psycho-Oncology.* 2008;17(11):1121–1128. http://doi.org/10.1002/pon.1322

9. Hui D, De La Cruz M, Mori M, et al. Concepts and definitions for "supportive care," "best supportive care," "palliative care," and "hospice care" in the published literature, dictionaries, and textbooks. *Support Care Cancer.* 2013;21(3):659–685. http://doi.org/10.1007/s00520-012-1564-y

10. Center to Advance Palliative Care (CAPC). State-by-state report card, 2015. https://reportcard.capc.org/).

11. Lewis JM, DiGiacomo M, Currow DC, Davidson PM. Dying in the margins: understanding palliative care and socioeconomic deprivation in the developed world. *J Pain Sympt Manag.* 2011;42(1):105–118. http://doi.org/10.1016/j.jpainsymman.2010.10.265

12. Reinhard, S, Feinberg, L, Houser, A, Choula, R. Valuing the invaluable 2015 update: undeniable progress, but big gaps remain. AARP report.

13. Policies and payment system to support high-quality end-of-life care. Pizzo R, Walker D, et al. *Dying in America.* Chapter 5, Policies and Payment Systems to Support High-Quality End-of-Life Care. Institute of Medicine. 2014.

6

THE STORY OF ANNIE

GRATITUDE AND FAITH

Betty R. Ferrell

Snapshot Reflection: A Story of Grace Through Suffering

For centuries, humanity has been attempting to reconcile the existence of cruelty and injustice with the idea of a loving and merciful God. Theologians and philosophers have written brilliantly but esoterically about the concept of *theodicy*, describing how religion provides unique explanations that offer comfort and meaning for individuals as they come face-to-face with suffering and death. For Ms. Annie Dickens, however, there was no need for abstract philosophies or intricate religious doctrines to help explain and guide her through suffering into death. All that she needed was firmly implanted into her heart, a heart that was fortified with unyielding faith. There was nothing elaborate or fancy about her faith. It simply flowed from a purity of loving God, no matter what and no matter how extreme the sufferings. And for Ms. Dickens, the physical sufferings were severe.

Annie was living in the county nursing home, where her joyful spirit directly contrasted with the belligerence of her disease. As her disease progressed, Ms. Dickens was told she had six months to live, but she lived for two more years. Over the ensuing 24 months, she experienced steady physical decline and severe body-wasting. Her final months of life were spent bedridden. She struggled with pain, discomfort, and shortness of breath. Her multiple diseases—chronic obstructive pulmonary disease (COPD), lung cancer, peripheral vascular disease—led to an agonizingly slow trajectory of physical deterioration. She was jaundiced and emaciated, her lips were cracked, and she had trouble with even the slightest physical movement.

But ask Ms. Annie how she was doing in the midst of all of this and, without fail, she would say that she was just fine—a response that seemed incongruous with her physical condition. Disease had enveloped her body, and her discomfort and pain were obvious. Yet, her spirit was always optimistic and full of hope. She never complained or expressed bitterness over what was happening to her. Instead, her prevailing attitude was one of appreciation. When I asked what she felt grateful for, she stated there were many reasons to be thankful. "I am grateful to you," she said to me. Please let me set the record straight in this regard: I was doing nothing spectacular; I was simply showing up with a tape recorder and camera so one day I might be able to tell a bit of her story. Even so, she appreciated that someone cared about her story and was willing to listen to it. She was also thankful for a volunteer with the palliative care team who would regularly visit a few times each week. These visits reassured her that she mattered and that others cared enough to spend quality, unhurried time with her. She was grateful for the care she received in the nursing home. She was so derailed by her disease that she could not take care of herself, and she appreciated the work of the nursing attendants, nurses, and doctors who took care of her. Ultimately, her deepest source of gratitude was reserved for God. "God saw fit to put me here," she would say. The doctors, nurses, social workers, volunteers—even myself—were part of God's plan to take care of her during this difficult time. She believed this without doubt or hesitation.

Annie's body was crippled with disease but her spirit remained resonant and full. God was her dominant source of strength. She offered up prayers and loving thoughts constantly and trusted that He would—at the end of the day, upon her last day—make all things well. She felt blessed that God was taking care of her, and this enabled her to face her physical sufferings with calm and peace. She lifted up her struggles with confidence that soon God would shepherd her home to blissful and eternal reward. There was nothing contrived or elaborate about this belief. Instead, her faith was as simple as it was strong, pure as it was unwavering. With God's presence comforting her, Ms. Annie Dickens endured physical suffering that few can imagine and confronted death with a spirit of gratitude, dignity, and determination that can only be described as remarkable, even enviable.

A Special Observation

The majesty of her spirit and faith triumphed over inconceivable suffering caused by her decaying body.

Take-Home Lesson

The story of Annie declares the dignity and grace of the human spirit in the midst of extreme suffering. It shows how social support comforts throughout the illness experience. Her narrative is an example of the healing power of spirituality and human caring. From her end-of-life experience, we learn that dying is far less about matters of the body than it is about matters of the person. We also discern that when a person is well attended throughout the dying process—her emotional, social, and spiritual needs being fulfilled—her suffering is eased, and she is deeply comforted.

—David Wendell Moller

INTRODUCTION

Gratitude and faith: These two concepts are overwhelming messages from the story of Annie. Her legacy reminds us as health providers of the need to transform our vision of those we serve from that of people who are sick and broken, to an understanding of their wholeness amidst an experience of illness, even as they await death. This story resonates strongly with me as a nurse and researcher whose work has focused on suffering and quality of life (QOL) concerns in advanced disease.

Our research at the City of Hope National Medical Center over the past 20+ years has been guided by a conceptual model of QOL.[1-3] This model views QOL as encompassing domains of physical, psychological, social, and spiritual well-being. These domains can be evaluated separately, but are inextricably intertwined. As in the story of Annie, physical symptoms impacted spirituality; psychological and spiritual concerns overlapped intensely; and social well-being, evidenced in Annie's life through her relationships with the volunteer Sally and David as the researcher, were all essential aspects of her wholeness—her quality of life.

I have reflected on the story of Annie and the lessons she provides for us. I have applied the QOL model to provide some perspectives on this story of gratitude and faith.

PHYSICAL WELL-BEING

Over the past three decades, there has been growing recognition of the enormous impact of physical symptoms on quality of life.[4-6] Patients with serious illnesses experience symptoms involving multiple organ systems, and this experience of physical symptoms often leads to whole-person suffering. Pain, fatigue, nausea, diarrhea, constipation, dyspnea, and cough are but a few common symptoms. Numerous studies have documented that patients with advanced disease often experience 10–20 physical symptoms, most which are rated as moderate to severe in intensity.

Symptoms are physiological and most often have distinct pathology and biological mechanisms. Yet it is the understanding of the person experiencing the symptoms that should guide our practice. Annie's dyspnea can be explained by the pathophysiology of her lung cancer, yet her lived experience of dyspnea can only be understood by embracing what dyspnea meant to her in light of her faith in God, response to knowing her life was ending, and gratitude for being in an environment surrounded by compassionate caregivers.

> I was particularly moved by this stark contrast between her horrendous physical status and her radiant psychological state.

In our symptom research over the past many years and studies, we have come to understand how little we know about a patient's symptoms or physical well-being if we rely only on assessments of symptom intensity. Hearing "my pain is a 6 out of 10" is important clinical information, yet it provides only a limited view of the patient's physical well-being and far less about overall QOL.[5-7] We have come to understand, as have many other clinicians and researchers, that another critical dimension of our assessment is *symptom distress*.

Symptom distress, measured also on a 0–10 scale or "distress thermometer," captures the degree to which symptoms impact the person and create suffering.[8] Annie's experience of moderate to severe symptom intensity was profoundly influenced by her faith and psychological response to her overall situation.

The story of Annie and consideration of her physical well-being raises for me the concept of vulnerability. We often categorize patients whose circumstances are similar to

Annie's, such as those who are elderly, ethnic minorities, homeless, or poor, as vulnerable. This designation of them as vulnerable serves an important purpose many times, as it helps us to identify those most in need or those who are likely to experience negative or distressing events, thus giving us an opportunity to respond to and even prevent negative sequelae.

However, Annie's life also gives us pause to consider this notion of vulnerability. She exhibits many characteristics common in our classification of vulnerability, yet she also expresses many strengths, primarily her faith and gratitude, which greatly mute her vulnerability. Exploring the concept of resilience has offered valuable opportunity through the literature to understand how people in overwhelming circumstances survive and often live with quality.[9-11]

Annie's story reminded me of a patient I cared for, now more than 25 years ago, in my role as a home health nurse. The patient, Florence, was in her 80s and lived in a low-income public housing center. She had multiple medical problems, including severe diabetes, hypertension, cardiac disease, pulmonary disease, and arthritis. Florence was fiercely independent and insisted upon remaining in her independent-living apartment rather than moving to a nursing home.

Florence was full of life, vibrant, funny, passionate, and even mischievous. As her disease raged and her body was so devastated, her spirit prevailed. Florence remained committed to "high fashion," full makeup, and her "dime-store jewelry" each day. She continued smoking and enjoying her "evening cocktails" and had a "boyfriend"—a man who lived nearby and was deeply committed to her. Florence and her boyfriend lived separately to avoid loss of her government-provided income, but they defied the housing rules and had many late-night rendezvous in the senior living center.

I cared for Florence over two years, during which time her physical disease and symptoms seemed to take over her body. Over these months, she had myocardial infarctions, strokes, became blind, had decubitus ulcers, infections, and became wheelchair-bound. I also felt as if she was "disappearing," as she had a series of amputations, beginning with amputation of a foot, but progressing to full-leg amputation.

Throughout the two years, despite a constant trajectory of physical decline, Florence's spirit remained fully alive. She had no religious affiliation but was full of the spirit of living, ever passionate, happy, positive, and unshaken by multiple crises and physical devastation.

After one visit, I was particularly moved by this stark contrast between her horrendous physical status and her radiant psychological status, I could not resist asking Florence to help me understand her response to illness. I confronted her, asking, "Florence, I have watched you over two years as you have faced so many crises, symptoms, amputations, and setbacks. Yet you always are happy. Tell me, what is your secret?"

This blind, elderly, "vulnerable" woman before me was absolutely silent, seriously considering my query. And then she revealed her "secret" with two words: "Clear conscience." And then again she was silent.

Clear conscience—the ability of the whole person, the psychological and spiritual, to trump all the physical devastation of disease. She was living her life in her own way and without regret and that provided great comfort.

> Her relationships with her professional caregivers were her family and connection to life.

PSYCHOLOGICAL WELL-BEING

Psychological well-being encompasses the overall patient experience of coping with illness, and it often includes psychological symptoms such as anxiety or depression.[12-14] This domain of QOL also includes issues such as the patient's fears of the future. But psychological well-being also includes the patient's strengths, supports, and as Annie relates, "the ability to take one day at a time" (Figure 6.1).

In Annie's story, we also hear a recurring theme of dignity. She is able to maintain her personhood and to be intact as a whole person capable of finding meaning in each day. Annie's story also contains an intense message of her faith. She says that she "gives it all to God," and, in reading these words, we can almost sense the burdens of her illness and symptoms lifted as she "gives up" her suffering. Significant work in recent years within the field of palliative care has applied dignity therapy and meaning-making interventions.[15-17] The purpose of these psychotherapeutic interventions is to help people with advanced, life-threatening illnesses reduce their existential distress and to help them to discover some meaning or purpose to what they are confronting and suffering.

> It is not difficult to imagine how any person enduring Annie's circumstances might well have a story to tell of great suffering, psychological distress, and disintegration.

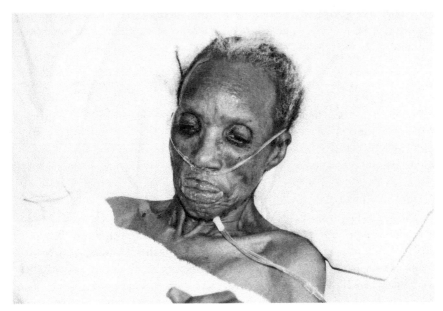

FIGURE 6.1 In the midst of unimaginable pain and suffering, Ms. Annie expresses gratitude to all of those who cared for her.

There is also deep meaning in this woman's philosophy of living "one day at a time." Through focusing only on one day—and very importantly, not seeing each day as a burden to be endured, but living in gratitude for each day as a gift—she lives her remaining life with deep faith and meaning, maintaining integrity and dignity. It is not difficult to imagine how any person enduring Annie's circumstances might well have a story to tell of great suffering, psychological distress, and disintegration. But Annie chose to accentuate the positive elements in her life and not focus on the devastation encompassing her body.

As healthcare professionals, we often reflect on what we learn from our patients. We would do well to grasp Annie's philosophy of living "one day at a time" for our own goals of care. What can we do today to make this day less distressing for the patient? What can I do with one more day of my practice that will instill a sense of gratitude for me that parallels this woman's gratefulness for her life?

My speculation is that Annie's psychological well-being was greatly supported by caregivers who knew her as a person, not just a patient. The volunteer Sally offered time to read scripture to her and to simply be present. The visits from David allowed her to share her life story, her legacy as a woman who had faced illness with faith and gratitude. There is an abundance of literature supporting the association between finding meaning in life and a decrease in suffering.[18-24] In telling her story and sharing her faith, Annie's life had meaning, and she not only received the support of others, she gave of herself in return. In this process, she was recognized as wise, as having a life worthy of sharing, of leaving her mark, and teaching others. Each opportunity to give filled her with spiritual richness. Ultimately, Annie addressed her lack of fear and capacity to find meaning while facing death by "giving it all up to God."

As healthcare professionals, we thrive on a philosophy of doing, "fixing," intervening, and prescribing within a biological model of cure. Psychological concerns are rarely "fixed," however. At best they are heard, honored, and respected; sometimes healed but not "fixed." Annie's ability to utter the words "I am not afraid of dying" is a testament to the holistic care and support that maintained her status as a living person.

SOCIAL WELL-BEING

Palliative care has been built on a philosophy of caring that acknowledges the patient in relationship with others. We often think about *social well-being* only in terms of patients with family members fully engaged in their lives and their care. But what about the "un-befriended," those dying alone, the homeless, those estranged from their families, or increasingly, those who are elderly and who have the mixed blessing of having now survived all their loved ones and are alone in their journey.[25-29]

For Annie, her relationships with her professional caregivers were her family and her connection to life. It is important to note how she valued the presence of Sally in her final days. This was not simply a few interactions by a volunteer. It was a relationship. It is also of note that Annie's closest relationship was with her God. God was a constant companion who filled her with His presence and supported her through her burdens. Acknowledgement and celebration of this relationship is second to none for Annie. It not

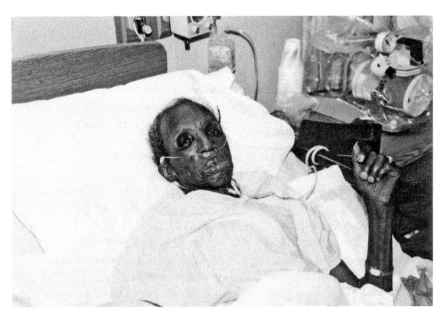

FIGURE 6.2 "I have to do this for Him," Ms. Annie affirmed.

only gave her comfort. It provided purpose and meaning in being able to share it with others.

SPIRITUAL WELL-BEING

So often in clinical practice and in research, spirituality is seen as a very abstract concept, too personal to define, and is an area of concern only when other needs are met. For Annie, spirituality was present in every day of her life, woven into the fabric of her being. Faith was the means by which she coped with illness and lived her life (Figure 6.2).

Annie fortunately received care in which her spirituality was recognized and honored. She was vocal about her beliefs, but often patients are more reserved, often not sharing their spiritual needs unless probed by a clinician or seen by a chaplain.

There is significant literature that has documented how infrequently spiritual needs are assessed and even less frequently are spiritual needs included in the plan of care.[19,30-36] Consensus recommendations have been made for palliative care programs to promote improved quality of spiritual care as an essential aspect of patient-centered care.[37]

Was Annie suffering? She told us of her experiences at the end of life—her symptoms, her awareness of dying, her place as a person very alone in the world. But she also spoke of her gratitude, her burdens handed over to God, and the blessings of this phase of life, born from her relationship with God and the compassionate care she was receiving.

Box 6.1 Tenets of Suffering

1. "Suffering" is described as a loss of control, which creates insecurity. Suffering people often feel helpless and trapped, unable to escape their circumstances. Those who suffer feel vulnerable and uncertain about the future.

2. In most instances, suffering is associated with loss. The loss may be of a valued object or relationship, or of some aspect of the self, whether a role or the loss of some aspect of the physical body. The loss may be evident only in the mind of the sufferer, but it nonetheless leaves a person diminished and with a sense of brokenness.

3. Suffering is thoroughly individual and intensely personal.

4. Suffering is accompanied by a range of intense emotions. Sadness, anguish, fear, abandonment, despair, and a myriad of other emotions may occur. This range of feelings is sometimes referred to as "emotional pain."

5. Suffering can be deeply linked to a recognition of one's own mortality. When threatened by serious illness, people may fear the end of life. Conversely, for others, living with chronic illness may cause a yearning for death.

6. Suffering often involves asking the question "Why?" Illness and loss are often seen as untimely and undeserved threats. Suffering people seek to find meaning and answers for that which is unknowable.

7. Suffering is often accompanied by spiritual distress. Regardless of their religious affiliation, individuals experiencing illness, injury, or threat often feel a sense of hopelessness. When one's life is threatened, there may be a self-evaluation of what has been lived and what remains undone. Becoming weak and vulnerable and facing mortality causes one to reevaluate one's relationship with a higher being.

8. Suffering is often an expression of the angst associated with separation from the world. Individuals often express intense loneliness and yearn for connection with others. This may be a highly ambivalent and confusing concern, because the same suffering person may also feel intense distress about dependency on those who are present.

9. Suffering is not synonymous with pain but is closely associated with it. Physical pain is closely related to psychological, social, and spiritual distress, which intensifies the physical experience. Pain that persists without meaning becomes suffering.

10. Suffering occurs when the individual feels voiceless. This may occur when the person is unable to give words to their experience or when their screams are unheard.

Ferrell BR, Coyle N. The nature of suffering and the goals of nursing. New York: Oxford University Press; 2008.

SUMMARY

My colleague Nessa Coyle and I wrote "The Nature of Suffering and the Goals of Nursing."[4] In this work, we outline 10 tenets of suffering, depicted in Box 6.1. As in this analysis of Annie, exploration of the dimensions of QOL help us to plan care that addresses all dimensions of QOL. Annie's needs at one level were clear and not so complex. At another level, they were revealed as quite complex as we came to know the depth of her faith, her life story, and how much she was physically enduring. It is this kind of knowledge, that which reveals the life story of our patients and how they cope in the midst of suffering, which should direct our care for them.

REFERENCES

1. Ferrell BR, Wisdom C, Wenzl C, Schneider C. Quality of life as an outcome variable in the management of cancer pain. *Cancer.* 1989;63:2321–2327.
2. Ferrell BR, Wisdom C, Wenzl C, Brown J. Effects of controlled-release morphine on quality of life for cancer pain. *Oncol Nurs Forum.* 1989;6(4):521–526.
3. Padilla G, Ferrell BR, Grant M, Rhiner M. Defining the content domain of quality of life for cancer patients with pain. *Cancer Nursing.* 1990;13(2):108–115.
4. Ferrell B, Coyle N. The nature of suffering and the goals of nursing. *Oncol Nurs Forum.* 2008;35(2):241–247.
5. Fink R, Gates R. Pain assessment. In: BR Ferrell, N Coyle (Eds.). *Oxford textbook of palliative nursing.* 3rd ed. New York: Oxford University Press; 2010:137–160.
6. Borneman T, Brown-Saltzman K. Meaning in illness. In: BR Ferrell, N Coyle (Eds.). *Oxford textbook of palliative nursing.* 3rd ed. New York: Oxford University Press; 2010:673–683.
7. Barkwell DP. Ascribing meaning: A critical factor in coping and pain attenuation in patients with cancer-related pain. *J Palliat Care.* 1991;7(3):5–10.
8. National Comprehensive Cancer Network: Distress Management Guidelines. At www.nccn.org/professionals/physician_glsf_guidelines.asp (last accessed March 30, 2011).
9. Lethborg C, Aranda S, Kissane D. To what extent does meaning mediate adaptation to cancer? The relationship between physical suffering, meaning in life and connection to others in adjustment to cancer. *Palliat Support Care.* 2007;5(4):377–388.
10. Lutha SS, Cicchetti D. The construct of resilience: implications for interventions and social policies. *Dev Psychopathol.* 2000;12(4):857–885.
11. Park C, Edmondson D, Fenster J, Blank T. Meaning making and psychological adjustment following cancer: the mediating roles of growth, life meaning and restored just world beliefs. *J Consult Clin Psychol.* 2008;76(5):863–875.
12. Barraclough J. ABC of palliative care: depression, anxiety, and confusion. *BMJ.* 1997;315(119):1365–1368.
13. Durkin I, Kearney M, O'Siorain L. Psychiatric care in a palliative care unit. *Palliat Med.* 2003;17:212–218.
14. Miovic M, Block S. Psychiatric disorders in advanced cancer. *Cancer.* 2007;110:1665–1676.
15. McClain CS, Rosenfeld B, Breitbart W. Effect of spiritual well-being on end-of-life despair in terminally ill cancer patients. *Lancet.* 2003;361:1603–1607.
16. Breitbart W. Reframing hope: meaning-centered care for patients near the end of life. Interview by Karen S. Heller. *J Palliat Med.* 2003;6(6):979–988.
17. Chochinov HM, Hassard T, MaClement S, et al. The patient dignity inventory: A novel way of measuring dignity related distress in palliative care. *J Sympt Manag.* 2008;36(6):559–571.
18. Coyle N. The hard work of living in the face of death. *J Pain Sympt Manag.* 2006;32(3):266–274.

19. Balboni TA, Vanderwerker LC, Block SD, et al. Religiousness and spiritual support among advanced cancer patients and associations with end-of-life treatment preferences and quality of life. *J Clin Oncol.* 2007;25(5):555–560.

20. Skalla KA, McCoy JP. Spiritual assessment of patients with cancer: the moral authority, vocational, aesthetic, social, and transcendent model. *Oncol Nurs Forum.* 2006;33(4):745–751.

21. LeFavi RG, Wessels MH. Life review in pastoral care counseling: background and efficacy for the terminally Ill. *J Pastoral Care Council.* 2003;57:281–292.

22. Puchalski CM, Dorff RE, Hendi IY. Spirituality, religion, and healing in palliative care. *Clin Geriatr Med.* 2004;20(40):689–714.

23. Sulmasy DP. *The rebirth of the clinic: an introduction to spirituality in health care.* Washington, DC: Georgetown University Press; 2006.

24. Puchalski CM. Honoring the sacred in medicine: Spirituality as an essential element of patient-centered care. *J Med Person.* 2008;6:113–117.

25. Cacioppo JT, Patrick W. *Loneliness: human nature and the need for social connection.* New York: W. W. Norton & Company; 2008.

26. Karp N, Wood E. *Incapacitated and alone: health care decision making for the unbefriended elderly.* Washington, DC: American Bar Association Commission on Law and Aging; 2003.

27. Kushel MB, Miaskowski C. End-of-life care for homeless patients: "She says she is there to help me in any situation." *JAMA.* 2006;296(24):2959–2966.

28. Podymow T, Turnbull J, Coyle D. Shelter-based palliative care for the homeless terminally ill. *Palliat Med.* 2006;20(2):81–86.

29. Hughes A. Poor, homeless, and underserved populations. In: BR Ferrell, N Coyle (Eds.). *Oxford textbook of palliative nursing.* 3rd ed. New York: Oxford University Press; 2010:745–755.

30. Williams BR. Dying young, dying poor: A sociological examination of existential suffering among low-socioeconomic status patients. *J Palliat Med.* 2004;7(1):27–37.

31. Brown AE, Whitney SN, Duffy JD. The physician's role in the assessment and treatment of spiritual distress at the end of life. *Palliat Support Care.* 2006;4(1):81–86.

32. Taylor EJ. Prevalence of spiritual needs among cancer patients and family caregivers. *Oncol Nurs Forum.* 2006;33(4):729–735.

33. Lawrence RT, Smith DW. Principles to make a spiritual assessment work in your practice. *J Fam Pract.* 2004;53(8):625–631.

34. Hodge DR. A template for spiritual assessment: a review of the JCAHO requirements and guidelines for implementation. *Social Work.* 2006;51(4):317–326.

35. Peterman A, Fitchett G, Brady MJ, et al. Measuring spiritual well-being in people with cancer: The Functional Assessment of Chronic Illness Therapy–Spiritual Well-Being Scale (FACIT-Sp). *Ann Behav Med.* 2002;24(1):49–58.

36. Taylor EJ. *What do I say? Talking with patients about spirituality.* Philadelphia, PA: Templeton Press; 2007.

37. Puchalski C, Ferrell B, Virani R, Otis-Green S, Baird P, Bull J. Improving the quality of spiritual care as a dimension of palliative care: the report of the Consensus Conference. *J Palliat Med.* 2009;12(10):885–904.

7

MR. AND MRS. WHEELER
LIFE ON THE BRINK

Robert Arnold

Snapshot Reflection: A Story of Endless Struggle

Dying from stomach cancer in his mid-50s, Bill Wheeler was dominated by feelings of anger and despair. His story—filled with physical suffering, social isolation, and bitter mistrust of his healthcare providers—is an example of the consequences of personal and economic disempowerment throughout the dying process.

To get to know Mr. and Mrs. Wheeler is to come to understand that, even in the best of circumstances, there was precious little comfort in their lives. Each day they faced hardship and struggle, living in a deteriorated neighborhood where prostitution, drug-related activity, and signs of gang presence were visible. Their rental home was shabbily furnished, the one exception being the large-screen rental television that dominated the space used as the living room. Whenever I would ring the doorbell for one of my regular visits, they would rush to turn on the lights. These lights would not be used when they were home alone, the reason being that they could not afford to do so. Thus, typically, hour after hour, they would sit and live in a nearly-dark environment in which the television was their main source of lighting. As if this were not depressing enough, roaches could be regularly seen climbing walls throughout the house. In brief, it is not exaggerating to say that the atmosphere of their home was dingy, somewhat dirty, and utterly lacking in aesthetic appeal.

There was little available to lift up the Wheelers as they struggled and lived in these circumstances. The clunker car they drove was unreliable, and they had nothing in the way of fancy clothing or so-called luxury items. After struggling to meet monthly expenses, they had no discretionary income that could be used for entertainment and diversion. And as weighed down as they were by these daily difficulties, the situation worsened when Bill got seriously sick.

He had not been feeling well for a while and had been experiencing stomach distress. His job afforded no health benefits, so he did not have a private care physician. Rather, he was dependent on the safety-net system of care. In particular, he relied on the emergency room (ER) of the public hospital for his healthcare needs, as do many urban poor.

The frequent ER visits for Mr. Wheeler and those like him who lack health insurance was a very expensive proposition for an overburdened safety-net system without sufficient resources. Every test conducted and every visit would result in an unreimbursed expense for the hospital. While of course safety-net hospitals and clinics receive government and grant funding, overall, that support is insufficient to meet the complicated needs of the patients they serve. As a result, when he would arrive at the ER, Mr. Wheeler would be seen only from the point of view of emergency medicine. He never received appropriate follow-up referrals and in-depth tests that could have identified the cause of his stomach problems sooner. Lacking personal empowerment, health literacy, and financial resources, he was unable to insist on a timely and comprehensive work-up. The consequence for him was an extremely late diagnosis of stomach cancer. Mr. Wheeler understood that the late diagnosis was the result of his being poor, lacking health insurance, and being dependent on a safety-net system with inadequate resources. And he became very angry about all of this.

Anger was the dominant emotional state with which he wended his way through nine months of battling cancer. He was angry that his disease had been diagnosed so late. He had been feeling awful, losing weight, and repeatedly showing up at the ER. Yet despite the weight loss and complaints of stomach distress, he never received the type of care that most affluent and empowered patients would have received. He also knew that with earlier diagnosis and treatment, things could have been different and his life might have been saved. He recognized and was haunted by the fact that, because of the late diagnosis, he was doomed to die from the cancer. He understood this death sentence was directly related to being poor and uninsured, and about that he was inconsolable.

At the point when he was finally diagnosed, his disease had progressed so much that there was little to offer him. The decision was made to enroll him in a clinical trial so he began a course a course of experimental chemotherapy. A couple of months into the treatment, poor communication on the part of doctors led him to the mistaken belief that he was in remission. Some of the cancerous lymph nodes had shrunken temporarily and, prompted by Mr. Wheeler's need for good news, the oncologist overemphasized how well the medicines were working and how well he was doing. In fact, because of the horrible communication, he came to the mistaken conclusion that his cancer was in remission, and that was far from being the case. The false hope that emerged stimulated moments of emotional relief for him but in the end became a great disservice as his hopes crashed and the illusion of cure could no longer be maintained. As a result, he became increasingly resentful and mistrusting of his physicians and the healthcare system, and this distrust remained unabated until he died.

His anger intensified the more things deteriorated in his life. His wife, Evelyn, was diagnosed with lymphoma, bringing more distress into an already chaotic situation. Family, friends, neighbors, and members of his church were scarcely present throughout this time, and he felt an acute sense of social and spiritual isolation. The resulting emptiness dragged him even further down, and it became his constant companion. In addition, we cannot forget that physically he felt awful most of the time. He lived with nausea and vomiting, often had severe stomach pain, and, in the midst of it all, even suffered a heart attack. Adding to his problems was very late enrollment in hospice—a byproduct of his mistaken belief that he was in remission. As a result, he received less-than-optimal management of his pain and other distressing symptoms.

From the first time I met Mr. Wheeler, I asked myself the question: "If I were in his shoes, would I be angry as well?" The answer would always be "yes." Heck yes, I would be. Mad as hell! Late diagnosis, mistrust and suspicion, isolation and abandonment, unrelieved physical suffering—yes, this would make me very angry indeed.

My self-reflection, however, was merely theoretical. After all, I inhabited a very different world than he did. My education served as a vehicle for empowerment, and my employer provided health benefits. My life was such that it would be unlikely for me to become so entangled in a downward spiral of inadequate care and associated despair. I would have had options.

Mr. Wheeler, however, had little recourse. He was dependent upon a system that failed him and upon its physicians, whom he distinctly mistrusted. He had no other options as to where to receive care, and his sufferings were little relieved. He lived in isolation, with depression and disheartenment shaping his view of the world and his relationship to it. The bottom line is that while disease was destroying his body, the burdens of poverty, inattention to his needs, and lack of concern for all he was enduring were also destroying his spirit.

This devolution of body and spirit continued unabated throughout illness into his death, leaving him feeling bitter at the injustice of it all.

A Special Observation

Bill and Evelyn Wheeler were systematically beaten down by illness, poverty, and their tension-filled relationship with the public hospital system.

Take-Home Lesson

The narrative of Bill Wheeler expresses his sense of betrayal and neglect. There was a great divide between the life experiences of Mr. Wheeler and his caregivers. His providers saw him as angry and difficult, which he was. Yet, in their relationship with him, they failed to understand *why* he presented himself that way. He was angry that his late diagnosis was related to being poor and uninsured. He resented that his doctors did not communicate with him effectively. He felt they misrepresented things, failed to listen attentively, and disregarded his suffering and needs. As a result, he became deeply mistrusting and suspicious. In addition, the decision to treat his cancer aggressively, despite its advanced stage, ultimately led to shattered hope, greater anger, and late enrollment in hospice. His experience is a declaration of failure—a failure of the healthcare system and the broader community to ease the suffering of someone who desperately needed help. The result is that Mr. Wheeler went to his death feeling neglected and uncared for. Perhaps no greater sense of abandonment can be experienced.

—David Wendell Moller

INTRODUCTION

Frustrated. Angry. Overwhelmed: After reading the narrative "Life on the Brink: Mr. and Mrs. Wheeler," a flurry of emotions whirls through my mind. Each fans the flame of the next. I am frustrated that millions of Americans lack access to care and that Mr. Wheeler has no continuity of care. I am angry with a healthcare system that is so chaotic the right hand does not know what the left is doing. I am overwhelmed by the task of building trust with a patient who perceives injustice and mistreatment in every encounter with the medical system. The deck is stacked against me.

As Mr. Wheeler, Mrs. Wheeler, the oncology team, and the primary care intern each express desperation, I am drawn into the abyss. There is no curative treatment for the metastatic cancer that eats away at Mr. Wheeler. Even before he had cancer, his life was difficult. He had no money and little support. Navigating the world of medicine is daunting. In addition, he is suffering from both his cancer and its treatment. The treatment that he receives makes his physical symptoms worse than before his diagnosis. Neither he nor his physicians have access to palliative care that might improve his symptoms as well as provide the psychosocial support he needs. I dread turning the page.

Mr. and Mrs. Wheeler's frustration runs deep. Mr. Wheeler hates the county healthcare system yet remains dependent on it for his cancer treatment. Mrs. Wheeler struggles with her husband's wish to die at home and her fear of independently providing 24-hour care without medical expertise.

The medical team also is overwhelmed. The primary care intern attempts to provide thorough medical care to two complex patients based on a biopsychosocial model while being criticized for inefficiently managing clinic time. The oncology team dances between maintaining a patient's hope and discussing bad news.

My anger builds. Multiple targets merit wrath. I rail against the medical system that reimburses physicians for procedures and treatments but not for talking to and supporting patients. I shake my fist at Mr. Wheeler for not sharing his frustrations with the medical team. My brain shouts expletives at the doctors who demonstrate such lack of skill in talking with a terminally-ill patient. I'm irate that a patient had to choose between pain control and mental clarity. But most of all, I'm enraged by the massive amount of suffering present in the pages.

The enormous challenge of any attempt to improve the situation is overwhelming. Could the actions of any individual physician change the course of Mr. Wheeler's case?

Although there are seemingly insurmountable obstacles to caring for the urban dying poor, presence and communication may light the path. In her book *My Grandfather's Blessings*, Rachel Naomi Remen writes:

> Sometimes when a life of service has taken us to the fringes of human experience, what we find there is so overwhelming that our hearts can break. One might think that compared to the size of the problem what we do means nothing. But this is simply not the case. When it comes down to it, no matter how great or how small the need, we can only bless one life at a time.[1]

By focusing on the individual patient, physicians can overcome feelings of hopelessness and helplessness. *Presence*, the act of being "cognitively, emotionally and existentially open" and engaging in another's experience in the current moment, helps physicians build trusting relationships with patients.[2] Skilled communication allows these relationships to thrive and deepen.

Unfortunately, both Mr. and Mrs. Wheeler's experiences highlight the acute absence of both skilled communication and presence in their medical providers. Multiple examples of miscommunication between Mr. Wheeler and Mrs. Wheeler and their healthcare team occur during Mr. Wheeler's illness. Although we may not be able to fix the problems of poverty and a chaotic health system, we can improve the care of individual patients. The purpose of this chapter is to empower physicians to act incrementally to effect change, one patient at a time. I will use the narrative "Life on the Brink: Mr. and Mrs. Wheeler" to highlight examples of poor communication, outline principles of effective communication, and discuss how these practices may improve the care and clinical outcome of patients like Mr. Wheeler.

> Mr. Wheeler hates the county healthcare system yet remains dependent on it for cancer treatment.

I am not so naïve as to think that applying a cookbook of communication principles is enough to remedy the broken healthcare environment. However, in vulnerable populations, such as the urban poor, the negative impact of poor communication is magnified due to inadequate resources, low literacy, and mistrust of the medical system. Good communication allows physicians to demonstrate respect and acceptance for patients who often feel cast aside. It allows patients to feel that their voices have been heard, and may empower them (and their clinicians) to do the best they can in their current situation.

In this chapter, I will present evidence-based communication guidelines when they are available in the medical literature. If there is no research-based evidence to support a specific strategy, I will report recommendations based on expert consensus. I will focus on the topics of breaking bad news, discussing prognosis as a specific type of bad news, and maintaining patient and family hope through the trajectory of illness. For each of these topics, I will first discuss methods for optimal communication between physicians and patients, and then reflect on how (mis)communication impacted Mr. and Mrs. Wheeler.

GIVING BAD NEWS

Both Mr. and Mrs. Wheeler receive bad news regarding new diagnoses of malignancy. Consensus guidelines suggest breaking bad news using a stepwise approach: setting the stage, eliciting understanding, providing information, addressing emotion, and checking for understanding.[3-5] The following paragraphs will discuss each step.

Setting the stage requires ensuring privacy, minimizing interruptions from pages or telephone calls, allotting adequate time for discussion, and clarifying with the patient any additional people he or she would prefer to be present during the discussion. In the narrative, a physician asks Mr. Wheeler if anyone is accompanying him during his hospitalization. As Mr. Wheeler notes, "He seemed like he's like, you know, a caring doctor. He says, 'Is there anybody down here smoking or somebody here with you today?'" Although Mr. Wheeler appreciates the physician's attempt at setting the stage, being told about a new diagnosis of metastatic malignancy in isolation exacerbates his anxiety and forces him to worry about how he will convey the information to his wife.

> Skilled communication allows these relationships to thrive and deepen.

Prior to giving bad news, it is important to determine the extent of the patient's prior knowledge on the subject. The patient's perception of his or her illness provides scaffolding

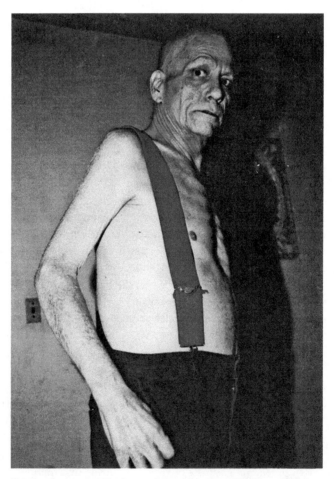

FIGURE 7.1 "We have been cast aside, disregarded and forgotten about," a mournful Mr. Wheeler declares.

upon which the physician may add new information and clarify misunderstandings. One recommended technique for providers to glean the patient's perspective is "ask–tell–ask."[6] Using this technique, healthcare providers ask patients what other providers have told them regarding their disease, give information building on what the patient knows, and then ask the patient about their questions or concerns to confirm understanding.[7] Unfortunately, this did not occur during Mr. Wheeler's multiple physician encounters, leading him to believe that the medical team was withholding information from him: "I think there is something wrong with my stomach these doctors won't tell me." Directly asking Mr. Wheeler about his concerns might have resolved this problem (Figure 7.1).

After eliciting the patient's understanding, it is helpful to negotiate the content of medical information to be discussed. Patients have varying preferences regarding the specificity of information given and its method of delivery. Asking patients if they are detail- versus big picture-oriented allows the physician to tailor his or her communication strategy to the patient. Mr. Wheeler has a clear preference: "I told him not to hee-haw around it" and voices frustration when he is told medical information in vague terms: "Next time I see him I am going to ask him point-blank how long I have."

After negotiating the method of delivery and content of information to be delivered, the physician should provide information simply and without jargon. Words such as *malignancy* and *metastasis* can confuse patients.[5] Also, providers should be prepared to repeat or reframe information to solidify patients' understanding. Unfortunately, Mrs. Wheeler's hematologist presents her diagnosis using medical jargon—"I think we do not have absolute proof right now that the type of lymphoma we are dealing with is one of those slow-rolling, indolent lymphomas," which limits the information she can take away from the discussion. Mr. Wheeler's physician gives him the mistaken impression that his cancer is in remission by saying, "It looks like the medicine is doing what we want," when, in fact, the effect of chemotherapy was a non-clinically significant decrease in the size of cervical lymph nodes.

The transfer of medical knowledge from provider to patient is complicated in the urban poor population by patients' low health literacy and lack of resources.[8,9]

Healthcare literacy refers to an understanding of written or spoken medical information, and those with less education or lower income status are more likely to have poor health literacy than their counterparts.[10] In general, African Americans have a lower rate of health literacy than white patients do, which may account for some of the racial disparity in health outcomes.[11] Low health literacy is associated with decreased understanding of illness, increased incidence of chronic illness, poorer intermediate disease markers, and less-than-optimal use of preventive health services.[12] An inability to understand medical information leads to an impaired ability to negotiate the healthcare environment and thus to substandard medical care and poorer health outcomes.

> The negative impact of poor communication is magnified due to inadequate resources, low literacy, and mistrust of the medical system.

Limited resources for independent research into medical conditions also restrict patients' ability to negotiate the healthcare environment. Patients often use the internet to seek information on disease management, connect with others who suffer from a similar condition, and communicate with their physician. Multiple studies have investigated the rate of internet use for health among Americans and its relationship to demographic variables. A 2004 study published in the *Journal of the American Medical Association* reported that approximately 20% of the US population used the internet for healthcare in 2001. Patients with higher education levels were more likely to use the internet.[13] Although the impact of internet use on clinical outcomes is unclear, patients who engage in online searches for medical information report that the information helped them understand their condition, gave them confidence to talk to a physician about concerns, improved their decision-making ability, allowed them to take better care of their health, and improved communication with their physician.[14] Patients who are unfamiliar with or without access to technology are at a disadvantage in the healthcare system. Given the lack of other resources, these patients are highly dependent on their interactions with their physicians (Figure 7.2).

The next step in breaking bad news is addressing the emotion that conveying bad news engenders in patients. This action normalizes the patient's feelings, develops trust between the physician and patient, allows the patient to feel accepted, and increases the likelihood of the patient's expressing further concerns. Mrs. Wheeler's expression of worry about the impact of her diagnosis of lymphoma and proposed treatment plan— "I can't stand pain" is an empathic opportunity for her hematologist to further explore her concerns. Physician responses such as, "Tell me more," or "What else worries you about this diagnosis?" would be helpful in exploring and alleviating her anxiety. The intern providing Mrs. Wheeler's primary care attends to her emotion by normalizing her feelings: "It's okay, you can cry. Don't be embarrassed. . . ." On the other hand, Mr. Wheeler did not feel that his doctor understood what he was experiencing: "She was just

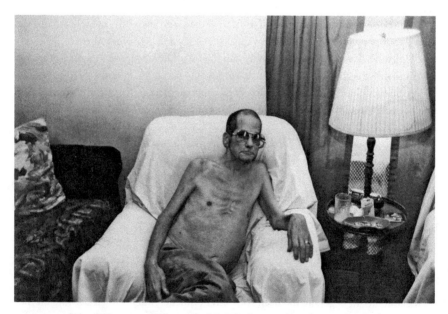

FIGURE 7.2 "They lied to me again," an angry Mr. Wheeler complained.

rude. Everything she said, there was something rude about it . . . hateful . . . when you get treated that way you want to get out of here." Emotional handling of patients in vulnerable populations is crucial because these patients often mistrust physicians and the healthcare system at large. Trust occurs when one party is vulnerable to another[15] and is based on the expectation that the physician will work in the patient's best interest.[16] Trust in physicians relies on the domains of competence, honesty, confidentiality and loyalty or caring.[17] A longitudinal survey of 246 breast cancer patients in 1998 found that in the six months following diagnosis, informational and decision-making support contributed to patient trust early in a disease course, while emotional support helped maintain trust later in the disease process.[18]

Before closing a bad-news discussion, physicians should check for understanding to avoid patient misinterpretation. For example, a physician may instruct the patient, "Tell me what you are taking away from this discussion" or ask "What will you tell your spouse about this discussion?" Regrettably, this does not occur during the conversation in which Mrs. Wheeler discovers she has lymphoma. When Mrs. Wheeler's hematologist pauses to note the large amount of information relayed, Mrs. Wheeler states, "I'm understanding." However, she is not asked to repeat back the facts of the conversation. Subsequently, she is unable to later explain her diagnosis other than "cancer," unable to clarify the meaning of indolent, and unable to explain why surgery wasn't an option for her.

PROVIDING PROGNOSTIC INFORMATION

Providing prognostic information is a form of giving bad news; thus, similar guidelines apply for how to discuss prognostic information. For example, a physician has to determine what and how much information the patient wants about her prognosis. To do this, a physician might inquire, "What kind of information do you want about the future?" or, "There are a couple of ways I can answer your question, so tell me which would be best for you. One way I can answer is to give you some statistics—the average time a person with this cancer at this stage lives. Or, I can talk about the worst-case scenario and the best-case scenario. Or sometimes people are thinking about a specific event in the future, like they are hoping to live until their anniversary. Which one of these would be the most helpful?"[19]

When giving information, it may be helpful for physicians to convey the inherent lack of specificity in prognostications.[19] Physicians may communicate uncertainty in prognostication with statements such as: "I can tell you about how long someone with your type of cancer lives. But some people live longer than I think, and others live shorter than I expect. I can't tell you exactly what will happen to you."

Despite the uncertainty, clinicians should be as honest as possible. The data suggest that physicians typically overestimate how long they expect a patient to live when talking to patients (compared to what they actually believe is the prognosis). This is a form of avoidance and does not allow the patient to accurately plan for his or her future.

Finally, while it is unclear whether it is better to use quantitative or qualitative prognostic information, typically, ranges are given—hours to days, days to weeks, weeks to months—rather than a specific number of weeks or months.[3]

Although not asked his preference regarding how much prognostic information he would like to be given by his physician, Mr. Wheeler states, "Next time I see him I am going to ask him point-blank how long I have." In response, his physician states, "We never expected you to live this long, and for patients with your type of tumor who live as long as you have, the average survival is two to five years." This seems optimistic, and frankly is ultimately misleading, given that the doctor subsequently referred Mr. Wheeler to hospice care, which requires the physician to certify a prognosis of six months or less for enrollment. This discrepancy contributed to Mr. Wheeler's feeling that they were not being forthright with him adding to his sense of mistrust and disempowerment.

As commonly occurs in practice, Mr. Wheeler is referred to hospice late in his disease course. The median length of stay for a patient enrolled in hospice is 26 days, with many referrals ordered in the last hours of life.[20] Late enrollment to hospice decreases the length of time that patients and caregivers may benefit from nursing, social work, or clergy support. This is especially relevant in patient populations without financial and social support, where hospice may serve as a safety net by delivering medications, providing durable medical equipment to ease the burden of caregiving, providing respite care for exhausted family members, and providing emotional and pastoral support for both patients and families. Mr. Wheeler was only enrolled in hospice for a few weeks.

> Emotional handling of patients in vulnerable populations is crucial because these patients often mistrust physicians and the healthcare system at large.

Physicians often express reluctance to deliver poor prognoses or bad news due to concerns that doing so may diminish a patient's hope. However, "many patients do not measure hope solely in terms of cure, but hope may represent achieving goals, having family and oncologist support, and receiving the best treatment available."[21] Effective communication correlates with improved patient adjustment to illness and decreased anxiety and depression.[22,23] In Mr. Wheeler's case, news regarding the effect of chemotherapy on his cancer caused him to believe "the medicines were working" and that he was on his way to "remission and a cure" when, in fact, no cure was possible given that, at diagnosis, as his oncologist had noted, "I'm afraid we got him too late in his disease process to be of any help to him." Once this discrepancy became apparent to Mr. Wheeler, he reacted furiously: "They should have told me the whole truth in the first place." Avoiding giving bad news, or offering premature reassurance, may decrease patient trust in the physician. Thus, despite physician concern that delivering bad news may diminish patients' hope, the opposite may be true. Good communication and demonstration of empathy may decrease patients' psychological morbidity and increase trust in the doctor–patient relationship.

PRESENCE

While the preceding communication skills are important, "being present" is also helpful. *Presence*, also referred to as *mindfulness* or *bearing witness*, describes being focused on the moment and listening without focusing on "fixing." It requires authenticity: "being before doing."[2] Presence includes the use of compassionate silence, which has a "moment-by-moment character that patients can experience as a profound kind of being with, standing with, and contact in a difficult moment."[24] Presence may also refer to the sense of security physicians develop for patients and families. Activities such as regular contact, anticipation of problems and rehearsing responses, and offering encouragement and hopefulness, as well as traits of consistency, dependability, and availability coalesce in creating this environment.[25] Imagine the impact of a doctor being willing to walk with Mr. Wheeler through his ordeal, someone willing to bear witness and act as a trusted advisor. Would the presence of a physician willing to listen to Mr. Wheeler's whole story, appreciate his perspective, and offer empathy have allowed him to feel heard? It is impossible to know, but one can appreciate a missed opportunity for Mr. Wheeler and a powerful tool for physicians in future encounters.

IMPROVING COMMUNICATION IN CRITICAL ILLNESS

As physicians consider interventions to improve communication between providers and urban poor patients, we must consider changes on both societal and individual levels. For example, interventions aimed at providing educational resources for underserved populations might include outreach efforts or technology training in local settings such as churches and libraries. Visual aids such as videotapes or illustrated brochures rather than printed text may improve patient understanding and knowledge among those with low health literacy.[12] Efforts to increase trust in the medical system may focus on engaging community members, as "trust is generated and maintained through repeated interactions in a long-term relationship"[16] in community affiliations.

On an individual level, physicians need both skilled communication abilities and an open-minded attitude in order to excel in caring for the dying urban poor. Although medical education has historically focused on teaching knowledge and skills, the educational framework has recently expanded to include attitudes. Leaders in medical education have begun to recognize effective communication as a method of demonstrating cultural competence by showing empathy, exploring socioeconomic issues, and addressing bias.[26] In 2007, the Accreditation Council for Graduate Medical Education (ACGME) approved common requirements for residency training programs based on a competency structure. Currently, communication skills and professionalism are two of the six core competencies in which trainees are required to demonstrate proficiency prior to graduation. Proficiency in communication, defined by the ACGME as "effective information exchange and teaming with patients," and in professionalism, defined as a "commitment to carrying out professional responsibilities, adherence to ethical principles and sensitivity to a diverse patient population"[27] are instrumental in caring for vulnerable populations (Figure 7.3).

Effective teaching of communication skills requires a practice-based approach. Intensive experiential communication training that exposes learners to didactic material on specific interviewing skills and allows them to interview standardized patients with observation by trained facilitators allows physicians-in-training to hone communication skills prior to entering independent practice.[28,29] Adding these sessions as a required part of clinical training adds weight to the importance of skillful doctor–patient

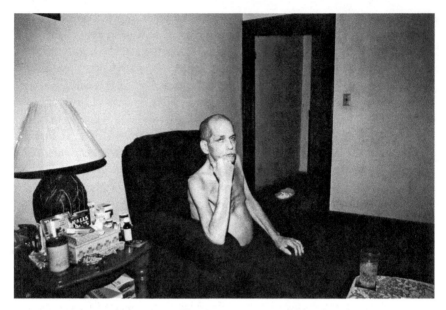

FIGURE 7.3 Despair and anger remained his constant companions throughout dying.

communication. This focus on teaching and evaluating specific communication skills during training will continue to improve physician–patient communication.

Changing physician attitudes requires a gradual approach throughout undergraduate and graduate medical education. Tenets of professionalism, including mindfulness, empathy, and self-reflection, are teachable skills. Self- and peer-evaluations used as adjuncts to traditional evaluation of medical trainees may help develop mindfulness and recognition of the impact of one's actions on others.[30] Curricular interventions such as structured reflection or the narrative-medicine technique of parallel charting, wherein trainees describe their emotional reaction to caring for ill and dying patients, may help trainees develop empathy and capacity for reflection.[31,32] Additionally, students and residents look to educators as role models who set a standard for professional behavior, so continued faculty development in this area is crucial.

The narrative "Life on the Brink: Mr. and Mrs. Wheeler" starkly portrays the negative impact of poor communication between the healthcare system and the urban poor. Through the examples of Mr. and Mrs. Wheeler's interactions with physicians and medical staff, one can appreciate multiple missed opportunities for dialogue and understanding. These interactions demonstrate how effective communication, awareness of the power of physician presence, improved cultural competence, and patient-centeredness may improve the care of vulnerable populations at both the system and individual level.

REFERENCES

1. Naomi Remen R. *My grandfather's blessings: stories of strength, refuge, and belonging.* New York: Riverhead Trade; 2000.

2. Risdon C, Edey L. Human doctoring: bringing authenticity to our care. *Acad Med.* 1999;74:896–899.

3. Girgis A, Sanson-Fisher RW. Breaking bad news: consensus guidelines for medical practitioners. *J Clin One.* 1995;13:2449–2456.

4. Lee SJ, Back AL, Block SD, Stewart SK. Enhancing physician-patient communication. *Hematol Am Soc Hematol Educ Prog.* 2002;464–83.

5. Baile WF, Buckman R, Lenzi R, et al. SPIKES—A six-step protocol for delivering bad news: application to the patient with cancer. *Oncologist.* 2000;5:302–311.

6. Back AL, Arnold RM, Tulsky J. *Mastering communication with seriously ill patients. balancing honesty with empathy and hope.* New York: Cambridge University Press; 2009.

7. Evans WG, Tulsky JA, Back AL, et al. Communication at times of transitions: how to help patients cope with loss and redefine hope. *Cancer J.* 2006;12:417–424.

8. Lo S, Sharif I, Ozuah PO. Health literacy among English-speaking parents in a poor urban setting. *J Health Care Poor Underserved.* 2006;17:504–511.

9. Fiscella K, Williams DR. Health disparities based on socioeconomic inequities: implications for urban health care. *Acad Med.* 2004;79:1139–1147.

10. Gazmararian JA, Baker DW, Williams MV, et al. Health literacy among Medicare enrollees in a managed care organization. *JAMA.* 1999;281:545–551.

11. Bennett CL, Ferreira MR, Davis TC, et al. Relation between literacy, race, and stage of presentation among low income patients with prostate cancer. *J Clin Oncol.* 1998;16:3101–3104.

12. Berkman ND, DeWalt DA, Pignone MP, et al. *Literacy and health outcomes. Evidence Report/Technology Assessment No. 87 (Prepared by RTI International-University of North Carolina Evidence-based Practice Center under Contract No. 290-02-0016).* AHRQ (Agency for Healthcare Research and Quality) Publication No. 04 E007-2. Rockville, MD.

13. Baker L, Wagner TH, Singer S, Bundorf MK. Use of the internet and e-mail for health care information: results from a national survey. *JAMA.* 2003;289:2400–2406.

14. Murray E, Lo B, Pollack L, et al. The impact of health information on the internet on the physician–patient relationship: patient perceptions. *Arch Intern Med.* 2003;163:1727–1734.

15. Goold SD. Trust, distrust and trustworthiness. *J Gen Intern Med.* 2002;17:79–81.

16. Corbie-Smith G, Thomas S, St. George DM. Distrust, race and research. *Arch Intern Med.* 2002;162:2458–2463.

17. Hall MA. Researching medical trust in the United State. *J Health Org Manag.* 2006;20:456–467.

18. Arora NK, Gustafson DH. Perceived helpfulness of physicians' communication behavior and breast cancer patients' level of trust over time. *J Gen Intern Med.* 2008;24:252–255.

19. Back AL, Arnold RM. Discussing prognosis: "How much do you want to know?" Talking to patients who are prepared for explicit information. *J Clin One.* 2006;24:4209–4213.

20. Quill TE. Is length of stay on hospice a critical quality of care indicator? *J Palliat Med.* 2007;10:290–292.

21. Sardell AN, Trierweiler SJ. Disclosing the cancer diagnosis. Procedures that influence patient hopefulness. *Cancer.* 1993;72:3355–3365.

22. Roberts CS, Cox CE, Reintgen DS, Baile WF, Gibertini M. Influence of physician communication on newly diagnosed breast cancer patients' psychological adjustment and decision making. *Cancer.* 1994;74:336–341.

23. Fallowfield L, Hall A, Maguire GP, Baum M. Psychological outcomes of different treatment policies in women with early breast cancer outside a clinical trial. *BMJ.* 1990;301:575–580.

24. Back AL, Bauer-Wu SM, Rushton CH, Halifax J. Compassionate silence in the patient–clinician encounter: a contemplative approach. *J Palliat Med.* 2009;12:1113–1117.

25. Billings JA. Feeling secure. In *Outpatient management of advanced cancer.* Philadelphia, PA: Lippincott; 1985. Chapter 5.

26. Betancourt JR, Green AR, Carrillo JE, Park ER. Cultural competence and health care disparities: key perspectives and trends. *Health Aff.* 2005;24:499–505.

27. Accreditation Council on Graduate Medical Education. Outcome Project. 2001. At www.acgme.org/outcome/comp/compMin.asp (January 28, 2011).

28. Back AL, Arnold RM, Tulsky JA, et al. Teaching communication skills to medical oncology fellows. *J Clin Oncol.* 2003;21:2433–2436.

29. Wagner PJ, Lentz L, Heslop SD. Teaching communication skills: a skills-based approach. *Acad Med.* 2002;77:1164.

30. Epstein RM. Mindful practice. *JAMA.* 1999;282:833–839.

31. Charon R. Changing the face of medicine. At https://cfmedicine.nlm.nih.gov/physicians/biography_58.htm (accessed Jan. 28, 2011).

32. Charon R. Narrative medicine: a model for empathy, reflection, profession and trust. *JAMA.* 2001;286:1897–1902.

8

THE LIFE AND DEATH OF LUCILLE ANGEL FROM PRIMARY CARE, CHAPLAINCY, AND PALLIATIVE CARE PERSPECTIVES

Rachel Diamond, Rev. Robin Franklin, and Timothy Quill

Snapshot Reflection: A Story of Rising from the Ashes of Poverty

Lucille Angel died at the age of 63. The last 48 hours of her life were extraordinarily beautiful. The preceding year was full of illness, uncertainty, loneliness, spiritual confusion, and estrangement from her church.

Church played an important role in Mrs. Angel's life. In the years before getting so sick she served as church secretary while her husband was a deacon. Her faith in God was a guiding light, enabling her to endure many of the tribulations she faced living in rural and urban poverty. But faith is not an easy thing in such circumstances, and it especially was put to the test in the time after her beloved husband died and when she received a diagnosis of terminal lung cancer. In her grief, she began to feel anger toward God, and she struggled to maintain her faith. In her confusion, she drifted away from her church involvement, but she never abandoned her belief that God was with her and would see her through this difficult time. Although she hoped for visits from her pastor and members of the congregation, none materialized. The result was that this deeply faithful woman grieved the death of her second husband and confronted the ending of her own life in isolation from her church and spiritual community.

On the other hand, her daughters, despite being troubled by their own hardships of living in poverty, rearranged their lives to be with her during the last weeks of life. Their caretaking was stunning. They created a 24-hour vigil around her bedside, providing tender physical care as well as spiritual support. In knowing that their dearly-loved mother felt the sting of her pastor's abandonment, they arranged for him to visit the day before her death. They welcomed him joyously and graciously into the home, not judging him for his prolonged absence. Despite the fact that he stayed for only a few minutes and appeared uncomfortable, his visit was meaningful to the Angel family, and they were thankful.

Mrs. Angel directly confronted the matters of her funeral and burial before her death. Like many urban poor, she wanted "to be put away well." But she had two major concerns. First, her family refused to engage in any conversation about funeral arrangements. They were emotionally unprepared to accept her death, and, in their fear and discomfort, they stridently avoided the topic. The second concern revolved around the lack of empathy displayed by the funeral director at the time of her husband's death. Mrs. Angel had unfortunate memories of waiting an excessively long time for the funeral-home attendants to arrive. And once there, she felt that they had displayed little compassion and hurried to remove the body. She wanted to make sure her daughters did not encounter the same problems.

Thus, in her remarkable strength, Mrs. Angel prearranged and prepaid her funeral so when the time of her death arrived, her daughters would be spared the burden of making funeral and burial arrangements. When the time of her death did come, her daughters were grateful. They spoke about how "peaceful" Mrs. Angel looked at her well-attended funeral, commenting that "Mama looks so beautiful" and "Her hair is starting to come back."

Despite their successful orchestration of continuous care at the bedside and good memories of the funeral, Mrs. Angel's death hit her daughters quite hard. The lack of supportive rituals and open conversation before and after her death left them each struggling emotionally to reconcile themselves to the death of their mother. The fact that they could not afford the price of a headstone for her grave exacerbated their struggle and even generated some feelings of guilt.

Mrs. Angel's experience is a story of confusion, neglect, isolation, and abiding love. It provides a glimpse of the harshness of living in rural and urban poverty. It reveals the devastating impact of domestic violence on the soul of a person, and the immorality of indifference toward its occurrence. Yet it declares a remarkable spirit that is found within her and her beloved family. Her story, as she neared the end of life, provides a glimpse of what is essential for a peaceful and meaningful death. It demonstrates how huge the need for spiritual care is and how difficult that sometimes is to achieve. It declares the utter importance of mindful presence and supportive presence. It shows the importance of the funeral as a therapeutic ritual and illustrates the healing power of love throughout dying into death.

A Special Observation

Out of the ashes of poverty-driven chaos and suffering, the spiritual strength of Mrs. Angel and the unshakable love for her daughters prevailed.

Take-Home Lesson

In this narrative, we witness many of the decisions that play out in illness and death. Mrs. Angel questioned *why* this was all happening. She never understood why the husband she adored lay dead in the cemetery while the "hoodlums" roamed free in front of her house day and night. She didn't understand why she was dying at such a relatively young age. In response, she became angry at God and wondered if she was being punished for some reason. She then felt ashamed and would berate herself for becoming angry at the Holy One she loved and trusted so much. She shrieked in horror when her hair fell out, becoming disappointed in herself for such vanity. She was angry at her doctors, who she felt communicated poorly about her treatment and what she could expect. She then sought to understand and forgive, recognizing that "they are only human" and doing the best they can. Her body was utterly cannibalized by disease. But her faith in God ultimately withstood the test of her sufferings, and her daughters' love and caregiving never wavered.

—David Wendell Moller

We will be dividing this chapter into three parts, each of which will view Mrs. Angel's life and death from a separate lens. The first part will view her story from the perspective of a primary care physician who might be involved in all medical aspects of her life from birth to death. The second part will explore the religious and spiritual dimensions of her life from the perspective of a hospital chaplain. The third part will view Mrs. Angel's life from a palliative care perspective, with a particular focus on the times where she faced serious illness. Although there will be overlap, we hope to illustrate some of the potential and limitations on each of these approaches when the patient's medical problems are complicated by significant poverty. Each section will further divide her life into three phases: (1) her early life when she was a young mother mired in an abusive marriage; (2) her middle life, when socially, although not economically, her life had improved but she faced increasingly complex medical problems; and (3) the very end of her life.

PRIMARY CARE PERSPECTIVE

During Lucille's early life, she experienced significant betrayal and disappointment from those she expected the most from, including her own physicians. The victim of brutal physical abuse at the hands of her first husband, she had the courage, in a time when a woman's silence was admired, to report this abuse to her family doctor. The risk she took in naming this kind of violence was significant, but in response to her candidness and bravery, her physician remained silent and apathetic. Lucille spoke of her understanding and expectations of the doctor–patient relationship at this time—which unfortunately focused on pathology and treatment rather than relationships and mutuality. Despite this abandonment, she didn't seem to voice much anger towards the situation or her doctor. Rather, her response was more of a sardonically defeatist acceptance. In this regard she, too, was a product of her time, when the biopsychosocial model for conceptualizing medicine had yet to be developed[1] and patriarchal medicine was the norm. In Mrs. Angel's case, much of the power dynamic between her and her family doctor was established even before any interaction took place—disparate knowledge bases and socioeconomic statuses made her vulnerable, and, while gender and race weren't explicitly mentioned, one might venture a guess that neither might have been the same as her own. Mrs. Angel's acceptance of her suffering during this time was an adaptive mechanism, not having any other real choice in the matter. Modern-day physicians are charged with looking at a patient holistically to help them not just accept suffering, but transcend it if possible. This may be done by trying to address whatever threat the patient perceives to their integrity or by listening to and validating the feelings of suffering, and jointly searching for creative solutions.[2]

Another factor working against Mrs. Angel was that the role of the physician in addressing domestic violence was not so established as it is today. It wasn't until the late

1970s that the US Surgeon General recognized violence as a priority for focusing preventative medical measures[3] and in the 1990s that domestic violence was more specifically
given a spotlight when Congress passed the Violence Against Women Act.[4]

Despite her tribulations, Mrs. Angel did what so many of us do in difficult situations—
she looked for elements in her life she could control or have some influence. For her, this
was taking care of her children and keeping up with routines such as going to church.
Ultimately her husband left her and her children, freeing them from the cycle of abuse.
As a female physician, I find this inner strength Mrs. Angel displayed both inspiring and
tragic. She found a way to remain functional in other roles in her life and didn't let her
husband strip her of her identity entirely. On the other hand, she had nobody to help her
realize her potential for happiness or self-worth. There is a maddening silence during this
period devoid of family, friends, religious leaders, or entrusted physicians, all of whom
could have had a significant impact on her quality of life at the time.

> She experienced significant betrayal and disappointment from those she ex-
> pected the most from, including her own physicians.

In the second phase of Mrs. Angel's life, she experienced tragic losses and vulnerability once again, with the death of her second husband occurring around the time of
her stroke and cancer diagnosis. Her primary care physician presented her with some
choices about how to approach her malignancy: she could have surgery or start chemotherapy, with the third option going unspoken; specifically, opting for no treatment
and dying sooner. We often see patients being given "choices" that we tend to think of as
positive. In many circumstances, however, it is just choosing among the "least terrible"
options, which may seem like no real choice at all. In addition, with medical science and
technology being as advanced as they are, navigating complex choices as a patient can be
foreign and overwhelming without the guidance of a physician. Mrs. Angel responded to
the question of therapy choices in a way that may very well have been frustrating for her
medical team but probably was the only way she could manage, which was doing nothing
at all. Perhaps to protect herself and her family, Mrs. Angel avoided disclosing her diagnosis to her family or talking to a specialist. She did this out of love as she did not want
to burden her husband during his time of being seriously ill with the worry about her
having received a cancer diagnosis. In addition, one might imagine that her capacity for
experiencing or confronting loss was exceeded, and she could only mourn one thing at
a time because the grief and anger about the loss of her husband was all-consuming. She
was dealing with him and did not have the personal resources to address the severity of
her own situation, a situation that was probably also fueled by denial and anger that such
unthinkably bad things were continually happening to her.

One might wonder how much Mrs. Angel's primary care physician pushed for her
to come in for an appointment, or to see a subspecialist. One would hope that she wasn't
casually lost to appropriate follow-up planning and that there were discussions about
the potential consequences of delaying therapy. It is also possible that this physician may
have had only generalized knowledge about Lucille's medical condition and had been un-
equipped to deal with the complexity of her illness. It is also conceivable that the primary care physician was so overloaded with the demands of seeing so many patients that

adequate time could not be devoted to sifting through the complex medical, social, and emotional issues that were challenging Lucille. Devoting the amount of time Mrs. Angel may have needed to work through her inner conflicts about treatment may have been impossible. Her physician's lack of expertise in such matters may have precluded the necessary information from being conveyed and a recommendation from being delivered. This brings up the struggle of responsibilities and boundaries that many primary care physicians face: When is it our professional duty to make recommendations, versus referring to a specialist to do so? How hard should we hound a patient for follow-up, and when should we take a step back and allow competent adults to make their own decisions, even if they might be detrimental to their health? It is important for physicians to know their own professional limits and when to rely on alternative resources to provide patients with the best care possible. In addition, they must be able to separate themselves to a degree from their own biases and identify the difference between a "bad" choice and a choice that they wouldn't make for themselves.

Ultimately Mrs. Angel found her way back to her primary care physician (PCP) and opted out of surgery (in fact, she had waited so long that surgery was no longer an option). Her PCP responded to her decision with compassion, letting her know there were still options to prolong her life and reason to maintain hope. What a strong juxtaposition to her former family doctor, who turned a blind eye to her struggles with domestic violence, leaving her no options but abandonment and hopelessness.

When her cancer later proved unresponsive to chemotherapy, Mrs. Angel once again felt anger and betrayal. Even though it was now her own damaged biology that was betraying her, she blamed her oncologist. She questioned treatment mistakes and lamented unrealistic expectations she felt her oncologist had set for her. Once again she mourned loss and had to adjust her hopes and understanding of her own new reality. One way she sought to cope with all the change and loss was by maintaining some semblance of control and predictability in her everyday life. Mrs. Angel made her own funeral arrangements and, in subtler ways, maintained a sense of mundane normalcy by watching her favorite TV show, *Jerry Springer*, every day.

How do we see other patients maintain some control as disease ravages their bodies? Some do so in ways directly related to their survival: researching clinical trials, seeking second opinions, and/or pursuing any and all possibly effective (and often futile) life-prolonging therapies. Some maintain control by making their last wishes known through legal documents such as a living will or Medical Orders for Life Sustaining Treatment (MOLST), or by enrolling in hospice care. Some go to such lengths as to hasten their death with physician-assisted suicide or by voluntarily stopping eating and drinking. Mrs. Angel probably had limited access to hospice and palliative care services in her urban poor community where utilization rates are usually low. Studies have shown lower rates of hospice use for minority older adults than for whites across diagnoses, geographic areas, and settings of care. On the other side of the coin, a greater preference for life-sustaining therapies regardless of prognosis has been observed among African Americans and Hispanics compared to whites.[5] Mrs. Angel certainly exhibited her desire to prolong her life with chemotherapy, and a real sense of anger and betrayal with her oncologist when this goal proved unachievable. Regardless, she eventually ended up being enrolled in hospice near the end of her life. It would have been very interesting to have a better understanding of how she came to this decision, and with whom she had these delicate conversations about goals of care.

CHAPLAINCY PERSPECTIVE

From my perspective as a hospital chaplain, Mrs. Angel had an inordinate amount of pain in her life. Her life was unfair. God did put more on her than she could or should have had to bear, though I do not believe that God "puts" anything on us to create suffering. Yet, as I read her story, I am confronted with a view counter to my own. From the age of 18, when she entered into an abusive marriage of 20 years, until her death at 62, she maintained her faith and belief in a God who was right by her side regardless of her circumstances. And there was a lot that was 'put' upon her, enough to test the faith of most. Though there were instances when she asked "why" or "what more could happen," she hung on to her faith. It was the source of her life and strength. My guess is her life of faith developed in the love and socialization of what she described as a poor but loving family of origin.

It is important for the reader to know my frame of reference. I am looking at this story through the eyes of a 21st-century African-American woman who is an ordained Christian minister raised in New York City. I am also a hospital chaplain where my own faith is not important or essential to my job. In the role of chaplain, I must serve people from diverse faith backgrounds consistent with their chosen beliefs and practices rather than focusing on my own. I think that it is important to know the backdrop to my faith because it is different from Mrs. Angel's and therefore I am commenting on her life from my frame of reference. It is essential for readers to know that my response is influenced by my own experiences (Figure 8.1).

In the first phase of her story, we are introduced to an 18-year-old woman who has left her parents' home for the first time to start a family of her own. The history does not

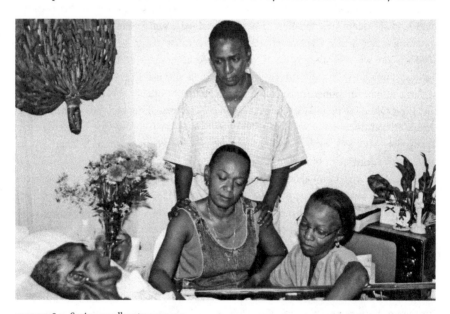

FIGURE 8.1 Saying goodbye to momma.

indicate when the physical abuse started, but it does note that the abuse was severe. Mrs. Angel attended church on a regular basis, and at some point, the abuse got so bad that she approached her pastor for advice, support, and/or consolation. The advice that she received was not to "antagonize her husband," as if simply trying to keep the peace would keep his fists or other chosen weapons at bay. Instead of the support and helpful guidance she could have used, she received advice that made her responsible for her own abuse, and which set her up for more victimization at the hands of her husband.

I will admit that I am surprised by the typical justifications for women to stay in abusive relationships. These often have both societal and religious origins. These reasons, which especially prevailed during the time in which she suffered the abuse, include affirming the sanctity of marriage, declaring that "divorce is bad" or that "the man is head of the household and it is the wife's place to submit." Was it Mrs. Angel's faith that caused her to stay? Was it secular social pressures? Or both? She freely admitted that she did not have a lot of choices, with mouths to feed and the need to keep a roof over their heads.

I could easily excoriate the pastor for his response during her time of crisis, but I also wonder if her faith helped provide some peace of mind in the midst of pain (spiritual, emotional, and physical) and ultimately abandonment when her abuser-husband left. My wish is that the pastor could have been a support to her in the midst of any decision to stay or leave. My wish is that there were people in the congregation who could have been there for her, though it is mentioned that Mike, her second husband, who was a deacon at the church, kept encouraging her to leave. Faith is not straightforward, as is demonstrated throughout Mrs. Angel's story. This woman's experience was characterized by significant ambivalence, anger, pain, and grief, along with a love for God. I admire her fortitude and ability to integrate disparate parts into a functioning and whole person.

As I read the next part of her story, I am reminded of the words from the last sentence in Psalm 30:5 in Hebrew scripture. This is not a direct quote from any of the versions of the Bible, but basically it says that *weeping may endure for a night but joy comes in the morning*. Her story indicates that she read the Bible, and her daughters continued to read it to her once she became unresponsive near the end of her life. Mrs. Angel read her Bible probably as a means of inspiration, habit, and solace. Though no reference is made to any particular part(s) of the Bible that were important to her, Psalm 30:5 was invoked in me as I read about her death. The Psalm acknowledges that suffering may occur throughout the night but reassures that the darkness of night will be relieved by the joys and light of the morning. So, out of the depths of despair, there will emerge cause for celebration. This was certainly true for Mrs. Angel. She endured suffering and loss throughout her life, and was weighed down by the burdens of poverty. She suffered the premature death of her beloved husband and lamented the drugs and violence that crept into her neighborhood. She ultimately endured significant deterioration of her health at a relatively young age. That said, she never despaired. She trusted in God and reveled in the love of her family and, for this reason, the night side of her life gave way ultimately to the light.

There is no way to understand how all of the hardships landed in this woman's lap. It was as if she lived under a perpetual dark cloud with small respites from incumbent stormy weather. The story of Job comes to mind. For readers who are not familiar with the story, it is a book in the Old Testament that relates the story of a man who is prosperous. He is not only prosperous, but attributes his wealth and good fortune to his faith in God. Job, through no misdeed of his own, progressively loses everything—his health, his family, and his wealth—but never his faith in God. Job speaks of his distress to his friends, who listen for a while; but soon they begin to be his accusers. They conclude that there was something Job must have done to invite the devastation into his life. Job faced unimaginable sufferings without wavering in his faith. While Mrs. Angel's faith was tested and shaken at times, she remained steadfast in her relationship with God.

Mrs. Angel never compares herself to Job, though later she does ask the *why is this happening to me* question. Her story does not indicate that she asked this as she cared for her husband, who began to deteriorate before her eyes and whom she watched writhe in pain because he refused to take the morphine that might have given him some relief. One of the saddest parts of this narrative is that the church community disappeared from sight as Mike got progressively sicker. It became harder for them to attend church, and eventually their church attendance fell off altogether. There were no visits from the pastor or from church members. There were no offers of respite help, bringing over meals, a listening ear, or a sympathetic shoulder. I suppose that, again, I need to be mindful of my judgments. I was not there. However, it is very difficult not to wonder why help did not come. The Christian tradition and other spiritual/religious traditions speak of visiting the sick and helping others. Furthermore, I am very used to activities such as visiting the sick and the simple offering of things like meals being a part of the African-American tradition. Mrs. Angel's story is proof that blanket statements about a group of people can be misleading. Each story has its own particular nuances.

As the second phase of her life comes to its conclusion, she is left to bear the burden of the death of her husband who brought her so much joy. As she enters into the last phase of her life, I would not say that she was over the experience of the death of her husband, but she found within herself enough energy to follow through with her desire to make a big Thanksgiving meal. She did so out of love for her family and an appreciation of the goodness of life. While going to the store to purchase what she needed for the meal, however, she had a stroke. The stroke left her with deficits on her right side and in lots of pain. It was also discovered that she was having trouble breathing upon her admission to the hospital. Her doctors performed follow-up tests and they also the presence of a spot on her lung, which may or may not have been related to her throat cancer.

In response to her stroke, Mrs. Angel asked, "Lord what else can happen to me?" In response to the spread of her cancer she was devastated, overwhelmed, and disbelieving. "How long, O Lord? How long?" I do not know the exact origin of this phrase, but I have heard it from the mouths of a number of African-American preachers and congregants in trying to make sense of situations similar to Mrs. Angel's. In the midst of all that was happening, however, there seemed to be a bright spot. Her doctor offered hope, assuring Mrs. Angel that it was not time to "give up" yet.

This phase is the longest part of Mrs. Angel's story. Dr. Moller's account in *Dancing with Broken Bones* takes us through her chemotherapy treatments and her desire to do them in the hospital because of the camaraderie she experienced with the staff. She liked them. He noted that she developed relationships with other cancer patients in the hospital and during doctor visits. Others told her that they were praying for her, and she prayed for them. Being concerned about the welfare of others was a quality that was pervasive in this snapshot of her life. She thought of and took care of others even in the midst of her own troubles. She did not address her own health in the midst of taking care of Mike because she did not want to burden him. She didn't even let her children know about her cancer diagnosis because she believed that they would tell Mike. Self-sacrifice can be a quality of those whose faith is strong. John 15:13 comes to mind and says that laying down your life for a friend is the greatest expression of love.

One thing that surprised me as I read her story was her ability to be angry with God. The Bible justifies righteous anger. This is anger that flares in relation to the mistreatment of others. This is anger at injustice. This is anger mostly on the behalf of another person. But anger at God? I do not want to make the blanket statement that anger at God is unheard of in the Christian church. There are ministers who understand this idea and make room for the expression of such feelings. However, I have also seen the other side in the church, and as I meet patients in the hospital. I have heard patients choke down their anger because they have been taught it is wrong or the idea does not fit with a loving and accepting God. Mrs. Angel was being open and honest in sharing this part of herself and despite her conflicted feelings she never stopped loving God.

There were times when she vacillated regarding the focus of her angry feelings at God. As noted in *Dancing with Broken Bones*, she was angry with God because of her husband's death. She was angry with God about the cancer diagnosis. She asked herself if she had done something wrong in her life to cause the illness to come upon her. She prayed to have God take her anger from her and claimed that God had answered her prayers. However, it is also noted that after stating God answered her prayers, she also said that *eventually* God would take the anger away. So, she lived in a process of praying for relief from her anger and with the contradictory belief that it had been relieved and that it would be relieved sometime soon.

Her feelings and behaviors were those of a person of faith doing battle with the real things that life had dealt her. Despite moving in and out of her angry feelings, she never severed her relationship with God. David Moller's words about this time of her life show this woman's unwavering faith and what I consider a real relationship with God. "Throughout her experience with cancer, Mrs. Angel felt even more connected to God than she usually did. Her relationship with God was dynamic, with ups and downs, but always in constant contact and communication."

My final comment on this story is about love. Love is not a topic that I personally often reference in sermons or other times when I speak. It is challenging to speak about love because for me it is more than flowers on Valentine's Day or the "normal" romantic pictures that the word invokes. Love like Mrs. Angel's is complex. But for her, love was also abundant. Before she had her stroke, she was in the process of preparing a big Thanksgiving dinner because this was normal for the family, and she wanted her daughters and grandchildren around. She kicked her daughter Joleen out of the house because this daughter stole from her. It was a hard step for her, and she felt extremely guilty after the fact. Love isn't always unconditional acceptance. Sometimes it requires setting limits on behavior. Mrs. Angel declared her love for her daughter by drawing a line in the sand regarding her stealing. In one incident, she agonized over the fact that Tawana had left the house during a Thanksgiving dinner so that Joleen could come home. There was tension between the sisters that went back to childhood, but even though Tawana could not be with Joleen she wanted Joleen to be able to be with her mother. Mrs. Angel's stance was, "They're sisters, all three of them are sisters and like I told them, I carried all three for nine months under my heart and I gave birth to all three of them and I love all three of them." She also loved Mike. She took care of him in "sickness and in health," and her grief was profound when he died. She made preparations for her own funeral and burial because she felt it would be too hard for her daughters to do so. All of this was done out of a commitment to loving her family.

Mrs. Angel's love seemed to be contagious. I want to suggest that David Moller "loved" her. Mike loved her and wanted her to get out of her dangerous first marriage. Her children loved her. They were at her side at the hospital, and they were at her side on a rotating basis in the weeks before she died. Even Joleen, who had been told to leave, came back to be a part of the bedside vigil that the sisters created to care for their dying mother. Tawana took care of her father, despite his history of abusing her mother, when there was no one else to do so. Was this obligation, or because there was no one else and she felt responsible? Was it some need to feel accepted by a parent who rejected her? Or was it because of a profound capacity to love, even in the midst of human imperfections, that she had learned from her mother? Not many details were given. In thinking about taking care of the type of father he was, I would personally have to think long and hard about caring for him.

Immediately upon her death, her daughters strained already very limited finances to call their extended family down South to tell them about their mother's death, and there were other bills that needed to be paid. As noted in *Dancing with Broken Bones,* it was nine months after their mother's death before they had phone service reconnected.

All of this brings to mind I Corinthians 13, which is a chapter in the Bible that speaks about love, and I include part of it here:

> [1]If I speak in the tongues of mortals and of angels, but do not have love, I am a noisy gong or a clanging cymbal. [2]And if I have prophetic powers, and understand all mysteries and all knowledge, and if I have all faith, so as to remove mountains, but do not have love, I am nothing. [3]If I give away all my possessions, and if I hand over my body so that I may boast, but do not have love, I gain nothing.
>
> [4]Love is patient; love is kind; love is not envious or boastful or arrogant [5]or rude. It does not insist on its own way; it is not irritable or resentful; [6]it does not rejoice in wrongdoing, but rejoices in the truth. [7]It bears all things, believes all things, hopes all things, endures all things.
>
> [8]Love never ends. But as for prophecies, they will come to an end; as for tongues, they will cease; as for knowledge, it will come to an end. [13]And now faith, hope, and love abide, these three; and the greatest of these is love.

I do not want to overly idealize Lucille Angel. No human being can live up to lofty accolades all of the time. However, her story does mirror this portrait of love. The day before she died, her missing pastor showed up to see her. Mrs. Angel was in a coma and in no condition to know that he was there. Yet her daughters welcomed his visit without rancor. Personally, I feel he did not deserve their graciousness. He had promised Mrs. Angel many months ago that he would stop by, and she was very angry as the months passed and he did not visit. Yet he made it to see her the day before she died. Maybe like many patients who hold on to life for the final child to fly in from out of town to say goodbye, she held on so that she could truly rest upon her pastor's arrival, even if she was never consciously aware of him coming. And that is precisely what her daughters prayed that she would receive upon her death. "Rest. Real rest. Mama," they prayed.

Faith is not straightforward, as is demonstrated throughout Mrs. Angel's story.

PALLIATIVE CARE PERSPECTIVE

One of the many striking aspects of Mrs. Angel's story was the relative absence of palliative care other than the witnessing author of *Dancing with Broken Bones*. As a matter of definition, palliative care involves the biological, psychological, social, and spiritual care of patients with serious illnesses, along with their families.[6] Palliative care is generally provided alongside any and all effective medical treatments, with special attention given to symptom management, assistance with medical decision-making, added patient and family support, and (when necessary) assistance with end-of-life decision-making. The lost opportunities to provide palliative care are evident throughout three phases of the narrative:

1. The early phase when she was mired in an abusive first marriage without any support to extricate herself;
2. The middle phase when she was first diagnosed with laryngeal cancer, then cared for her second husband during his prolonged illness and death, and when she subsequently had a stroke and was diagnosed with lung cancer; and
3. During the final phase of her illness when she was on hospice.

The specialty model of palliative care is predicated on the involvement of an interprofessional team of providers (physicians, nurses, chaplains, social workers, and others) with every seriously-ill patient and his or her family. There is growing evidence that the quality of care provided to and quality of life experienced by such patients is improved relative to those receiving usual medical care.[7] There are even some data to suggest that patients with advanced lung cancer (the illness that ultimately ended Mrs. Angel's life) who receive palliative care from the time of initial diagnosis live longer by an average of almost three months in comparison to those receiving usual medical care.[8] Unfortunately, there are not enough palliative care providers trained across the country to provide this kind of care to all such patients—they tend to be concentrated around major medical centers.[9] But even if there were, it may not be a good idea to always create a separate team of medical providers to break out this kind of comprehensive care from usual care.

An alternative would be to train all clinicians who care for seriously-ill patients to do the basics of palliative care as part of their usual job responsibilities, and then reserve the formal palliative care consultations for the more complex and difficult cases.[10] In this model, all clinicians who care for seriously-ill patients would be trained in the basics of pain and symptom management, and specialists might be called in for more difficult pain/symptom questions. All clinicians would be trained to present patients and families with the full range of treatment possibilities, including exclusively palliative approaches, along with recommendations about the best path, based on patient values and clinical probabilities/burdens of treatment,[11] while palliative care specialists might be called in to address requests for nearly futile treatment or address conflicts about how to proceed. All clinical teams and community chaplains would be trained to provide basic psychosocial and spiritual support for patients facing serious illness and their families, while palliative care chaplains might be consulted around a major crisis of faith. And finally, all clinical teams would help patients and families make the transition to hospice when necessary and provide ongoing continuity, while palliative care specialists might become involved when there is major family or staff conflict over the transition, and might take over the primary provider role when no one else is willing or able to step up.

Of course, as *Dancing with Broken Bones* repeatedly illustrates, if you happen to be poor and/or live in inner-city areas of this country, not only may specialty palliative care be absent, but access to primary care and to other subspecialists may be spotty at best. Many of these otherwise very dedicated clinicians who serve dying-poor patients have never been trained in basic palliative care domains, and helping someone like Mrs. Angel navigate the world of serious illness. With so little psychosocial support around her throughout her illness experiences even the most sophisticated and mature of palliative care clinicians and systems would be strained. In the following section, I plan to explore the three phases of Mrs. Angel's life covered in this narrative and see how palliative care might have improved her quality of life as well as her interactions with the medical system.

In the first phase, Mrs. Angel was a mother of three children living in rural poverty and being repeatedly abused by her husband. The doctor who saw her was willing to treat her physical injuries, but did not intervene in the larger pattern of abuse. Being complicit with such abuse in such dire circumstances tragically adds to the problem, but the options for adult protective services even in metropolitan areas are limited, much more so in rural America. Without the anchor of serious illness, specialty palliative care, even if available, would not have a meaningful role in such situations, but it is feasible that clinicians trained in primary palliative care might have been able to think more broadly about intervention options in response to this kind of overwhelming situation.

> Her worsening prognosis and disease progression led to anger not only at her doctors, but also at God.

The next phase of Mrs. Angel's life was where palliative care services (primary or specialty) might have made the biggest difference. Hopefully, the treatment team overseeing the radiation treatment of her initial diagnosis of oral cancer would be attentive to her symptom management during treatment, and perhaps they might have also identified her as someone at high risk for second cancers, given her smoking history. When her second husband became terminally ill, if he had been receiving hospice services, perhaps Mrs. Angel would have been identified as someone with major bereavement risks, given her past traumas and her and Mike's very close relationship.

When she later experienced a stroke, the medical alarm bells should have begun clanging for some kind of clotting problem associated with latent malignancy, and, shortly thereafter, she was diagnosed with lung cancer. During this time, communication with her clinicians, particularly around her prognosis, appears to have been less than ideal. Many clinicians have not been properly trained to have honest prognostic conversations with patients, and the norm is often to minimize or even not speak of the risks of recurrence or of not responding to first-line therapy, unless the patient specifically asks.[12] My guess is that this would have been a difficult conversation to initiate with Mrs. Angel as she may have felt that openly considering such matters could undermine her sense of hope and might even have worsened her odds of recovery. Yet when her disease was still progressing after two rounds of chemotherapy, she felt severely betrayed and angry at the doctors for in some sense "not doing their job."

How would a properly trained primary care clinician or oncologist approach these discussions? The most recent recommendations would be to "ask" before "telling," and then "ask" again to ensure understanding,[13] meaning that she might be asked if she would like to know the odds of treatment's curing her disease at the time treatment was being initiated. She might have not wanted to know this information, but even if the invitation to become informed was declined, she would at least have been informed that there was some significant possibility that treatment might not work. Would this have lessened the betrayal and anger she felt at the time of disease progression? Perhaps not, but at a minimum, she would have been given the opportunity to learn what the clinicians were really thinking. Many specialty clinicians believe that if they tell the truth about odds and prognosis, patients may seek care elsewhere.[14] Of course, poorer patients such as Mrs. Angel do not have the luxury of going to other treatment centers. Nonetheless, telling the truth about odds and prognosis with compassion should be the standard of care for all clinicians who care for the seriously ill, and the clinicians delivering such information must be prepared to respond compassionately to the inevitable emotions and need for support that are associated.[15]

If palliative care clinicians are the only ones to talk honestly about prognosis, it can become a self-fulfilling prophecy where a palliative care referral becomes a marker for a bad prognosis and/or the potential need for a hospice referral. Prognostic discussions can and should leave room for being an exception in terms of prognosis in both directions ("could be longer and could be shorter than we expect"), and the honest clinician will always try to prepare for what is most likely, while at the same time ("hoping for the best and preparing for the worst").[16]

In Mrs. Angel's case, her worsening prognosis and disease progression led to anger not only at her doctors, but also at God. The general discomfort that clinicians often have entering into discussions about poor prognosis is probably only surpassed by their discomfort with religious discussions, especially if they involve anger at God. Clinicians, including those who are palliative care–trained, are not adequately prepared to do spiritual or religious counseling, but they should be able to openly explore what the patient is thinking and feeling in religious and spiritual domains.[17] Open-ended exploration of these aspects of a patient's suffering in these domains by all clinicians should be standard of care—"Tell me more about" whatever it is the patient is experiencing. Lessening the aloneness of and bearing witness to these experiences are critical, but if some kind of spiritual or religious counseling is needed, this is outside the realm of most clinicians' expertise and should be conducted by clergy and/or chaplains if possible.

Sometimes this can be a "no-win" situation for patients because many religious advisors are not well trained to be present for those who are seriously medically ill. Mrs. Angel's minister was not present for her in any deep, personal, or lasting way, and when he did show up, he was in and out as quickly as possible. Nonetheless, her family was very forgiving and appreciative of his presence. The parallel between the lack of training and comfort of community clergy in addressing end-of-life spiritual and religious issues, and the lack of preparedness of community clinicians to engage with end-of-life medical issues, is striking. Unfortunately, the relative shortage of hospital-based chaplains is comparable to the shortage of palliative care–trained specialists, so community clergy and community clinicians should be trained in these basic skills as well.

POTENTIAL ROLE OF HOSPICE

Hospice is the premiere program to provide palliative care to terminally-ill patients and families in the United States,[18] but a disproportionately small number of African-American, Hispanic, and/or socioeconomically disadvantaged patients select hospice for the last part of their care.[19–21] This is in large measure because of hospice's requirement that one forgo disease-directed therapy and hospitalization in the future to be accepted into the program. For seriously-ill patients such as Mrs. Angel, who have had marginal access to medical care, it is difficult to trust that they are not being deprived of potentially effective medical treatment because of expense or some other kind of discrimination. Furthermore, some of the requirements to be accepted into hospice may not make sense to these patients, such as giving up on future hospitalization or having medical treatment for potentially reversible conditions. The mantra that hospice "neither hastens nor postpones" death may make no sense to many of these patients—"If easy-to-treat things might postpone my death, are you really not going to offer them to me?," they may think. And the fact that they have to rely on only one doctor, which in itself deprives them of access to the entire system of healthcare, also may not make sense, at least not without a lot of trust. Ironically, because many poorer patients do not have confidence in the system they may be deprived once again of having the highest quality care at the end of their lives (Figure 8.2).

On the positive side, hospice clearly can be a wonderful system of care for those who come to terms with their prognosis and accept that they are dying. It is a capitated benefit, so there are no added charges for services or medications or supplies that are provided, as long as they are needed to help palliate the main treating diagnosis. One also gets support from a multidisciplinary team that includes a physician, home care nurse, nursing aides, a social worker, volunteers, and chaplains. The home-aide support is limited, however, to two to four hours per day, which means that family has to provide the bulk of the care. In Mrs. Angel's case, her daughters were collectively able to provide 24-hour care at home, and the hospice team was able to support the daughters in working through some of their own issues around their mother's illness and their challenging past and present lives.

The issues faced by Mrs. Angel's family members were very complex, including one daughter with a serious drug-abuse problem that flared as her mother got sicker. Mrs.

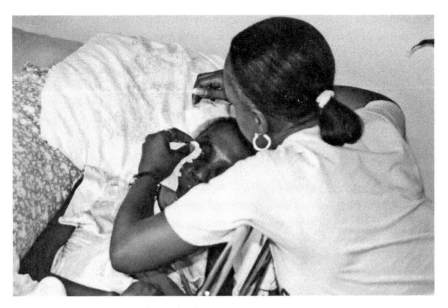

FIGURE 8.2 Tender mercy of a loving daughter.

Angel's first husband, the children's father, who had neglected and abandoned them throughout their childhood, came back on the scene debilitated with a serious illness of his own just as Mrs. Angel was also getting sicker and in need of ongoing care, and each parent was taken in by one of the three children. Although hospice lessened some of the economic burden of her final illness by paying for all medically-needed palliative treatments, Mrs. Angel's funeral and burial costs were not at all covered by hospice, so the family was even further impoverished by her care needs after her death. As Dr. Moller makes very clear in these narratives, there are no simple answers to these complex issues raised when poverty, serious illness, and alienation collide, but despite the associated chaos and losses, there can also be an opportunity for healing and coming together, as was experienced by this family. Mrs. Angel's story is not simple or unidimensional, and the odds are stacked profoundly against good care in these circumstances. Yet, through continued family presence and religious faith coupled with some medical support, there was the opportunity for crucially important healing moments, if not permanent transformation.

> There are no simple answers to these complex issues raised when poverty, serious illness, and alienation collide.

Hospice care at home during the final phase of Mrs. Angel's life gave the best opportunity for such healing to occur. Hospice attempts systematically to address the biological, psychological, social, and spiritual realities that patients and families face by giving access to interdisciplinary professionals as needed. But the suffering associated with real life and with real dying is not readily corrected—this suffering is still at times profound, and our abilities to compensate for, much less ameliorate, such losses are severely limited, even without the added burdens of serious poverty and family dysfunction. But, as illustrated time and again in these stories in *Dancing with Broken Bones*, profound suffering can be witnessed and acknowledged, ideally with continuous compassionate presence from chaplains, social workers, nurses, and physicians, and in doing so can lessen some of the aloneness that can be so profound and deep at this stage of life.

FINAL THOUGHTS

We end this chapter focusing on a paragraph on the first page of her story. David Moller wrote, "Rather than lament her sufferings, she spent much of her time during her final months being thankful for where her life was and reflecting on what she had done in the past." Telling her story caused her to reflect on her life, thinking about what she did, what she could have done in a different way, and what she should have done. No conclusion is drawn. It is likely that her thoughts were like the statement that appears in the telling of her story—*Everything happens for a reason*. Philosophically, it rubs us the wrong way, but it clearly helped Mrs. Angel survive as long as she did. We wish we could have known her.

REFERENCES

1. Engel GL. The clinical application of the biopsychosocial model. *Am J Psychiatry.* 1980;137:535–544.
2. Egnew TR. Suffering, meaning, and healing: challenges of contemporary medicine. *Ann Fam Med.* 2009;7:170–175.
3. Dahlberg LL, Mercy JA. The history of violence as a public health issue. *AMA Virtual Mentor.* 2009;11:167–172.
4. Dahlberg LL, Butchart A. State of the science: violence prevention efforts in developing and developed countries. *Int J Inj Contr Saf Promot.* 2005;12:93–104.
5. Johnson KS, Kuchibhatla M, Tulsky JA. What explains racial differences in the use of advance directives and attitudes toward hospice care? *J Am Geriatr Soc.* 2008;56:1953–1958.
6. Morrison RS, Meier DE. Clinical practice. Palliative care. *N Engl J Med.* 2004;350:2582–2590.
7. National Consensus Project for Quality Palliative C. Clinical practice guidelines for quality palliative care. *Kans Nurse.* 2004;79:16–20.
8. Temel JS, Greer JA, Muzikansky A, et al. Early palliative care for patients with metastatic non-small-cell lung cancer. *N Engl J Med.* 2010;363:733–742.
9. Meier DE. Variability in end of life care. *BMJ.* 2004;328:E296–E297.
10. Quill TE, Abernethy AP. Generalist plus specialist palliative care—creating a more sustainable model. *N Engl J Med.* 2013;368:1173–1175.
11. Quill TE, Brody H. Physician recommendations and patient autonomy: finding a balance between physician power and patient choice. *Ann Intern Med.* 1996;125:763–769.
12. Norton SA, Metzger M, DeLuca J, Alexander SC, Quill TE, Gramling R. Palliative care communication: linking patients' prognoses, values, and goals of care. *Res Nurs Health.* 2013;36:582–590.
13. Back AL, Arnold RM, Baile WF, Tulsky JA, Fryer-Edwards K. Approaching difficult communication tasks in oncology. *CA Cancer J Clin.* 2005;55:164–177.

14. Back AL, Arnold RM. Discussing prognosis: "how much do you want to know?" talking to patients who do not want information or who are ambivalent. *J Clin Oncol.* 2006;24:4214–4217.

15. Roter DL, Hall JA, Kern DE, Barker LR, Cole KA, Roca RP. Improving physicians' interviewing skills and reducing patients' emotional distress. A randomized clinical trial. *Arch Intern Med.* 1995;155:1877–1884.

16. Back AL, Arnold RM, Quill TE. Hope for the best, and prepare for the worst. *Ann Intern Med.* 2003;138:439–443.

17. Lo B, Ruston D, Kates LW, et al. Discussing religious and spiritual issues at the end of life: a practical guide for physicians. *JAMA.* 2002;287:749–754.

18. Morrison RS, Maroney-Galin C, Kralovec PD, Meier DE. The growth of palliative care programs in United States hospitals. *J Palliat Med.* 2005;8:1127–1134.

19. Lepore MJ, Miller SC, Gozalo P. Hospice use among urban black and white US nursing home decedents in 2006. *Gerontologist.* 2011;51:251–260.

20. Mack JW, Paulk ME, Viswanath K, Prigerson HG. Racial disparities in the outcomes of communication on medical care received near death. *Arch Intern Med.* 2010;170:1533–1540.

21. Zheng NT, Mukamel DB, Caprio T, Cai S, Temkin-Greener H. Racial disparities in in-hospital death and hospice use among nursing home residents at the end of life. *Medical Care.* 2011;49:992–998.

9

DYING POOR NEEDN'T MEAN DYING POORLY

INSIGHTS FROM A SAFETY-NET HOSPITAL
PALLIATIVE CARE PROGRAM

Gregory P. Gramelspacher and Richard Gunderman

Death is inevitable, but suffering is not. We must all look forward to the day when compassionate and skilled end-of-life care becomes such a part of the fabric of American communities and the American healthcare system that we won't need to request it—it will simply be offered when needed.
—Kathy Foley[1]

To most, poverty means living with fewer of the things that money can buy—no retirement savings, no car, and perhaps even no home and no food. But for many who experience poverty first-hand as a daily fact of life, it means more than struggling to live with less. It also means dying with less. For too many, it means facing terminal illness with reduced access to healthcare as well as diminished understanding and even compassion from the health professionals caring for them, most of whom have never been poor a day in their lives.

Many factors have led to the establishment of palliative care programs for the poor, including the availability of new sources of funding, the finding that good palliative care can reduce overall healthcare costs, and above all, the recognition that caring well for all terminally-ill and dying patients—whatever their socioeconomic status—is an essential part of good medicine. But many of the deepest insights into palliative care's mission to care for the poor lie in the stories of particular patients.

ALLEN: THE HARM OF FUTILE CARE

Allen was a 55-year-old man with advanced liver cancer who had suffered a seizure and was admitted to Wishard Hospital, the city of Indianapolis's former safety-net facility (which has recently moved into a new building and been renamed Eskenazi Hospital). Allen's initial workup by the medicine team revealed that Allen's liver disease was causing him to suffer episodes of low blood sugar, which were in turn precipitating seizures.

The team also learned that Allen lived alone in an apartment, had no job, experienced difficulty providing for himself, and had been steadily losing weight. His condition was so poor that he was unable to have more cancer-directed therapy, and before long, he was no longer able to care for himself. The medicine team caring for him in the hospital was concerned that he might die soon, so they decided to talk him about his code status—i.e., what he wanted those caring for him to do if at any point during his hospitalization he suffered cardiopulmonary arrest.

The intern on the team went to talk with Allen and asked him what he wanted the doctors to do. To everyone's surprise and consternation, Allen said, "Do everything." Thinking that his junior colleague had botched the discussion, the senior resident posed the same question and, not long afterward, so did the attending physician, but the result was always the same. Allen reiterated that should his heartbeat or breathing stop, he wanted the team to "do everything."

This placed the team in an uncomfortable position. Despite their best medical judgment, if Allen suffered cardiopulmonary arrest, they would have no choice but to subject him to a traumatic and probably futile resuscitation effort. Every evening, the intern dreaded signing out to colleagues who might be summoned to Allen's room to attempt to resuscitate him. After all, the probability that Allen would survive a resuscitation attempt was very low, and the likelihood that even if resuscitated he would survive long enough to be discharged from the hospital was considerably lower still. Even if he were to defy all odds and leave the hospital alive, his quality of life would be very poor.

To the team's surprise, however, before disaster could strike, the social worker on the service was able to place Allen in a local nursing home. The team members greeted this as welcome news, primarily because it extricated them from their dilemma. By transferring Allen's care to another facility, they had been able to sign off the case before he arrested.

The problem was that no one on the team could name the nursing home or the physician to whom Allen's care had been handed off. The team had given very little or no thought to what Allen's new caregivers would be doing for him, and they were simply grateful that they had managed to dodge the bullet of his resuscitation status.

Just two days later, though, Allen suffered a respiratory arrest at the nursing home, and its staff sent him right back to the hospital in an ambulance. He was admitted through the emergency department to the same intensive care unit and the same medicine team. The bullet had ricocheted back. Once again, Allen was their problem.

After eight days of aggressive, life-prolonging treatment, the team became convinced that there was no point in carrying on, despite Allen's expressed wishes that the doctors "Do everything." Judging that continued aggressive treatment was futile, they called in a clinical medical ethics consultant. As expected, the consultant saw matters the same way. After talking with the patient's daughter, he advised that the ventilator be disconnected. As soon as this recommendation was implemented, Allen died.

The concerns of well-off suburban patients, such as whether they are receiving the very best cutting-edge care and the "bedside manners" of their physicians, often differ dramatically from those of the poor, who wonder whether they will be able to get into the hospital—or even get to the hospital—at all.

Following these events, the ethics consultant reflected on what he had witnessed. From his point of view, the medical team had done as fine a job as possible managing Allen's acute medical problems and keeping his organs functioning. In other respects, however, they had done him an unfortunate disservice by failing to extend to him the care he truly needed in a more complete and deeper sense.

They had failed to call for help in a timely fashion, essentially waiting until their patient was moribund before asking some essential questions about the goals of care. Moreover, they had failed to have a meaningful conversation with their patient about what desires he had for end-of-life care. Part of the problem was their lack of understanding of how to have such a conversation, or who they could turn to for help in doing so.

They also failed to make the effort to understand their patient's life outside the hospital, especially what might be leading him to insist that, in the event of an arrest, they should "do everything." They knew that he was poor, but they had very little understanding of what his day-to-day life was like and what continuing to live meant to him. This made it difficult for them to grasp what he was really saying when he insisted that they "do everything." What did he view as alternatives, and what had the team done to educate him in this regard? The most important conversations had never taken place.

The ethics consultant decided to investigate Allen's medical history, which led to some important insights. It turned out that just four months earlier, during a visit with his primary care physician, Allen had said that, should his pulse or breathing stop, he did not want to be resuscitated. Unfortunately, the medicine team had never spoken with his primary physician, and no one knew that he had once answered the question very differently. What had changed?

It emerged that Allen had some important unfinished business in life. First, he really loved to fish, something he had not been able to do for months and to which he really wanted to return. No one had inquired about what brought him joy in life, and even if they had, none of them had any experience with fishing or how important it could be to someone. Second, Allen and his adult daughter had become estranged, and his feelings of guilt and hope for reconciliation made it difficult for him to let go. He did not want to die while they were still at loggerheads with one another. The team members were so focused on the complex medical issues that no one had taken the time to get to know Allen as a person. To the ethics consultant, it seemed clear that when Allen said "do everything," what he really meant was "Get me back to my apartment and give me one more chance to do what I love and what needs to be done."

The ethics consultant was not called during the first admission because the team perceived no "ethical" issue. They saw just a competent patient making a decision with which they happened to disagree. The team was operating with an excessive focus on acute medical care, one that prevented them from appreciating the longer-term questions and concerns that shaped their patient's perspective on the situation.

Allen's story illustrates a larger problem. Our healthcare "system" is often anything but. It often functions more as a collection of silos—inpatient care and outpatient care; decisions between the extremes of doing everything and doing nothing; therapy that aims at cure versus care whose primary purpose is comfort. And when it comes to the care of the poor, these defects are often magnified, in part because most of the resources needed for good care are harder to come by.

Allen was a glaring example of a patient whose care had not been well integrated. No one had ever talked with him about nursing home placement. His was just another case in which first-line, second-line, and third-line therapies had failed to produce a remission. One day the oncologist had simply told Allen that he had reached the end of the road; there was nothing more the cancer team could do for him.

Cancer patients like Allen see their oncologists every two or three weeks for months, often for years. Then, when all cancer-directed therapies have failed, the oncologist asks the social worker to make a referral to hospice, and the patient is told to return to the clinic only "as needed." In Allen's case, however, in no small part because he was poor, hospice was not readily available. Additionally, he could not call on family, friends, or any other network of support to assume responsibility for helping to care for him.

Sensing that their physicians' commitment to continued care is weakening, patients like Allen often ask themselves, "Why isn't my doctor scheduling a follow-up appointment?" "Who is my doctor now?" "Do I even have a doctor?" They often feel abandoned. And to the mind of a poor patient like Allen, one inescapable explanation is the fact that he cannot afford to pay for his care.

> Witnessing how differently rich and poor, black and white were dying had helped Carrie and Colleen see more clearly what dying really means to every human being and what truly needs to be attended to in order to ensure that patients can die with dignity.

Even among better-off patients, the referral to hospice too often takes place just weeks or even days before the patient dies. From the ethics consultant's point of view, such patients were receiving too little appropriate care too late in the course of their disease. Something needed to change. What, he asked himself, could be done to do a better job of following through on medicine's core commitments and to restore trust?

The ethics consultants' sentiments echoed those of Susan Block, who described the origins of palliative care in these terms:

> When I look back to the very beginning of this enterprise, what I remember most is a sense of something being really broken in the system of how we cared for the dying. There was no road map. No one really knew how to approach it. There were few real experts. We also sensed that doing things better was a very real possibility— that we could create a system that addressed the real needs of dying patients and families.[2]

And change it did. The cases of Allen and dozens of other similar patients convinced the ethics consultant that a new paradigm was needed. Too many doctors were so focused on therapy intended to produce a cure, or at least a plateau in the progression of the disease, that they were completely overlooking opportunities to relieve suffering. And such problems were especially acute for poor patients like Allen, perhaps in part because of the large chasm of culture and life experience that separates the dying poor from the health professionals charged with their care.

THE DYING POOR

Allen's story, like the stories of countless other patients, provides insights into the special challenges facing the dying poor and those who care for them. The concerns of well-off suburban patients, such as whether they are receiving the very best cutting-edge care and the "bedside manners" of their physicians, often differ dramatically from those of the poor, who wonder whether they will be able to get into the hospital—or even get to the hospital at all.

For many well-to-do patients, one of the greatest frustrations with receiving care at an urban hospital is parking—where to find it and how to pay for it. For Allen, however, parking was not an issue because he did not have a car. Instead, he had no choice but to rely on public transportation, a considerably more time-consuming and potentially exhausting prospect. Often a single bus transfer could add an extra hour to his journey, a burden on his time that doubled with the return journey home.

Today, most poor patients like Allen have mobile phones, but many do not have unlimited minutes, making each call a potential budget buster. Between automated operators and long hold times, a single call to a hospital or doctor's office can use up 20 or 30 minutes or more of talk time before the caller actually gets to speak with the person they are trying to reach. From the health professional's point of view, phone numbers and addresses for poor patients often change, which can make it difficult to reach them and their family members.

When an appointment needs to be rescheduled, clinic staff members often spend a considerable amount of time trying to reach a patient whose contact information has changed. After multiple attempts, they frequently give up. When patients who were never reached show up at the appointed time, they naturally feel frustrated when they learn that they have wasted the better part of a day getting to and from a cancelled appointment.

Allen's estrangement from his daughter highlights the differences in family and community life that often differentiate poor and better-off patients. Such estrangements can happen in any socioeconomic stratum, but poor patients—and especially the homeless—are often the most isolated socially. As a result, they cannot assume that, should they develop a serious illness, family and friends will be there to help care for them.

Even patients who do have family and friends nearby cannot always count on them. In many cases, family members are working two jobs, have substantial family responsibilities, or simply lack the disposable income necessary to drop what they are doing for a period of weeks, months, or years to care for a seriously-ill loved one.

Consider having enough food to eat. If one of the authors were facing a terminal illness, we are confident that our family, neighbors, and fellow parishioners in a faith community would spring into action, supplying home-cooked meals every day. Grocery shopping would be unnecessary, and we might even run out of refrigerator space. In contrast, patients like Allen have no one waiting in the wings to deliver casseroles day after day to their door (Figure 9.1).

Consider a patient who resembled Allen in many respects. He had just received the news that he had been diagnosed with terminal cancer. To his physician's surprise, he did so with complete calm, reacting not angrily or fearfully but with quiet reservation. When

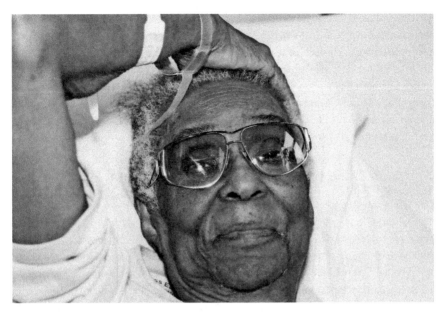

FIGURE 9.1 Dying poor needn't mean dying poorly.

his physician asked him how he could be so unfazed, the man replied, "Why should I get upset? This is just the fifth bad thing that has happened to me this week."

Coming from more-advantaged backgrounds where setbacks and catastrophes are considerably less common, many health professionals misjudge how poor patients will react to bad news. Considering such a prospect, they imagine how they would respond, shaking their heads at how terrible it must be to be poor and dying. But again and again, poor patients exhibit remarkable equanimity, in large part because their life-long experiences have taught them to expect bad news.

A number of older palliative care patients, particularly African-American men, have in the past been the victims of violent crime, including suffering gunshot wounds. When, having reached their 70s, they learn that they have cancer, they do not feel cheated. Why? Simply because, many have said, they never expected to live so long. Far from feeling unfairly punished, they are surprised that such bad news has taken so long to befall them.

When Allen and other patients are told that they have a serious medical problem, they feel—often quite rightly—that they have no choice about where to seek care. It never even enters their minds that they might go to one of the posh suburban hospitals. They take it for granted that their only refuge is the county's safety-net hospital.

When they arrive there, they typically do so not with a sense of entitlement, but with little more than hope—hope that there will be someone there who cares enough to take care of them. At a private hospital, a physician often takes ownership of the patient, but at a public facility serving the urban poor, many patients cannot say who their doctor is because this changes all the time. Medical students, residents, and attending physicians rotate on and off of services at regular intervals, and, too often, no one assumes ongoing responsibility for the poor patient.

The problems facing the poor and those who care for them can also be viewed as opportunities, which is just what the clinical ethics consultant who saw Allen decided needed to be done. He decided to attempt to start a palliative care service for the patients at the safety-net hospital. When the unmet needs are so great, he reasoned, almost anything a palliative care team could do would make a worthwhile difference. This line of thought also led to a dramatic change of course in his career. He shifted from general internal medicine and clinical ethics consultation to palliative care, becoming the safety-net hospital's first full-time palliative care physician.

PALLIATIVE CARE: ENHACING LIFE

One important step in making this new vision of caring for the dying poor a reality was the realization that palliative care is not a strictly medical issue. A good palliative care physician could contribute a lot, but providing truly comprehensive care to the dying poor would require a team of knowledgeable and dedicated professionals, including, among others, nurses, social workers, community liaisons, and chaplains.

A good nurse, for example, would play a crucial role helping to organize and coordinate the care of a dying patient, making sure that accurate contact information was available to both patient and physician, helping to remind patients of their appointments and prescriptions, and checking on patients and answering questions between appointments.

A good social worker would help patients keep the rest of their lives sufficiently well ordered to permit them to receive good medical care. It is all well and good to offer the latest diagnostic and therapeutic options to patients, but what good does it really do if someone cannot get a bus pass or lacks the money to buy food?

A community liaison would help to connect patients to resources in the community, including local faith communities, which in many cases play a crucial role in helping to care for dying patients on a day-to-day basis. In addition, for many patients, congregations represent one of their most important sources of fellowship and support.

From the very beginning of the palliative care program, the goal was to move dying patients out of the hospital and into the community because, ultimately, this is where they would receive the most humane and dignified care. To do that, however, the team needed to understand, become involved with, and depend to some degree on the community. The physicians couldn't do it alone, and neither could the hospital-employed members of the team. Only by calling on and trusting in the good will of family members, friends, and neighbors could patients receive truly comprehensive care.

For similar reasons, chaplains often play a crucial role. The palliative care physician soon learned to bring a chaplain with him to many family conferences. Often the participation of the chaplain dramatically improved the atmosphere in the room. For example, opening and closing such a meeting with a prayer helped to situate a difficult conversation in a larger and ultimately more fruitful context of meaning. Decisions needed to take into account not only acute medical needs but the sources of joy and meaning in the patient's life.

Of course, involving a chaplain in this way can be inappropriate if the team knows that a particular patient or family is not open to it. But when faith and spirituality are clearly important to those involved, the palliative care physician often saw benefits.

When everyone, including nonbelievers on the healthcare team, was joined in prayer, barriers typically represented by white coats and stethoscopes soon began to loom much less large.

One of the biggest practical hurdles faced by the palliative care program at Wishard Hospital was funding. Hiring physicians, nurses, social workers, community liaisons, and chaplains is not inexpensive, and at an institution where 40% of patients have no insurance and 60% are on Medicare or Medicaid, money is not easy to come by.

Philanthropy often played a crucial role. For example, the first palliative care social worker was funded by a one-year grant from a local community foundation. When the impact of her work was assessed at year's end, it turned out that she was actually paying for herself several times over, which persuaded the hospital to make the investment necessary to sustain such a position.

How could a social worker more than pay for her own salary and benefits? For one thing, when she determined that a patient lacked insurance, she knew the system sufficiently well to be able to obtain insurance for them, turning uncompensated care into at least partially-compensated care. Likewise, she could often help patients access care in less costly settings outside the hospital, again saving money for the publicly financed indigent care system.

Institutional responses are equally important. For example, discovering just how costly it is to care for dying patients in the intensive care unit helped to persuade the health system to invest in a community-based hospice facility for the dying poor, which has helped to reduce costs even further. Far more importantly, however, it has enabled many more poor patients to die with dignity.

The whole palliative care program at the safety-net hospital was founded as a result of an unsuccessful grant application. The palliative care physician had applied for funding from a large national philanthropy, but the foundation chose to fund a program in another state. Even to be considered for the funding, however, the safety-net hospital needed to commit to provide matching funds. When the grant did not come through, the palliative care physician was able to persuade the hospital to release the funds anyway, which turned out to provide sufficient resources to get the program up and running.

> Such patients, many of whom come from disadvantaged circumstances, often suspect that the hospital or health system is using palliative care as a ruse to avoid doing everything they can.

Programs such as the Open Society Institutes' Project on Death in America have helped to transform the culture of death and dying in the United States. Its Faculty Scholars Program helped promote more coordination and coherence in the care of the dying, in large part by providing faculty members with both tools and legitimacy needed to bring about change in the way physicians are educated to care for the dying.

By fostering a sense of community among health professionals dedicated to improving the care of the dying, the Project on Death in America stimulated more open and timely discussions among patients, families, and the members of healthcare teams.

In many cases, this made it possible to move the care of patients out of expensive acute-care settings and into more hospitable outpatient clinics and nursing homes.

Logically, the closer patients get to death, the more important palliative care becomes. Yet the key to providing excellent care is to begin building a relationship between patients and the members of the palliative care team early in the course of what could turn out to be a terminal disease. Patients need to think of their care from the very earliest stages with the assurance that they and their family will be well cared for right up to the moment of death and even beyond it.

The care of the dying, the members of the palliative care team realized, needed to be seen less as a medical problem to be managed by doctors and nurses and more as an existential problem to be shared with patients, families, friends, and often faith communities, without whom it could never be adequately addressed.

The question "What are we going to do if the patient requires resuscitation?" needed to be supplanted by new and different questions: "How and when is this person going to die?" "Where is this person going to die?" And perhaps most importantly of all, "When this person dies, who will care?"

In Allen's case, good medicine could not be defined simply in terms of managing low blood sugars, ventilators, or the circumstances of discharge from the hospital. Instead, it required the members of the palliative care team to help ensure that he did not die during an ill-advised, traumatic, and ultimately futile effort at resuscitation. It meant ensuring that he could die at home, or at least in a decent nursing home. And it required that the team caring for him would make the effort necessary to understand what he really meant when he said "do everything."

Taking good care of the patient required shifting the whole conversation to a different frequency. The essential questions were no longer technical or even medical but personal, social, and existential.

The palliative care physician was soon having very different encounters with patients and families, an increasing number of which were taking place outside the hospital, in patients' homes and neighborhoods. In one case, he was planning to visit a dying patient in the morning but learned that the patient had died overnight. Some physicians might have decided that their role was ended when the patient died, seeing no point in going on to make the visit. But the palliative care physician carried on, stopping by the family's favorite bakery for donuts and then spending over an hour sitting on their front porch reminiscing with them about their loved one.

What diagnostic and procedural codes apply to such a visit? Of course there are none. How much revenue does such a visit generate for the hospital and the health system? Of course it generates none. And what is the impact on the physician's own budget? He loses a few dollars and several hours of his time. Yet visits such as this, which revolve around display of human caring, often mean more to patients and families than the most sophisticated tests and therapies that modern medicine can offer, and it stands today as one of the professionally defining experiences that this palliative care physician will never forget.

At the safety-net hospital, the relative dearth of opportunities to generate extra revenue and income by performing more diagnostic tests and therapeutic procedures played an important role in the development of the palliative care program. At some private hospitals, particularly in posher areas, conversations in the physician lounge often focus on topics such as new car purchases and upcoming vacations. In the culture of the safety-next hospital, in contrast, staff members are less united by a desire to enjoy the finer things in life than by a commitment to caring for the poor.

Even the other hospitals in town are committed to the success of the safety-net hospital, in part because they do not want the patients whom it serves to show up on their doorsteps. The entire city understands the importance of the hospital, and local property taxes have long been high enough to enable it to keep fulfilling its mission.

These professional and civic cultures have created a fertile environment for the development of a palliative care program that serves the urban poor. The executive staff of the hospital is not always looking for an immediate financial return for every new initiative, and serving the needs of the poor is more or less taken for granted as an essential aspect of the institutional mission. In a sense, being a relatively poorly-funded organization has enabled the safety-net hospital to innovate and take risks that would have seemed impossible to many better-funded organizations.

COLLEEN AND CARRIE: PREPARING THE NEXT GENERATION

Despite these successes, the palliative care physician quickly realized that changing the practice of only one physician was not enough. More needed to happen. Changes needed to be made in the way physicians were educated, so that more patients could benefit from high-quality palliative care. He started by forming palliative care small groups in the medical school's first-year Introduction to Clinical Medicine course.

Every year, first-year medical students who asked to participate in the palliative care group had the opportunity to experience remarkable patient interactions. In their first week, pairs of students would accompany a palliative care team member to see a seriously-ill or dying patient in the hospital or clinic. In the second week, they would again accompany the palliative care team member to see the same patient, but this time in the patient's home.

Thanks to this new educational initiative, at the very same time that first-year students were dissecting a cadaver in the anatomy lab, they would be meeting and getting to know seriously-ill and dying patients, whom they would continue to visit at least monthly until the year was completed or the patient died. Instead of merely encountering a dead body, they would get to know patients as human beings as they made the transition from life to death. Many of the students found the experience transformative.

About a third of these students actually experienced the death of a patient in their first year of medical school. Even those whose patients did not die gained a more comprehensive view of how medical care fits into the larger context of patients' lives, right up to the time of their death. They met and got to know their patients at home. They learned how important it is to know not just the medical chart, but also the neighborhoods and communities where patients live. They talked with patients, not just about their symptoms and diagnoses and treatments, but also about their lives, the meaning of their stories, and how they wanted to live.

Consider two first-year medical students, Colleen and Carrie, who participated in palliative care groups. As a first-year medical student, Colleen was actually in the home and at the bedside of a dying patient during her second week of medical school. Carrie got to know a dying patient well over the course of her first year. Both found the experience so profound that, seven years later, as they were completing their residency training, they decided to pursue a new palliative care fellowship that had been established at the safety-net hospital. They were returning full circle to the field of medicine they had encountered in their very first days of medical school (Figure 9.2).

When Carrie was still in training, she was diagnosed with breast cancer, and her treatment slowed her professional progress. She eventually went into remission, but during her fellowship, it became clear to her that working in palliative care was too emotionally taxing. She was encountering too many patients like herself—young women in their 30s who had been diagnosed with cancer, some of whom were dying. She took time off from fellowship training in order to spend more time with her family. Several years later, she experienced an extensive recurrence of her cancer.

For six months, the palliative care physician spent nearly every Friday afternoon with Carrie, not as her doctor or former mentor, but as her friend. Despite excellent treatment, it became clear that her disease was progressing. When the palliative care physician recommended hospice, Carrie asked him if he would assume responsibility for her care.

Eventually, Carrie developed a malignant fluid collection around one of her lungs, which she decided not to have drained. She had had enough. Unfortunately, her condition worsened at a time when the palliative care physician needed to be out of town. So Colleen, Carrie's good friend from medical school days, took over for him. One palliative care student had become the palliative care patient, and another palliative care student had become that former student's palliative care physician.

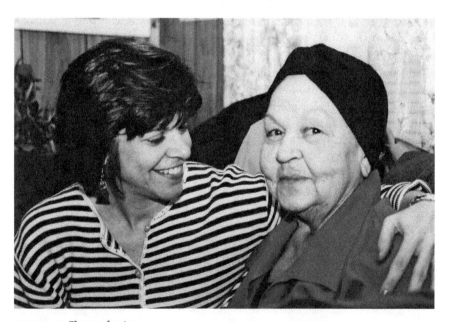

FIGURE 9.2 The art of caring.

When Carrie died at home, her family was by her side, and so was Colleen, her medical school classmate and palliative care physician. Although the members of the palliative care team could not prevent Carrie from dying, they had done the very best they could to ensure that she died on her own terms, surrounded by those who loved her.

Carrie's death was shaped by the experiences she and Colleen had shared in caring for the dying poor. From the very first days of their education, they had ventured beyond the walls of the hospital into the neighborhoods and homes of people they otherwise would never have encountered. They had seen what death looks like when stripped of many of the "bells and whistles" that come with affluence. They knew first-hand the difference between a death in which healthcare operates with a blank check, leaving no medical option—however remote the prospect of benefit—untried, and one that might be called a truly dignified and caring death, one in which the meaning of the patient's life remains front and center. The two classmates were united in the belief that the latter should be the overarching goal for Carrie and those caring for her.

Something similar could be said about their understanding of the effects of economic, ethnic, racial, and religious differences on the dying poor. Witnessing how differently rich and poor, black and white were dying had helped Carrie and Colleen see more clearly what dying really means to every human being and what truly needs to be attended to in order to ensure that patients can die with dignity. Underneath what turn out to be superficial differences lies a shared humanity that cries out for respect and compassion, no matter what a person's point of origin or station in life.

Following in the footsteps of the founder of the palliative care program, Colleen not only continues to practice palliative medicine locally but also plays an active role in attempting to improve the care of the seriously ill and dying on an international stage, particularly in Kenya, where the Indiana University School of Medicine has a longstanding AIDS initiative.

The first time Colleen visited East Africa, she was stunned to learn that the entire region was without morphine. It was not just that the poor or middle-class people could not obtain it—it was nowhere to be found. This situation was emblematic of why Kenya and neighboring countries had no choice but to embrace palliative care.

Simply put, palliative care is an ineluctable feature of Kenyan healthcare because, in many cases, local health professionals, clinics, and hospitals are unable to provide the expensive forms of therapy that are taken for granted in richer countries such as the United States. Here, many cancer patients receive very expensive courses of only marginally-effective chemotherapy that Kenyan people simply cannot afford. Moreover, many Kenyan patients present with quite late-stage, incurable disease. When the unavoidability of death is so undeniable, focusing less on forestalling death and more on dying well becomes a more natural perspective to adopt.

Colleen devotes several weeks of her vacation every year to Kenya, where she helps to try to enlarge and enrich local palliative care programs. She does it because, in essence, the world is a big place, and when people truly care about human suffering, it is only natural that some would go and devote a portion of their time to serving impoverished people in other parts of the world. We may never lack morphine, but that is no reason that poor people around the world cannot experience the same level of compassionate and dignified care that is sometimes lacking in even the richest of communities.

The experiences of Colleen, Carrie, and hundreds of other students represent a radical departure from how most medical students learn to understand and experience death. Just ask a medical student what happens when a patient dies in the hospital. Most will mention three things—ceasing resuscitation efforts, verifying the absence of vital signs, and writing a note to document death.

But death in the hospital is a much more complex event than this, and it should often be a profoundly different one, as well. What happens? A nurse usually washes the body. A toe tag is placed to ensure accurate identification. The patient's body is placed in a bag, and the bag is loaded onto a special cart with a false bottom. What appears to a layperson to be an unoccupied cart is in fact the covert way the dead are transported to the morgue.

> By communicating diagnoses, prognoses, and treatment options to patients and families in ways they can understand and helping them to find a life context that provides for authentic and meaningful choices, palliative care enables medicine to be truer to its best self by ensuring that it is well fitted to the story of each patient and family.

Most medical students have no idea where the morgue is and have never been there before. Nor do they understand the sorts of trials that await the family—notifying friends and loved ones, making arrangements with a funeral home, and actually attending the funeral. For most, it is not until the funeral that they will see their loved one again, and it is also the final time.

The point of this discussion is not to stigmatize medical students—to suggest that they are ignorant or have not made the effort to learn what they should. Instead it is to point out that an education in medicine, nursing, social work, chaplaincy, and so on that fails to provide a rich understanding of how death and dying are experienced by patients and families is omitting an important learning objective for all health professionals.

Often, not just medical students but also residents, fellows, fully-trained physicians, and many other practicing health professionals go about their work every day with serious gaps in their understanding and misapprehensions about these matters. They may, for example, let their ignorance speak in almost prejudicial terms by referring to palliative care professionals as members of the "death squad."

If there is one thing that Colleen, Carrie, and hundreds of other students have learned, it is that it would be a mistake to presume that palliative care is about throwing in the towel. Palliative care at its best is not a reactive, rear-guard, last-ditch-effort kind of medicine. Far from it: it often represents one of healthcare's most prospectively oriented and important opportunities to both enhance care and reduce costs. For many physicians, the care of the dying provides one of the best opportunities to remain true to the ideals of compassion and hope that drew them into medicine in the first place.

Palliative care provides physicians and other health professionals an opportunity to step outside of the healthcare "arms race," in which growing budgets, expanding facilities, and ever more sophisticated pieces of equipment are too often regarded as the most important signs of success. Palliative care costs money, but it can save even more by keeping patients out of the hospital and giving them the opportunity to opt out of additional therapies that offer little chance of success and high probabilities of prolonging suffering. Even poor patients deserve nothing less, and, ironically, it is in caring for the poor that health professionals perceive such possibilities most clearly.

Of course, like any type of medicine, palliative care and hospice medicine can also be practiced badly. It is a problem when anyone—even a palliative care physician—walks into a patient's room and talks about nothing but death, death, death. And let's face it, some patients do initially see palliative physicians as harbingers of death. They may resist the idea of hospice care for months, falsely believing that if they allow themselves to be transitioned to palliative care, they will be authorizing medicine to give up on them.

Such patients, many of whom come from disadvantaged circumstances, often suspect that the hospital or health system is using palliative care as a ruse to avoid doing everything they can, perhaps in order to save money. As Richard Payne has written:

> I have witnessed much ambivalence, sometimes outright hostility, and certainly difficulty in discussing the pertinent issues about personal choices and preferences for care with many of my terminally ill patients, particularly African American patients and families.[3]

The key corner to turn, from the standpoint of good palliative care, is to earn the patient's trust and make a clear and unmistakable commitment to non-abandonment. Patients must have good reason to believe that palliative medicine is not about death and dying but about life and living fully, right up to the day they die.

By communicating diagnoses, prognoses, and treatment options to patients and families in ways they can understand and helping them to find a life context that provides for authentic and meaningful choices, palliative care enables medicine to be truer to its best self, by ensuring that it is well fitted to the story of each patient and family. To be sure, in some cases, the patient's goal may be to live as long as possible, no matter what risks doing so might entail, but this turns out to be the exception rather than the rule.

Far more commonly, what patients and families are seeking is not the mere prolongation of life but the opportunity to make the most of whatever life remains to them. Above all, the appearance of the palliative care physician does not mean that the medical team has given up on the patient. Far from arguing for doing less, giving up early, and saving as much money as possible, palliative care physicians sometimes find themselves advocating for further diagnostic testing to clarify a diagnosis or prognosis, or promoting the option of more aggressive therapy in hopes of producing a remission in the patient's disease. The palliative care team is there to get to know and serve the patient, and its members will hang in there, no matter what.

PAM: A PATHWAY TO HEALING

Pam's story illustrates several of these key features of palliative care. First, Pam's palliative care physician found himself in the position of arguing for more rather than less therapy. Second, Pam was operating with a misperception of the costs, risks, and benefits of treatment. Third, over the course of her disease, Pam experienced a dramatic economic transition. At the beginning of her story, she had health insurance, but, as her disease progressed, she ended up uninsured and unable to pay for her care. Her story serves as an important reminder of just how fluid the boundaries between well-off and poor can be, an important lesson without which it may be difficult or even impossible to craft good health policy.

Pam was a woman in her mid-30s, an accomplished tennis player, married, with three children aged 5 to 15. Over time, she noticed progressive swelling in some of her lymph nodes. This led eventually to a biopsy that disclosed an incurable but treatable form of lymphoma. She saw an oncologist who suggested that she commence chemotherapy, but for reasons known only to her, she decided to wait.

And Pam kept on waiting. In fact, she never did go in for therapy, and, after several years had elapsed, she returned to the hospital much sicker, her disease having progressed to a much later stage. By that point, she had lost much of her energy, her job, and her health insurance. A once middle-class patient had become poor. When she presented at a suburban healthcare facility, where the staff quickly determined that she lacked both insurance and means to pay for her care, she was quickly transferred to the safety-net hospital.

When Pam arrived, it was necessary to drain cancerous fluid collections from around her lungs, and again a hematologist suggested that she begin chemotherapy. Again she declined. Bewildered, the hematologist requested a clinical ethics consultation.

An ethics consultant (not the one who became a palliative care physician) saw her and determined that her decision-making was not impaired, even though her decision was not one with which most health professionals or even most laypeople would agree. The ethics consultant suggested a palliative care consultation, something that would not have been available just a few years earlier, but by now the palliative care program was up and running.

The palliative care physician met Pam. Instead of launching into a discussion about chemotherapy options and survival probabilities, he talked with her about her kids, her tennis, and her life. Through this conversation, he learned that she had strong religious beliefs. In her mind, the choice of whether or not to take chemotherapy would indicate whether or not she believed that God would take care of her.

Pam also wanted to try several different alternative and complementary treatments, which she believed might be just as beneficial as conventional therapy and spare her many of its untoward side effects. In short, she stuck by her decision to decline chemotherapy. So she went home with hospice care, three catheters draining cancerous fluid from her chest and abdomen. The palliative care physician also had trouble understanding why she wouldn't take chemotherapy, but he did not waver in his commitment to standing by her, whatever she chose.

Conversations between Pam and the palliative care physician continued over many home hospice visits, in which Pam revealed that she had once had a friend with lymphoma who had agreed to undergo chemotherapy, but, in spite of her physicians' best efforts, she had died. It turned out that Pam feared that the same thing would happen to her. This, the palliative care physician concluded, was the most important reason that she was declining chemotherapy.

Many weeks later, Pam was hospitalized because a catheter in her chest had become infected. She was very sick and malnourished. During this hospitalization, she was talking with the palliative care physician one day when she asked her mother and husband to leave the room so that she could talk with him one on one.

When they were alone, she told him that she had changed her mind and was now willing to take treatment. Despite concerns that she was now too sick, her hematologist agreed to begin chemotherapy immediately. Once the infected catheter was removed, she required transfer to the intensive care unit on a ventilator.

Two lessons from Pam's care deserve to be highlighted. First, it took not hours or even days, but weeks before Pam felt comfortable enough with the palliative care physician to share with him the experience of her friend who had died of lymphoma. This is one example of how a long-term commitment to continuity of care can make a big difference. Second, it took weeks at home and another stay in the hospital before Pam could agree to take chemotherapy. Instead of badgering her, the palliative care physician simply kept talking with her about her family, her life, and her goals for her therapy. With time, she made the decision to proceed with it largely on her own. Patience is an important virtue in palliative care.

The next day, the palliative care physician came to the ICU to say good-bye, thinking that, because he was going to be away for the next week, it might be the last time they would see each other. Pam asked to have her restraints removed, so that she could write him a note. She wrote simply, "I ♥ you. Have a safe trip!"

Incredibly, Pam lived to hear about that trip. She responded very well to treatment and went into remission. Though she had once been knocking on death's door, over the years since, she has seen all her children graduate from high school. And she is now back to work and playing competitive tennis in a year-round league.

Over the years, Pam has helped to teach many medical students about dying. By sharing her story with small groups of palliative care students, she has explained how the experience of actually facing death helped her overcome her fear of death. In this case, palliative care did not bring the patient to a decision to accept death, but rather dissuaded her from the fatal decision not to undergo treatment. The palliative care physician's commitment to ongoing, deeply discerning conversations opened up possibilities for a new life.

Pam could also convey to them in especially engaging and memorable terms what it is like to be dying and poor. Unlike many other poor patients, Pam had once been reasonably well off, and the fact that poverty was new to her enabled her to see more clearly the nature of the transition she and her family had undergone. For her, poverty was not a timeless fact of life but a new condition into which she had fallen. Having once paid her bills and put food on the table relatively effortlessly, she felt what it was like to struggle do to so all the more acutely. Her perceptiveness and candor did a great deal to enrich the education of the medical students who had the opportunity to meet her.

And because of her longevity, many students had just this opportunity. Most palliative care patients actually die within a few months or years, limiting the number of students who can learn from their experience. In Pam's case, however, the patient survived for many years, and she was able to share her experience with students year after year. The vast majority of students who had the opportunity to meet with Pam did not choose to specialize in palliative care, but all went onward into their careers with an enhanced understanding of what it is like to be poor and dying.

Of course, the stories of Pam many other such patients have also helped to inspire students and residents like Carrie and Colleen to pursue careers in palliative medicine. These learners have recognized the important difference palliative medicine can make for patients and families, as well as the difference it can make for those who practice it. They have discovered the deep sense of purpose and fulfillment that can come from caring for the dying, and thanks in large part to the fact that the palliative care program is based at the safety-net hospital, they also gain a deeper insight into the plight of the poor.

SUMMARY

Palliative care physicians enjoy the opportunity to make a special kind of difference in the lives of patients, families, and communities. Through their experiences in the palliative care program at the safety-net hospital, many medical students and residents have learned to their surprise that the dying poor sometimes have access to better care than the dying rich do.

In recent years, a wealthy couple with a long history of philanthropy in the local community had learned enough about the palliative care program at the safety-net hospital to realize that they wanted their care to be directed by that team of palliative care professionals. In their minds, receiving the best care money could buy at a more luxurious hospital would not be enough, so they sought the best end-of-life care available, regardless of price. And they received the kind of care they hoped for. In the last decade of their lives, and despite advanced age and significant medical problems, together the two of them spent a total of one night in the hospital. They both died at home, with their family.

There is deep satisfaction in knowing that the experiences of dying patients and their families, the medical profession, and the healthcare system have moved a long way from the early days of palliative care. In the words of Susan Block:

> We've gotten ourselves a real field of palliative care and we are making things happen in that field. In some ways, we succeeded beyond our wildest dreams. In medicine today, our textbooks are different, teaching is different, the scientific literature is different. The field really is dramatically different than it was when we started.[4]

Today, the dying poor are not only receiving better care sometimes—as this story illustrates, they are also playing an important role in helping to illuminate what such care really looks like, and their experiences are helping to improve the care of dying patients in their community and throughout the world.

REFERENCES

1. Foley K. An open letter to the grantmaking community. In *Transforming the culture of dying*. New York: Open Society Institute; 2004:11.
2. Block S. Quoted in: *Transforming the culture of dying*. New York: Open Society Institute 2004:17.
3. Payne R. Quoted in: *Transforming the culture of dying*. New York: Open Society Institute 2004:51.
4. Block S. Quoted in: *Transforming the culture of dying*. New York: Open Society Institute 2004:65.

10

NOTES FROM THE TRENCHES ON SOCIAL INJUSTICE: RACE, CLASS, AND HEALTH DISPARITY

F. Amos Bailey

Too many die prematurely from preventable illnesses. Lucille Angel, J. W., and Cowboy, for example, had been smokers for most of their adult life. They died early in life.

The link between tobacco and death, particularly cigarettes, had become clear in the 1950s, and, by 1964, the evidence was robust enough for the Surgeon General to warn the public of the risk. In 1971, President Nixon announced the War on Cancer, and the National Cancer Institute (NCI) was founded. While there has been progress made in developing treatments for treating cancers (most notably in children), the impact of treatment on many cancers has been modest. Although the cancers that are attributable to tobacco use account for well less than half of the total cancers diagnosed each year, those cancers are more lethal, and at least half of cancer mortality is related to tobacco use. Working to reduce the rates of tobacco use and therefore prevent lung cancer and many other malignancies would clearly make the most sense from a public health approach. However, efforts that have been made to prevent the initiation of smoking and encourage smokers to quit have been stymied at almost every turn. And this is especially true in the context of urban poverty.

Public and policy decisions related to smoking cessation/prevention are an example of social injustice and unethical social practice. Those who were economically empowered and well connected politically worked to undercut and change the focus of NCI toward treatment rather than prevention. Well-funded tobacco lobbies fought a hard battle against efforts to reduce the extent of smoking through tax increases. After all, additional taxes would push up the cost of tobacco and threaten profits. Pharmaceutical companies also benefit from developing relatively ineffective medications for treatment of various cancers and then charging a high price for them. Why did Lucille in particular smoke? In part, it was a personal decision perhaps, but, also her community (black) and gender (women) were particularly targeted to begin smoking. Wellness and prevention are generally not supported adequately in our healthcare systems, and this support is even more of a rarity among lower socioeconomic classes. And the pleasure of smoking is an antidote to the stress and hardship of poverty, which makes it an attractive behavior for many seeking a bit of refuge.

> While they speak matter-of-factly about their deprivations in the rural South, they are almost uniformly grateful that they had food on the table.

Governmental policies that focus more on curing than on preventing cancer has had a heavy effect on poor and minority populations, such as African Americans. These groups smoked and continue to smoke at a much higher rate than the general population, and there is clear correlation between socioeconomic class and smoking rates. The tax base and benefits of large corporations were repeatedly placed above public health and well-being throughout much of America's history. Lucille and many others like her generally start smoking at a young age. She quit when her physicians told her to. This is when she was first diagnosed with laryngeal cancer; in many ways, it was too late. She went on to tragically have a stroke and then was diagnosed with lung cancer, from which she would ultimately die at a relatively young age.

So, although there is an increase in average life expectancy in the United States, the gains are quite unevenly distributed. The fact of the matter is that lower socioeconomic classes and minorities have had very modest to no increase in life-expectancy, in part due to risky health behaviors such as smoking.

While the percentage of smokers among all groups has declined throughout the country, there is much work that could be done to specifically reduce the use of tobacco among economic and racial minorities. While it is well known that tobacco use causes serious health problems, apparently that knowledge is not enough to address the problem. It would seem appropriate to work more intensely with members of these communities to develop strategies and programs to reduce the numbers of young people who begin smoking and help those who are smoking to quit successfully. With the recognition of the problem of "food deserts," the lack of stores that sell healthy foods as opposed to overpriced corner stores that specialize in junk food, efforts are being made to build a better infrastructure that supports healthier choices. One such example is that some drugstores and other establishments have quit selling tobacco or are making commitments to do so. Easy supply is important in the development of unhealthy habits, as smokers almost always begin their habit between the ages of 15 and 25. In this regard, it is critical for programs to locate health-promotion initiatives in local communities and to target young members of the communities. This effort might include schools, community centers, or churches and other faith congregations. It is also important to actively involve the lived example of role-model community members to help young people through their "youthful" decision-making during the most critical time for them, so they may stay free from tobacco use and go on to become lifelong nonsmokers. For those who have started smoking, stopping is difficult, but counseling and medications that could be available through community health clinics can make a difference. Using peer community counselors and health promotion with navigators should be considered. Navigators are being deployed in chronic and serious illnesses, but looking upstream for lifestyle modification is an important step to take to improve the health of the community.

In this regard, the prevalence of early death and unhealthy behaviors like those experienced by Cowboy, Mrs. Black, J. W., Mrs. Angel, Joe Noble, and so many others who live in poverty represents a failure of population health and is reflective of a persistent presence of inequity and injustice throughout American society. It also, sadly enough, reveals a lack of commitment and interest by the broader society to improve the health status of those who live at the margins of society.

RURAL POOR VERSUS URBAN POOR: DIFFERING FORMS OF THE SAME STRUGGLE

Living in poverty is always difficult, exhausting, and ultimately, dangerous. While going through the dying process in Northern and Midwestern cities, many urban poor reflect on their rural upbringing. They often do so with great enthusiasm. While they speak matter-of-factly about their deprivations in the rural South, they are almost uniformly grateful that they had food on the table. The context of rural poverty and its associated lack of opportunity and services, such as education and healthcare, led many to seek greater opportunity by moving to the cities. While this migration pattern goes on around the world, it was a particularly defining characteristic of the transition of American life throughout the second half of the twentieth century with respect to African Americans. In large numbers they migrated northward in the hope of a better life. Once there, however, they encountered new challenges that were connected to race and impoverishment and which were tethered to the dynamics of the urban environment.

There are some advantages to living in a rural setting. In the country, there is room for large gardens or small farms to supplement diet with subsistence-style farming. Also, there is the possibility to fish, hunt, or live off the land. Even heat for the house might come from the forest with basically free firewood. For the urban poor, however, routes to partial self-sufficiency are limited. While drug use/abuse is a plague in both rural and urban settings, addiction and drug dealing are more common in poorer pockets of our cities.

Joleen, Lucille Angel's youngest daughter, is involved in the drug culture, and this causes great emotional distress for Lucille as well as financial hardship. Lucille struggles to help her daughter and granddaughter, even while struggling with her own terminal illness. She takes them in and uses her own meager financial resources and Social Security Disability to support them all. She graciously states that she can make things stretch for them all. However, Joleen's attempt at sobriety is short-lived and mostly dependent on her staying at her mother's side to avoid temptation. She ultimately is tempted back to a street life and ultimately steals from Lucille when she is cashing her check. This breach in trust leads to a major rupture in their relationship and also Joleen's relationship with her sisters. Ultimately, they reconcile at the very end of Mrs. Angel's life, and Joleen shares the task of sitting in vigil with her mother with her sisters.

The point that Lucille's narrative drives homes, as do all of those presented in *Dancing with Broken Bones*, is that the harm of poverty is real and afflicts and injures both individuals and families in profound ways.

Many African Americans mistrust hospice because they view it as a means of denying services.

Addiction is often a barrier to symptom control in the home. If the patient or family has a history of substance abuse disorders, then safely using opioids for pain relief may be difficult. This issue looms even larger with growing awareness of the opioid abuse and addiction problems inflicting widespread damage on young people throughout the nation. In home hospice, strong opioids like liquid morphine and other medications have the potential for diversion from intended use, and this may give providers pause in utilizing these drugs for pain control. At the same time, these medicines must be available to patients to ease their suffering. Inasmuch as abuse of prescription pain medication is now recognized as a public health crisis, stricter controls are being put on these medications, and physicians may be less willing to prescribe them. While increase in awareness of the problem may reduce their illicit use, it also is also likely to make access difficult for palliative care patients who need medications even before entering a hospice program. It may very well be that, despite the good intentions of crafting greater controls around opioid prescribing to address the addiction crisis, patients may be left without adequate pain control as the pendulum swings from aggressive pain management strategies to a more-restricted approach. Even home hospice programs are seeing tighter controls, and it is not just people in poor and minority communities that will bear the brunt of these restrictions. However, the poor and marginalized may come under more scrutiny by providers due to unconscious biases and stereotyping. To be sure, there are real issues surrounding safety in a home with controlled substances. The very presence of the drugs can lead to abuse or diversion of medication intended for patients. I have visited homes were the patient has been sleeping with the medication in the bed with them to safeguard it. Providers are now being required to implement Risk Evaluation and Mitigation Strategies (REMS) for patient safety and hopefully public safety in response to the problem.

The response to the opioid crisis is legitimate. But raging pain and unrelieved suffering is never an acceptable option. So, it is critical that the needs of patients near the end of life not get lost in the burgeoning medical and societal interest in regulating the use of opioids.

In addition to the issue of diversion, fears of addiction or danger from pain medicine, particularly morphine, are barriers to pain treatment and relief. In relating the story of the death of her husband Mike, Lucille reports that he was in terrible pain from his cancer. He resisted taking the morphine that had been stationed in the home. He would turn to prayer and distraction to try to deal with his pain, rather than relying on the medicine. Lucille saw the great suffering that he had experienced, and almost certainly his suffering was particularly frightening as it prefigured what would happen to her in the not-so-distant future. Dramatically she recounts how, after Mike died, she threw the medication into the toilet in anger and frustration at his suffering and the suffering that drug addiction could bring.

Pain management for cancer is a frustrating problem. There is, in fact, good evidence that most patients with cancer pain, more than 90%, could have good pain control with the oral opioids that are currently available. However, the problem of pain control is more of a health services delivery issue than a need for new pharmaceutical agents. The barriers for adequate pain control at the end of life are present for all; however, the poor and minority groups have more difficulty overcoming the barriers. As mentioned earlier, resistance to using adequate opioids for pain control can be due to opiophobia of both patients and caregivers. Morphine is particularly feared because it is a medicine that is often given near death and is incorrectly thought to actually cause death, and this leads patients and families to underdose. The result is poor pain control that certainly negatively impacts quality of life and often quantity of life.

Other barriers can include the cost of pain medication, although after Lucille was referred to hospice, this would not be an issue as hospice pays for the medication. In addition, patients often get inadequate dosing from physicians who often have not been adequately trained in pain management. Federal and state laws that require frequent travel to the doctor to obtain a new prescription can become a barrier for many patients as they become weaker and it is more difficult to travel, as well as to absorb the cost of the travel. Many times patients pay friends and neighbors to drive them to medical appointments, adding to the financial and practical barriers. Finally, in general, pharmacies in low-income neighborhoods often do not stock commonly-needed opioids for cancer pain and for symptom management from all types of illnesses at the end of life. Pharmacies may have legitimate concerns that stocking these medications will make them targets for robberies. That is understandable, but the consequence is that patients in these areas may be underserved.

Home hospice is a program that can help overcome most of the barriers to pain control at the end of life. The home hospice program can provide education for both patients and caregivers that can help them assess and treat pain safely and effectively. In addition, fears about availability and proper use of opioids can be eased by the hospice nurse who serves as an advocate and ensures that the pain medication is titrated, present in the home, and does not run out at a critical time. However, not all patients are referred to home hospice. In fact most are not. For those who are referred it is often so late in the disease course that it is a fairly short stay. And the rates of home hospice use in minority communities have been historically low compared to other groups.

Barriers to enrolling minority patients into hospice are myriad. However, some issues are not found only in minority populations, but are also problems with hospice in general. One issue is the "terrible choice" of hospice care. This refers to the fact that, in almost all settings, the patient, in order to enroll in hospice care, must forgo other forms of treatment for the primary diagnosis. This is often viewed as an obstacle that leads to late referral. Ideally, hospice care would be available on basis of need, not this "forced choice." Ironically, in our work at the Balm of Gilead at Cooper Green Hospital in Birmingham, Alabama, the lack of insurance among the poor allowed us more flexibility in treatment plans, and we often continued some disease-modifying treatments while transitioning to home hospice care. Later in my work at the VA in Birmingham's Safe Harbor program, we allowed veterans to continue to try disease-focused treatment and simultaneously use home hospice to support them. Some would continue treatment throughout the course of their illness, and others would ultimately decide that the burden was greater than the benefit. However, this open-access approach to hospice care meets the needs and preferences of patients better.

Hospice and palliative care providers often overvalue quality of life and don't put enough value on quantity. You can't have quality with no quantity. This mismatch in expectations is an ongoing cultural-competency issue. Many African Americans mistrust hospice because they view it as a means of denying services because of the requirement that active, curative treatment be stopped. When working with the Balm of Gilead, the Birmingham Area Hospice, which was formed in the health department, had minority staff who were integrated into the hospital-based palliative care team. They were not so rigid about mixing hospice support and ongoing medical treatment. As we sought to develop of process for combining ongoing treatment with supportive care in the VA system, we discovered that there was the need for educating home hospice agencies that some veterans may be comfortable being "traditional" hospice patients and forgo all curative treatment. But others would be best served by being offered the choice to continue receiving active treatment while enrolled in hospice. Clearly, this approach flies in the face of the traditional model of hospice care and took some getting used to. Some nurses and agencies could be flexible around this, while others could not. This way of expanding choices near the end of life is important for us to consider, as the model provides an opportunity to reshape the delivery of hospice care in a way that would be more trusted and valued by minority communities.

> Many urban poor see themselves as survivors.

Mistrust of the healthcare system is confounded by ongoing health disparities in access and outcomes. Certainly it is not difficult to understand how home hospice and palliative care may be viewed as another way to deny access to services and helpful care for those living at the margins. In addition, when hospice and palliative care programs promote themselves as ways to save healthcare dollars, it is easy to understand how a person having lived at the margins throughout life might feel that the cost savings are coming at his or her expense. So, in summary, the "terrible-choice problem," lack of open-access hospice care, and concern that healthcare cost savings will be on the backs of the neediest are both perceived and real issues that undermine the effectiveness of care near the end of life for vulnerable populations (Figure 10.1).

Even beyond class and racial considerations, not all terminally ill patients will accept hospice care, as ours is a death-defying society. While these patients would in fact be eligible for hospice admission based on their prognosis, their refusal to enter into hospice leaves them with less-than-optimal care and unfulfilled needs. Their care would be improved from additional support that provided supportive services, similar to hospice but without the regulatory restrictions, provided in the home. This type of care can also be integrated into clinics and acute care hospitals as part of palliative care consultation services. Three randomized control trials (RCTs) of early integration of palliative care into cancer care demonstrated improvement in survival and control of symptoms. In 2010, Temel and colleagues reported in the *New England Journal of Medicine* that the impact of palliative care services, provided at the time of diagnosis for patients with stage 4 lung cancer (the same condition Lucille Angel and Cowboy died of), demonstrated that pain control and symptomatic depression were much less common in patients who received palliative and supportive care from the time of diagnosis onward. Even more startling was that survival was on average 12 weeks longer in the group that received palliative care services (in conjunction with standard treatment) from the time of diagnosis.

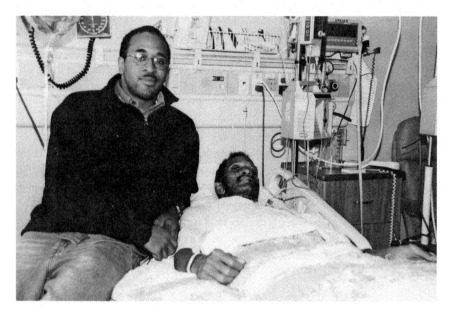

FIGURE 10.1 Compassionate care requires understanding who the patient is as a person.

An essential take-home point is that better pain and symptom control results in increased survival as well as improved quality of life; in fact, the increase in length of survival is tied to improved quality of life. Since then, Bakitis and colleagues and Zimmerman and colleagues have published RCTs of early palliative care interventions delivered in clinic, by phone, and by interprofessional teams that demonstrated improved symptoms, quality of life, and other patient-centered outcomes. Thus, the issue going forward is to devise ways of expanding access to palliative care services to more patients. If palliative care was a drug or treatment as opposed to a service it would seem likely that its widespread adoption by the healthcare system would be readily embraced.

One approach could be to base eligibility for palliative care services, including hospice care, on functional status and/or diagnosis rather than on prognosis. Prognosis is difficult to predict, and many patients need and could benefit from palliative care services long before they are referred and/or are eligible. Another possible intervention is to provide open-access hospice care, in which patients can access hospice and chemotherapy or other disease-modifying treatments simultaneously. Some private healthcare plans have adopted programs for patients who need palliative care services but do not need or desire the services of a hospice program. Innovative programs such as consult services, outpatient clinics, and home-based primary care programs are being pioneered in numerous healthcare systems. The limiting factor for these programs may be the difficulty of funding these services in a fee-for-services environment, since some of the more successful programs have been pioneered in the VA and health maintenance organizations (HMOs), which have a capitated reimbursement system that is more open to these kinds of health service innovations. A third barrier is likely to be the limited workforce of physicians and mid-level providers available to meet the need for increased palliative care services or even greater length of stay in hospice, if the demand were there.

COMMUNICATIONS

One of the recurrent themes in *Dancing with Broken Bones* is the apparent misunderstandings patients have regarding their illnesses. Mrs. Angel didn't seem to understand whether her cancer was primary lung cancer or recurrence of a laryngeal cancer. J. W. lived with misunderstanding that his "cancer was low," and Mr. Wheeler believed the deception that he was in remission, ultimately leading him to greater mistrust and despair. These misunderstandings often provoke anger and resentment and impact patient and family trust in the healthcare system as a whole.

In part, the issue may be that patients and families desire to hear a story or narrative that is different from what their physicians are trying to communicate. Denial can be a useful coping mechanism, and certainly hope and optimism are important in facing illness. Many urban poor see themselves as survivors. Mrs. Angel, for instance, had been a survivor of physical abuse by her first husband, poverty, discrimination through her life, and ultimately of her first cancer. Why should she not be a survivor now? J. W. survived and got along despite the odds being stacked against him. So why should he not beat his cancer? And Mr. Wheeler hoped for a miracle. So, why should it not be happening with his treatment?

> Ultimately, it is the work of providers to help patients and families understand which goals are reasonable and achievable and which ones are most important.

While physicians have been shown to be overly optimistic in their prognostications and communication, patients hear and interpret what they want as well, as did both Mr. and Mrs. Wheeler. Weeks and colleagues reported in the *New England Journal of Medicine* that about 75% of patients with stage 4 lung and colon cancers, which are incurable, thought that the chemotherapy that they were receiving had the potential to cure their own cancer. This "Lake Woebegone effect" may be hardwired into us, especially in a culture that is aversive to and fearful of death.

However, cultural competency and basic communication skills about difficult situations can be taught and learned by physicians in training. Programs such as Oncotalk are training more oncologists in basic communication skills. Often these programs use a variation on Ask-Tell-Ask in which the patient is asked to tell the healthcare provider their understanding of their illness, then the clinician corrects and expands on the patient's understanding, and then finally asks the patient to repeat back to the clinician the new information that was shared.

Basic concepts such as not using medical jargon, avoiding euphemisms, and ensuring that patients understand the purpose and intent of treatment, curative or palliative, is important in building a provider–patient alliance. It is important to maintain hope, but not false hope. Lucille was bitterly disappointed when she found that her cancer was progressing despite chemotherapy, and the illusion that her treatments were potentially curative could not be maintained. Mr. Wheeler was bitterly disillusioned. And J. W. was left in a state of confusion and uncertainty. Each were let down not because of a lack of caring among providers but because of an absence of comfort and proficiency.

Having a goals-of-care conversation with patients and families is an important skill that healthcare providers need to learn in order to be effective when meeting the complex needs of their patients. This is more than using a six-step system to share bad news or the Ask-Tell-Ask techniques. These tools are important, but not sufficient to meet the need. In a goals-of-care conversation, the provider should ask the patient to share with the team what their hopes and dreams are for their care and for their life. People naturally can still have a desire for the cancer to go away or their dementia to resolve, even when they know this is something that is unlikely to happen. Ultimately, it is the work of providers to help patients and families understand which goals are reasonable and achievable and which ones are most important. Invariably there will be tradeoffs, and some goals will take priority over others. Goals-of-care/goals-of-life discussions are crucial and underutilized. Cultural-competency issues are critical, as the values of the patient and family must lead this conversation and be the basis for developing specific goals of care, and will do so in ways that reflect the uniqueness of the individual and his or her background. But this requires cultural competency, or, as Dr. Moller phrases it, cultural humility on the part of providers. In this regard, it is important to train providers to check their own biases and cultural preferences and to be honest but supportive throughout their relationship with patients and families.

> There is great underuse and underdevelopment of hospice and palliative care, especially for vulnerable populations.

One of the goals of palliative care is to always have a positive plan of what can be done to improve quality of living for both patients and families facing serious and life-limiting illness. One of the important tools is reframing the meaning and parameters of hope. Lucille, again for purposes of illustration, can hope for a cure for her lung cancer but may understand that her doctors can't achieve that for her. She can work with her healthcare team to have good symptom control and work with her family to be at home, rather than in a hospital. She can hope to bring her daughters together, help them, teach them, remember, and be remembered. Her hope is not just to live longer, but to live on in the life and memory of her children and all that she touched.

She wanted to continue to give back even unto the end of her life. Planning her own funeral, reuniting her family, and being part of a project that would lead to Dr. Moller's writing a book that would be in part about her experience, were ways of remaining empowered. Lucille continued to make a contribution and transcend her own death in the legacy that she built while dying.

RELIGION: STRENGTH AND WEAKNESS AT THE END OF LIFE

Many African Americans are religious men and women. Lucille Angel was a spiritual woman, as were Mrs. Black and Annie. J. W., despite his imperfections, was profoundly spiritual and his faith in a loving God gave him great sustenance. While individual people can be spiritual, religious, or both, many African Americans have been raised in the

African-American Baptist tradition. This tradition places great emphasis on having a personal relationship with Jesus. This relationship is often tested throughout the lives of the urban poor and especially in the last months of life, when struggles of living in poverty are exacerbated by the sufferings surrounding the experience of dying. Church plays an important part in their lives, and faith provides meaning and purpose to their suffering in life and throughout dying. One of the enduring themes in this religious tradition is deliverance from oppression and, ultimately, empowerment.

Many of the rituals of the black church are about deliverance. "Swing Low, Sweet Chariot" is a coded expression for deliverance from slavery. "We Shall Overcome" became an anthem a hundred years later for deliverance from racism during the Civil Rights movement. Lucille looked for and ultimately did find deliverance from her abusive husband in her church. After she was divorced, she married Mike, who was by all accounts a wonderful husband to her. Mike and Lucille had been very active in their church, but with his illness and ultimately death, and then Lucille's own cancer diagnosis, they were not able to remain active in that community. As is often the case when people become ill and are no longer able to participate in the communal life of their faith, congregational support fell away. Mrs. Brown recaptured that support by telephone connection to a prayer community. Annie sought it in her own prayerful ways. Some faith communities may have special ministries of the clergy and lay members to visit the sick and shut-ins. However, it usually takes a formal organizational commitment and leadership to maintain these kinds of services, and not all faith communities have those in place. Many inner-city faith communities are underresourced and lack the capacity to consistently tend to the sick and dying in their homes.

Since they are often an important resource and institution, it is important to nurture faith communities' capacity to reach out and maintain connections to those who are most in need. Some may be too small to support these kinds of programs alone. But if organized into groups, they can share the responsibility of providing for those in need in the community, with both practical and spiritual support.

There are several examples of programs to strengthen the religious community's support of their community's health. One is Stephen's Ministry, which trains committed lay religious individuals to be a source of support for the sick and is modeled on St. Stephen, who was martyred for his faith and work. Stephen's Ministry is a lay caregiving ministry that supplements pastoral care. The program teaches lay persons to provide one-on-one care for individuals who need and are receptive to this kind of support. The confidential caregiver and care-receiver relationship, usually conducted by weekly visits, may continue for months or years. Other programs include Parish Nursing and Care Team Networks. Care Teams are organized and trained to support a community member in need, while Parish Nurses work as health resources to their congregations. All of these kinds of programs are volunteer-based and are difficult to maintain, even in well-resourced congregations. So, the challenges in the context of urban poverty are even greater. Many religious communities serving poorer neighborhoods are overwhelmed by the needs of their congregations, and regrettably, the needs of the terminally ill may receive far less attention than would be optimal.

Although deliverance and a personal relationship with a loving God are important theological concepts for believers, sometimes doubt and questioning arise. While Ms.

Annie Dickens never wavered in expressing her faith, Mrs. Angel shared her doubts, anger, and associated shame with Dr. Moller. Rabbi Kushner wrote a book called *When Bad Things Happen to Good People,* which was in part about his experience of having a child who died from progeria. It is reported that more than one person had asked him why he did not write *Why Bad Things Happen to Good People.* He said, "The book would be very short; I don't know." In fact, this was the question that Lucille struggled with: Why was this happening to her? How would she be delivered from this illness? How could this be the work of a loving God? Why did she not always feel the presence of God? There are in fact no definitive answers to these questions, but it is an understandable part of the human condition that anyone facing such trials would ask these kinds of questions. She longed for her minister to come see her to talk with her, yet he didn't come during her time of existential and spiritual struggle. Instead, she worked these things out in her own mind and in her conversations with Dr. Moller. When finally the minister did come, it was only for a few minutes of prayer. Being unconscious at the time, she never even knew he had finally arrived at her bedside.

Many ministers in the Southern Protestant traditions have little or no formal theological training or education. They are called to ministry and are often self-taught. However, even clergy who have gone to seminary training often find it difficult and uncomfortable to counsel their own congregation members when they are facing a terminal illness. Chaplains, who have been through a clinical pastoral-education program, are more likely to have developed skills to support people in their own search for spiritual comfort and to be at peace while dying. Lucille, ultimately, seemed to make peace with her illness and her coming death in conversations with Dr. Moller, both an outsider and an insider with whom she could feel more comfortable sharing her fears, doubts, and anger with God. This was something that she probably did not feel comfortable sharing with her family and even with her minister, if he had come to see her.

Clearly there is much room for education, training, and programmatic development to help clergy, communities of faith, and their lay members be better equipped to meet the needs of those in the community who are struggling in the throes of dying.

FINAL THOUGHTS

The work of our group at the Balm of Gilead was "organic" palliative and hospice care that grew out of our attempt to provide standard medical care for cancer patients and for those with HIV/AIDS. From our work with home-hospice programs, we saw how patients who were discharged from the hospital thrived physically, as well as psychosocially and spiritually. The goal was to provide this opportunity for healing, not to be confused with being cured, for all of our seriously-ill patients; not just those in the last days or weeks of life.

The goal was to make the hospital and clinic more like the gold standard of care that we observed in the home for hospice patients, including those who were still actively being treated for their disease. We sought a different approach than forcing patients into the "terrible choice" of hospice care when they were not ready to make "that decision." We found that patients and families began to trust us when we listened to their priorities and when we offered them a broader range of treatment options. So, for example, a very sick person could come to our unit and begin very simple, symptom-focused treatment, and after a few days they would stabilize. At this point they may ask, "Can we do this at home?" And our response would be, "Yes! Let's work on this together to show you how this might be done." We always assured them that the Balm of Gilead would remain a safe place for them to return to if things got too difficult at home.

The director of the Birmingham VA Medical Center noticed what we were doing at Cooper Green Hospital with the Balm of Gilead and invited us to implement this approach with their patients. This is when and where we started Safe Harbor. Both the Balm of Gilead and Safe Harbor strove for early integration of palliative care into all possible settings and diseases. We actively, in this model, sought to relieve patients and families of the burden of having to make the "terrible choice" of hospice care when they were not ready to do so.

Nationally there is great underuse and underdevelopment of palliative and hospice care, especially for vulnerable populations. Very few patients actively seek these services on their own. Instead, they are dependent on whatever the culture of care at a particular hospital is, or even the predispositions of individual providers. The patients who are at the core of this book were constrained by the economics of where they received care. Ironically, if one had the "misfortune" to be reliant on the safety-net services of Cooper Green Hospital, one could expect to be routinely referred to palliative care if necessary. The same was true for the patients in *Dancing with Broken Bones*, as they were being cared for in a hospital with an award-winning palliative care program. But not all essential, safety-net hospitals have such fully-developed programs, the result of which is that the quality of end-of-life care for the urban poor is widely inconsistent.

Home-hospice services can provide comfort, peace, and reconciliation. It is true, at least theoretically, that hospice care is available to a vast majority of Americans. The quality, however, may be variable. Just as urgent a problem is that timely referral is often variable and many times lacking. Because of late referral and mistrust of hospice among the poor and racial minorities, there are striking deficiencies in care for this population. Work needs to be done in educating providers and the broader community about this problem.

The stories in *Dancing with Broken Bones* remind us that, while we treat diseases and seek to relieve distressing symptoms, we also care for people. Patients are far more than their illnesses. In order to provide comprehensive, person-centered care, it is important to respect the utter uniqueness of each patient as an individual. This requires that physicians and other healthcare professionals not only learn the science of medical treatment, they must learn the art of caring. This requires getting to know patients. And that requires time: time that may not be available in the busy clinical pace of the hospital and under economic pressures to see large numbers of patients. It also requires that providers stretch themselves beyond the comfort zone of clinical focus. This may mean understanding the ways and practices of different cultures. It means guarding against our own prejudices and unconscious biases. While these can be very difficult tasks, they are imperative if we are to improve quality of and access to care. This may require that we meet patients and families as human being to human being, sometimes across a racial and economic divide, and muster the courage and commitment to inquire about their lives, who they are, and what is important to them in life, illness, and dying.

If we commit to deepening our commitment to the underserved and developing our own skills in cultural humility, we will make great strides in advancing the cause of caring for the most vulnerable in a way that will actualize the hopeful message of a time-honored African-American spiritual:

> There is balm in Gilead,
> To make the wounded whole.

11

NOTES FROM THE TRENCHES IN THE SHADOWS: LIVING, DYING, AND CARING AT THE MARGINS

Kimberly Curseen and Tammie E. Quest

What does it mean to care for a person? The word *caring*, as an adjective, is defined as "displaying kindness and concern for others." As a noun, it means the work or practice of looking after those who are unable to care for themselves, especially the sick and the elderly. In medicine, the focus on caring for others is a primary and important guiding principle. However, in today's society, there exist numerous barriers for those in the medical profession to provide optimal care for patients who live at the margins of society. This is due in part to society's social structure, which more often than not places limits and conditions on the distribution of its resources. Whenever a society assigns and grades status to individuals based upon their position and ability to contribute, life becomes difficult for those who are unable to achieve the status norms. Those who suffer with illnesses that interfere with the ability to make conventional contributions (such as adding wealth and products and contributing productively) are blocked from optimizing and fully reaping the benefits of society. While many people with physical limitations have made and will continue to make tremendous contributions to society, their ability to contribute, as well as the contributions they have made, may not be fully recognized. In the context of access to medical care, patients belonging to populations that may be marginalized have a particularly difficult time navigating the healthcare system.[1]

There is growing research focusing on how poverty and low socioeconomic status commingle with race in influencing health status. Health insurance coverage and access to healthcare are impacted by race and socioeconomic status, all of which are relevant to health outcomes. For providers in the trenches who care for patients at the margins, the dilemma is how to provide quality care within the limitations of our current healthcare system—a system that is not fully designed to meet a majority of the needs of this patient population.[2] When providing care for these patients, medical providers must determine not only what is *medically appropriate* for their patients, but also what is *medically possible,* given the existing economic and healthcare constraints for this patient population. With respect to medical providers, there may be barriers resulting from the providers' lack of familiarity with cultural differences and/or the providers' ability to overcome any biases, implicit and explicit, as well as their willingness to develop empathy for the population they are choosing to serve. Medical providers have to overcome their own implicit bias when caring for a patient who has been marginalized and who is often pejoratively judged through pre-existing stereotypes. In many cases, providers may not even consciously be aware of the biases they have. But, nonetheless the consequence of unconscious stereotypes is real for patients and includes the reinforcing of discriminatory attitudes and practices which erect barriers to healthcare for these populations. For this reason, it is important for medical providers to be self-aware of how implicit bias may be affecting their decision-making and interaction with patients. Even healthcare professionals who routinely work with marginalized populations can be affected by implicit bias, which is why self-awareness and education in this area is important for everyone.[3]

The importance of addressing healthcare disparities has been recognized on the national level. The US Department of Health and Human Services' (DHHS) Office of Minority Health has developed programs at the healthcare system and community levels to educate and promote cultural competency. Much of the healthcare disparity research focuses on race and ethnicity, but the need for education and research stretches beyond these narrow categories.[4] For example, in a recent review article, it was stated that 3.5% of Americans identify themselves as lesbian, gay, or bisexual, and 0.3% identify as transgender (LGBT). This means that there are 9 million people in this group. LGBT youth are at increased risk for depression/anxiety, substance abuse, social mistreatment, isolation, suicide, and other health comorbidities. In addition, these Americans often receive poorer quality care that is a direct result of the lack education on how to appropriately meet their unique needs. People who live at the margins can also be the victims of direct and institutional bias as well as unconscious negative stereotyping, both of which serve to exacerbate their marginalization. In short, individuals who are not part of the mainstream such as criminal offenders, the mentally or physically disabled, the poor, or sufferers of addiction are a part of a group of people who live at the fringes of society.[5,6] And as such they are often viewed and treated differently from those who pass the test of "social normalcy."

Providers who care for those patients who face the greatest challenges in life can find their work very rewarding, as caring for the "least among us" is one of the highest forms of service to humanity. But special skills and understandings are essential if the care of patients is to be optimized. Thus, for those providers who serve in the front-line trenches and provide care for marginalized populations, it is important that practical mentorship, support, and guidance be available. With proper resources and development of skills in culturally-competent care in serving diverse and vulnerable populations, providers can step beyond merely identifying problems and attend to how they can be successfully resolved.

The desire to be helpful and to care for people in need is a driving force for many who enter the medical profession. However, providers who repeatedly encounter barriers that interfere with the mission of providing quality healthcare run the risk of experiencing despair and burnout over time.[4,7] The inability to both understand these barriers and develop strategies to overcome and/or manage them can erode a provider's empathy over time. They often feel overwhelmed by the enormous challenges presented by marginalized patients and are haunted by concern that they might making a sustainable difference in their lives. They can be frustrated by poor decisions patients make, including a lack of adherence to treatment. This is where cultural awareness is brought into play. It helps advance appreciation of the difficulties and obstacles patients face and why they behave as they do. It serves to generate compassionate understandings about people who are clearly different from us and that is an essential foundation for the development of empathy. Ultimately, empathy is paramount in providing quality care for patients living at our society's margins,[8] but it is a professional quality and encompasses a set of skills that must be actively mastered.

IN THE TRENCHES: STANDING IN SOLIDARITY WITH ANOTHER

What does it mean to be "in the trenches?" A trench is a narrow ditch dug by troops to provide a place of shelter from enemy fire. *Trench* in the archaic sense of the word means "to border on or encroach on." Defining this is important because, when we speak of being in the trenches, it implies that we are not only close to the patient, but that we are also fighting both with and for the patient against whatever barriers may exist. Being in the trenches implies that there is teamwork between provider and patient in pursuit of common goals, which defines collaborative decision-making in a pure sense. Being *entrenched* with someone also implies that there is a mutual understanding between both parties. This understanding also requires that both provider and patient guard against any outside stressors that might inhibit the patient in reaching their goals.

There is sacrifice embedded in the concept of being entrenched, which could pose challenges to the concept of boundaries between provider and patient, as the sacrifice may not be exclusively professional but spill over into the realm of the personal. The extent to which providers may be willing to sacrifice in becoming entrenched with their patients will determine the level of comfort they will experience in doing so.[9]

When considering the concept of becoming entrenched, providers should reflect on the following questions: (1) What does it mean to fight for a patient? (2) What is my responsibility, and how far is too far to go in order to help a patient? (3) What am I willing to sacrifice both professionally and personally? These are the difficult questions that providers who work in the trenches are faced with daily. Often they are challenged to navigate their daily tasks without a professional roadmap to guide them, and they must deal with the complexity that results from shifting patient needs, societal norms, and personal priorities and values on their own.

The following composites of patient profiles illustrate, in a practical way, some of the many issues faced by providers who work in the trenches while serving their patients.

LIVING AT THE MARGINS

Ms. D lived in a shotgun-style house in what is considered the "poor side of town." Her small house had a kitchen in the back and bedroom in the front, which had to be entered and walked through in order to reach any of the other rooms. Ms. D, in trying to manage her health problems, called a home-based medical program seeking in-home medical care and personal care as well. She had Medicaid for insurance and was not elderly. People under the age of 65 usually qualify for Medicaid in most states if they are receiving Supplemental Social Security income (SSI) or their income is below the federal poverty level. Typically, Medicaid does not require that any of their personal income be diverted for skilled-need care that is delivered in the home, as can be case with the elderly in facilities for long-term care. This means she might qualify for in-home, community-care programs which could be very helpful to her both economically and healthwise. But it is also likely that she, and others like her, might not even be aware of this resource being available. Despite the benefit that would accrue for her, it is also important to note that Medicaid for disabled, elder folk living at home does not cover basic living costs such as room and board.[10] Those needs would have to be supported in other ways.

Ms. D's situation was rather dire. She was bed-bound and morbidly obese. She suffered with severe pain in her knees, which was exacerbated by her obesity. Ms. D also had a history of lupus, deep venous thrombosis, heart failure, and was pre-diabetic. (Like so many poor she endured excess morbidity.) She had a doctor but was no longer able to keep her routine appointments, and her doctor's office would no longer fill her medications. If she had to attend a doctor's appointment, she required an ambulance, which was painful both emotionally and physically to her, as well as expensive. Ms. D lived with her developmentally-delayed adult son and teenaged daughter. Ms. D was fearful of how she would be treated by medical professionals, anticipating that she would stigmatized by their judgments. Because of this shame-inducing worry she had delayed seeking medical care. It was very important to her that her medical providers understood that she had once been a productive and working member of society, but she did not trust that they would recognize that in her. Exacerbating the situation is the fact that Ms. D had undergone surgery and, as a result, developed major depression. Throughout this all she experienced a financial downturn from which she had not been able to recover. Ms. D's situation was indeed complicated, and she had multiple care needs that didn't fit neatly into traditional models of care.

> Medical providers have to overcome their own implicit bias when caring for patients who have been marginalized.

Yet despite all that was going on, she found within herself the resources to become an advocate for her health. She was able to articulate her needs and request primary medical care treatment in her home. Her hope was that, along with assistance in personal care, physical therapy, and weight loss, she would be able to reintegrate into society. Her goal was to be able to leave her home and to become more functional as a mother to her daughter and son. She remained optimistic about the future and felt that, with some help, there was still time for her to reclaim her life.

Ms. D accepted a visit from a home-based palliative care physician who was willing to perform a home assessment. However, when the palliative care physician agreed to take the case, their administrator questioned whether she was an appropriate patient. The administrator expressed the following concerns: (1) that her goals might not be aligned with palliative care, (2) that the program lacked the infrastructure to support her, (3) that she would require more effort than one provider could provide, and (4) that she needed primary care and not palliative care.

Field Note

When assessing, consider not starting with the patient's goals, but begin by first assessing and identifying the patient's needs. It is difficult to formulate goals when the patient's needs have not been addressed. In addition, assisting with a need (which is external) may earn the patient's trust so your patient may feel more free to share his or her goal (which is internal) with you as their provider.

Many programs for in-home care have limitations. For example, "concierge" medicine had limited availability in Ms. D's area and did not accept Medicaid, while in-home care practices in the area were linked to veterans, elderly, and dual-eligible (patients with both Medicare and Medicaid). Neither her prognosis nor her goals were aligned with hospice care, and she was unable to leave her children for any type of inpatient program or facility. Ms. D's income was less than $1,000 a month, but she wanted to make sure that we understood that she was not a charity case and that she didn't want multiple people in her home or anyone prying into her affairs. Ms. D expressed her feeling that she had faced enough judgment.

Ms. D and her family lived at the periphery of society and existed in a constant state of insecurity, in which any new challenge could further destabilize their family unit and financial situation. While Ms. D's personal care was important to her, the care of her family was of primary importance, and any decision that she would make not only needed to take into account the impact on her personally but how it would affect her family. Her young daughter and son and could not remain in the home alone if she was not present, and she did not want her children to be burdened with her personal care or with her death. Ms. D had no reliable family members to act as her proxy, and she had lost most of her friends when she became homebound. For providers to "be in the trenches" with Ms. D, it would be required of them to extend their effort to include being in the trenches with her family as well. Thus, whatever decisions were to be made about the treatment and care of Ms. D' they would need to take into account her social and family situations.

For patients such as Ms. D, interprofessional teams are the ideal way to approach their care. However, these services must be available and accessible, and with Medicaid programs varying from state to state, what may be applicable and accessible in one area may not be applicable and accessible in another. When funding is questionable or unstable for state-run programs—such as Medicaid programs that are designed to help people receive services within their homes—then solutions that could lead to a patient's independence are also questionable and unstable, resulting in patients living year-to-year with uncertainty as to what support they will continue to receive.[11]

Patients such as Ms. D are at risk for early mortality. But her immediate challenge was to find a way to live with her chronic illnesses while maintaining a desire to recover functional status and restore some of the quality of her previous life. In order to provide care for a patient like Ms. D, providers must understand and be willing to accept *her* goals. Although her situation appeared dire and she was very ill, both her quality of life and length of it were important to her. It would therefore be essential to approach Ms. D's care through this lens.

It is crucial for providers who care for patients who live economically marginalized to possess a basic understanding of Medicaid, including its limitations in their state. In addition, for all patients who are vulnerable, it is important to avoid presenting plans that are not possible to achieve logistically or which do not fit into their needs and goals of life. It is also important for providers to be cognizant of the available resources in the local community, especially if their medical practices are unable to provide the interprofessional care that is required for optimal results. The relationship with home health companies, community resources, emergency medical services, hospitals, and charitable organizations can be used to create an interprofessional team for patient support, even when formal relationships do not exist. Interprofessional collaboration for complex patients can improve care and reduce costs. Collaboration across healthcare systems for complex patients also improves care and reduces cost by creating unique inter-professional teams.[12]

Field Note

Invest in the community you are practicing in and develop relationships wherever you can. You never know when they will come in handy. Be careful not to burn your bridges.

Caring for Ms. D started with listening to her story and developing a rapport. Providers should spend the necessary time to understand how patients have come to their current situations, while reinforcing a commitment to partnering with them in delivering their care. In Ms. D's case, this also meant accepting the limitations that she placed on what she was willing and not willing to do. Her medical team should not view her preferences as barriers to treatment but as parameters in which to work, and should think creatively about how her goals can be achieved within the parameters she set. Taking the time to build affinity with her allowed Ms. D to become confident of her caregivers' intentions and to reconsider her parameters of decision-making if she could see that it might help her reach her most-important goals. Developing trust in the relationship on both sides is of primary importance.

The next part of caring for her was to take time to identify her current available resources and then to determine her eligibility for other available and necessary resources. While Ms. D's palliative care team did not have the services of social worker, they did have very good relationships with home health social workers from different agencies whom they could call upon to assist in clarifying appropriate resources that were available to her and find out how to best make them accessible. Holistic understanding of her needs allowed her medical team to provide more-comprehensive care. They ordered home health for physical therapy along with the skilled professionals needed for blood draws and wound care. Through this multidisciplinary approach, Ms. D's care was enhanced with a whole new team that became invested in her welfare and goals. Because of the team's ability to leverage community resources, they were able to facilitate access to care such as radiology and labs. They also gained insight and developed strategies to specifically order what was needed, while still being in compliance with Medicaid regulations. Another important intervention for Ms. D was having her team pay careful attention to her medication formulary so as to ensure that no gaps in her prescription medications existed. All of this embodies a coordinated effort. It is a complicated but necessary process in the care of economically-vulnerable patients and one that extends beyond the biomedical model and draws into play care of the whole patient including taking into account her social circumstances.

Through the team's continued process of rapport building, Ms. D became open to developing advance-care plans for herself and also for her children in the case of a catastrophic event that would leave her severely debilitated or at the end of her life. A local parish was made aware of her situation and "adopted" her family and helped to bridge the gaps of food supplies and ease some of the burden of her financial insecurity. The parish also provided Ms. D and her teenage daughter with a social outlet, providing a sense of fellowship and support which proved very important to them. The social worker from the home health agency was able to assist Ms. D in accessing state resources available for her developmentally-disabled son which proved to be quite helpful.

Field Note

When it comes to needing resources, ask: don't tell yourself no, let someone else do that. Give people the opportunity to rise to the occasion. If they don't, you are no worse off than you were before.

This example demonstrates how providers who are not only medically savvy but also logistically and resource savvy can provide excellent care to vulnerable patients. It is important, however, to realize that not all problems can be solved by the medical provider. Thus it is essential to engage the collaboration of interprofessional team members who serve both within and outside of their medical system. This collaborative approach can make a dramatic difference in a patient's life.

In short, the challenge is to reframe a patient's obstacles to care into logistical problems yet to be solved. To be in the trenches with the patient requires tenacity and a willingness to be persistent in the face of barriers, along with skills in accessing resources that reach beyond medical treatment to care of the whole person.

Field Note

It may not always work out in your favor, but then again—it may. Don't be afraid to think outside of the box.

DYING AT THE MARGINS

As providers, when we contemplate how we would want our patients to experience death, an ideal situation would encompass the following elements:

1. The patient will understand and accept their prognosis.
2. The patient enjoys excellent family support.
3. The patient willingly enters into hospice with loving support from family members and friends and dies gracefully, fully aware of and accepting their transition.

4. Following death, the patient will be remembered for their good qualities and their unique contributions.
5. These elements occur within the confines of a safe and stable environment, whether it be in a home, hospital, or inpatient hospice unit.

A provider who is able to witness the patient's experience and benefit from these elements is likely to be encouraged and motivated to care for dying patients. There can be great reward and meaning in doing so. However, for many patients, this ideal is not going to occur. The journey for many patients, especially those who live marginalized and disempowered, is complicated and may be fraught with unique suffering and conflict throughout the process of dying. Providers serving in the trenches with these patients face many challenges. They may struggle with the injustice, inequity, and frustration that are all too often manifested in the lives of these patients. Providers also often have their own biases and their values may be challenged in a way that proves uncomfortable and sometimes even frightening when they are required to enter into the chaos that surrounds the lives of patients and families.

Mr. T had end-stage heart failure and stage 4 lung cancer. He has a history of illicit drug abuse, particularly cocaine, which he had continued to use during his treatment. As his disease progressed, it became clear that pursuing aggressive treatment would no longer be the best approach. He had been told by his oncology team that he was no longer a candidate for cancer therapy. Mr. T had declined an automatic implantable cardioverter defibrillator (AICD) and was not a candidate for other advanced cardiac therapies, nor did he desire them. Consequently, palliative care was called to manage his symptoms and to discuss his options.

Mr. T expressed that he wanted to go home, but he was not sure if he could since he was currently homeless, but he thought that his mother might be willing to take him in. He explained he was open to hospice care, but he didn't want them to dictate how he was going to live. Mr. T explained that he had used cocaine as well as other drugs for a very long time and had no desire to stop using them. His plan was to continue to use cocaine recreationally if and when he chose to do so. He also expressed his preference not to be confined to the house and stipulated that, although he was willing to live with his mother, he wanted the freedom to come and go as he pleased. Mr. T was experiencing severe pain in his left thigh and wanted it to be managed with medication so he could be more active.

While he understood he was going to die and expressed his desire to be a Do Not Resuscitate (DNR) patient, Mr. T did not want to sign any papers attesting to his wishes, even if that meant that he might undergo cardiopulmonary resuscitation (CPR) if he had a sudden heart attack. He wanted his daughter to become his healthcare agent, even though they had been estranged since his release from prison following his conviction for sexual assault. Mr. T also stated that he would refuse to go to a hospice unit under any circumstances. He also shared that he was an atheist and would get angry with any reference to God or a higher power. Additionally, since he did not renew his Medicaid, he was currently uninsured and therefore a "self-pay" patient.

His medical oncology team faced many challenges. First, Mr. T's living situation was not secure, and although he continued to stay in the hospital, discharging him to a shelter or to the street was not an ethical or humane option for them. However, the team was receiving pressure from the hospital, which was concerned about costs and length of stay, to discharge him. And the patient himself wanted to get out.

> Being in the trenches . . . implies not only that we are close to the patient, but also that we are fighting both for and with the patient against whatever barriers may exist.

If hospice would not assume the provision of care for Mr. T, the challenges faced by the palliative care team included the following:

1. Whether the team could manage the symptoms of a patient who had no payer source for clinic visits.
2. Whether the team could manage the symptoms of a patient who was not likely to be compliant.
3. Whether the team could manage the symptoms of a patient who declared he was going to use illicit drugs—cocaine and marijuana, etc.—if he chose, but who also required pain control.
4. Whether the team could address the needs of a patient who had limited support in the home. (Could they be his sole provider without a supporting in-home agency?)

Hospice was challenged by several concerns: (1) assuming the financial burden of his care; (2) concern for staff safety, the reason being related to his history of assault and drug use; (3) limitations that he was placing on the care to which he would agree; and (4) instability of the home situation and caregiver support therein. As a result, the wisdom and appropriateness of continuing to provide care for him was questioned by multiple staff members.

This patient composite of Mr. T presents multiple challenges for any care team. When presented with patients such as this, providers may benefit from a reexamination of the roots of what it means to provide end-of-life care. When reviewing the definitions of palliative care and hospice care, there is no provision that predicates care based on the patient's morality, personal disposition, or history. Both definitions focus only on the needs and goals of the patient and the ability of both palliative and hospice care services to help support these patients and their families' goals.

Field Note

It's called "palliative care and hospice care." Not "palliative and hospice care for super-awesome wonderful people who have values that align with our own." The definition of palliative care implies that we take all comers and that treatment must be compatible with their goals and values, not ours.

The medical oncology team chose to discharge Mr. T because being discharged was consistent with his wishes, and he had made it clear that he did not want to die in the hospital. He also shared that he experienced difficulty when being confined and that he experienced this during his hospitalization. Despite pressure from the administration, the medical team did not rush Mr. T's discharge, however, until they could be certain that services and plans for his safety outside the hospital could be secured. Several meetings between administration and the team became necessary, but the team did not relent until a safe discharge could be arranged. During his hospitalization, it was also discovered that Mr. T had an outstanding warrant for his arrest stemming from a parole violation. After this became known, the team reached out to the court system and was able to secure compassionate release for him.

Field Note

In a hospital system, you cannot be forced by administration to do something that would be either medically inappropriate or result in harm to your patient.

The palliative care team had a particularly difficult time with this case. They managed his pain very aggressively in the hospital, but reached a decision that if Mr. T was discharged, they could not safely prescribe opioid therapy if he remained unmonitored. They would be willing to write him daily prescriptions but insisted that he no longer use cocaine. The team spent a great deal of time with him developing a rapport, and because of that budding relationship he reluctantly agreed not to use cocaine. Although unenthusiastically, he accepted the concerns they expressed regarding the harm that cocaine use would cause for him given his congestive heart failure. Mr. T was open about his marijuana use and desire to continue using it, and the team felt the benefit of treating his pain outweighed the risks. They aggressively looked for hospice agencies that would accommodate him, but decided that they would manage his care as an outpatient if no other arrangements could be made. The plan was to see him as a "charity case" and to have their social worker explore methods for reinstating his Medicaid. The team social worker was very proactive, and in addition to helping him fill out his forms, made sure the forms were delivered to the proper agencies.

Field Note

Some patients, in order to access resources, may require a significant amount of assistance, especially if their health literacy is low. It is important for patients to be motivated to locate their own resources, but in some instances, that may not be possible.

A hospice agency was eventually located and agreed to take Mr. T on as a patient. It was a religious-based hospice, and they struggled with his being an atheist as well as with his criminal record. In an effort to more effectively address these issues, staff who were willing to accept his values and belief system were specially hand-picked to work with him. Staff would arrive at his home in groups of two, and if he was not at home, they would usually be able to locate him under a local bridge. They agency provided support for his mother, including assistance with utilities when she required it. Mr. T eventually developed a good relationship with the hospice chaplain, who was able to attend to his spiritual needs despite his not being religious. The chaplain learned of his struggles with depression/anxiety and his attempts to chemically cope. He revealed a trauma the chaplain kept confidential. This relationship was significant for both of them. One out of four people will suffer from a mental condition in their lifetime, and it is estimated that 1 million people die by suicide every year. Depression is a cause of disability and the third leading cause of the "global burden of disease." Mental illness for many cultures carries stigma, which forces patients to suffer in silence and discourages them from seeking treatment. Society often marginalizes these individuals. Society also criminalizes their illness, with patients ending up in the criminal justice system instead of receiving treatment for their underlying condition that may be driving the criminal behavior. This leads to further marginalization, earlier mortality, and excessive morbidity.[13] Addressing mental symptoms should be as much of a priority as addressing physical symptoms.

Patients have a right to choose their beliefs and treatment course. However, medical providers also have a right to remove themselves from a case if they believe that they cannot provide appropriate care due to the patient's beliefs and choices. In such instances, medical providers should remove themselves from the case while attempting to identify alternate providers that are willing to manage the patient within the parameters of their values. Just as we accept our patient's values, it is equally important to be accepting of our colleagues' and, if at all possible, avoid placing them in situations that they feel may compromise their values (Figure 11.1).

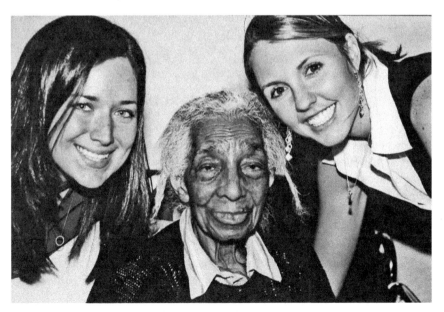

FIGURE 11.1 Caring at the margins must involve learning skills in cultural humility and competence for the next generation of providers.

Field Note

When assigning patients who have difficult social situations, consider thinking carefully about the individual you pair them with from your staff. Thoughtful matching of patients with providers is not giving in to prejudice or bias. Rather, it is caring for your patients where they are. This can be a hard pill to swallow.

Mr. T had collapsed in the middle of the street and became very delirious toward the end of his life, when he was often attempting to escape the confines of his home. Although Mr. T had continuous care, gaps existed, and he was able to leave home during one of those unmonitored times. Mr. T did not die at home as everyone had hoped, but in the hospital ER. Attempts were made at resuscitation, although he did not want this. The reason being that he had previously refused to sign a DNR, his mother refused to honor his wishes or to make a decision, and his hospice nurse was informed that they could not take her word for his expressed wishes in any event. Hospice, through a donation, cremated him. Although the hospice team expressed the view that they had done a good job in working with Mr. T within the parameters he defined for them, it is worth noting that Mr. T never expressed gratitude and was often hostile and angry and was occasionally threatening to the nurses. However, the chaplain, who knew him better than other hospice team members, believed that Mr. T was grateful toward the end.

Field Note

When you are caring for patients, the reward is in the job that you are doing. While it is wonderful when patients are accepting, they are not required to be grateful, graceful, or even kind. Find fulfillment in the work itself and renewal and support outside of it. You will last longer.

CARING AT THE MARGINS

Miss B was a young adult woman with cerebral palsy. She was cared for by her mother at home. She was bed-bound, with contractures and frequent seizures, minimally verbal, had a percutaneous endoscopic gastrostomy (PEG) tube, and required total care. She lived in the home with her mother, her sister, and her sister's children. The family struggled financially a great deal and moved frequently because their home environments became insecure. The latest home they lived in had rotting floorboards, but they were told if they "fixed it up," they might have an opportunity to buy it later. The family often had other family members and friends floating in and out of the home. Miss B's sister, along with her brother-in-law, intermittently lapsed with methamphetamine use. The matriarch of the family, Miss B's mother, was a recovering addict and had been sober for more than 20 years.

Miss B was on hospice care because her family was told that she was not likely to survive because of her frequent seizures, recurrent infections, progressive weight loss, and generalized decline in the previous several months. Her mother accepted that her daughter's prognosis might be less than six months. Ms. B's mother had repeatedly expressed that if her daughter were actively dying, she would want her to be kept comfortable. Her mother also insisted on providing her with excellent, dedicated care, which included strict management of her medications, personal care, and treatment of reversible acute medical issues. Upon entering the home, providers saw there was disarray except for the area where Miss B resided. Over her hospital bed, there were toys hanging from the ceiling. Her linens were clean, and stuffed animals lined the bed. Her mother talked to her constantly and looked for any signs of recognition. She bathed Miss B daily and meticulously turned her every two hours, usually with assistance from her other daughter and her grandchildren. While the family often appeared to be in chaos otherwise, when they were discussing or caring for Miss B, they were united, reasonable, and reliable.

Field Note

The attention and care the patient receives may not always be reflected in the condition of their home environment. Before making judgments concerning the living conditions of the patient, investigation is required.

I brought a medical student to her home for a home visit, and as we walked in, their five dogs jumped all around her feet. There was a toddler without shirt or shoes watching TV while seated on the floor. Once again, the house was in disarray, and there was plywood on the floorboards to reinforce them. During our visit, her mother was very excited and stated that Miss B tried to communicate and seemed to recognize the toys. Although I had never seen her do this, on this visit I did see her for the first time appear to attempt to communicate intentionally by gesturing to the toys and by tracking me as I examined her. This was a remarkable moment, and we were all very happy. Her mother shared that she had communicated these incidents to her hospice nurse for two weeks, but the mother was the only one who had witnessed it, and she was very happy that we had witnessed it as well.

Both the mother's and the family's whole life revolved around Miss B. Her mother stated that caring for her brought out the best in her family and Miss B held them together. Her sister stated that she was one of the reasons the sister tried to stay sober. Miss B's mother said that she had been told since her daughter was born that it might be better for her to either be institutionalized or be allowed to die and that the mother's efforts to engage with her were futile. Over the years, the mother expressed how she enjoyed and found rewarding the interactive times she spent with her daughter. However, as her daughter aged, these times became fewer and fewer.

Field Note

Quality of life is subjective and is measured by the individual patient and the family. The lives of people can have great meaning even if they are not able to physically make traditional contributions to society. The existence of a person in her family unit carries importance beyond what she may be able to physically contribute. Even if we are not able to recognize anything meaningful in someone's existence, this should never imply that meaning does not exist. It is important to learn your patient's and family's values since they are the true measures of quality of life. Coming to terms with this concept can be difficult when it differs from your definition.

When we were leaving the home, I asked the medical student what he thought of the visit. He looked at me, very distressed and explained that he didn't realize people actually lived like that. I realized that I had prepared him for what he would medically see, but I did not realize that I needed to prepare him to witness poverty. Although I was hoping that he would see the resilience of the family, he could not see the patient beyond the living situation. He had not been prepared for what he was going to experience. He went on to ask how I could face going into homes like that every day. He also wasn't sure why she was on hospice care with a tube feeding and with the family so intent on her living.

In caring for patients who are seriously ill, developing empathy is an important part of that care. *Empathy* is defined as "the ability to understand and share the feelings of another." People from all walks of life enter the medical profession with a wide variety of experiences. Even if we have a strong desire to provide compassionate care to others, this does not necessarily mean that we will all possess abilities to empathize with our patients, especially when faced with populations that we have not previously encountered. However, the capacity to empathize with others is a skill that can be taught.[8] A new model for empathy—referred to as the Empathic Choice Model—views empathy as an active decision versus a passive emotion, which means empathy is a skill that can be taught and we can choose to be empathic and not rely on our base instincts.[14]

Miss B's story highlights the importance of education concerning populations who are living at the margins of society and who are vulnerable. It would be wrong to assume that everyone will interpret a common experience the same. In medical schools, there is a push to teach empathy, communication, collaborative decision-making models, and diversity. This education is important in the development of empathy.[15] There is a study that demonstrated the value of using mindfulness training to enhance empathy. Incorporating this type of training into medical and allied health education may be a good tool to prepare students for the diverse patients they may encounter.[16]

Being in the trenches with patients and other caregivers while working collaboratively toward patient's goals is a fantastic experience. However, it is equally important to be cognizant of the many difficulties to be encountered. In caring for patients who are marginalized, the highs and lows of being a medical provider for this population can be extreme because of the circumstances surrounding their medical and social situations. Practicing principles of collaborative decision-making, along with developing skills to better understand and to empathize with them serves to complement the technical aspects of medical care. Educating the next generation of medical providers on how to step out of their comfort zone and engage a diversified population of patients will ensure that patients have providers who are willing to be in the trenches with them for the days to come.

REFERENCES

1. Napier AD, Ancarno C, Butler B, et al. Culture and health. *Lancet.* 2014;384(9954):1607–1639.
2. Smith DA, Akira A, Hudson K, et al. The effect of health insurance coverage and the doctor–patient relationship on health care utilization in high poverty neighborhoods. *Prev Med Rep.* 2017:158–161.
3. Chapman EN, Kaatz A, Carnes M. Physicians and implicit bias: how doctors may unwittingly perpetuate health care disparities. *J Gen Intern Med.* 2013;28(11):1504–1510.
4. Jackson CS, Gracia JN. Addressing health and health-care disparities: the role of a diverse workforce and the social determinants of health. *Pub Health Rep.* 2014;129(1 Suppl 2):57–61.
5. Hafeez H, Zeshan M, Tahir MA, Jahan N, Naveed S. Health care disparities among lesbian, gay, bisexual, and transgender youth: A. *Cureus.* 2017;9(4):1184.
6. DeMeester RH, Lopez FY, Moore JE, Cook SC, Chin MH. A model of organizational context and shared decision making: application to LGBT racial and ethnic minority patients. *J Gen Intern Med.* 2016;31(6):651–662.
7. Fleming MD, Shim JK, Yen IH, et al. Patient engagement at the margins: health care providers' assessments of engagement and the structural determinants of health in the safety-net. *Soc Sci Med.* 2017;183:11–18.
8. Bohns VK, Flynn FJ. Empathy gaps between helpers and help-seekers: implications for cooperation. *Emerg Trends Soc Behav Sci.* http//digitalcommons.ilr.cornell.edu/articles. 2015.
9. Chin MH. Movement advocacy, personal relationships, and ending health care disparities. *JAMA.* 2017;109(1):33–35.
10. Johnson RW, Lindner S. The adequacy of income allowances for Medicaid home and community-based services. https://www.urban.org/sites/default/.../adequacy_of_medicaid_hcbs_allowances.pdf. 2017.
11. Khatutsky G, Wiener JM, Greene AM, Thach NT. Experience, knowledge, and concerns about long-term services and supports: implications for financing reform. *J Aging Soc Policy.* 2017;29(1):51–69.
12. Hardin L, Kilian A, Spykerman K. Competing health care systems and complex patients: an inter-professional collaboration to improve outcomes and reduce health care costs. *J Interprof Educ Pract.* 2017;7:5–10.
13. Arboleda-Flórez J. What has not been effective in reducing stigma. In *The stigma of mental illness—end of the story?* New York: Springer; 2017: 515–530.
14. Cameron D, Cunningham W, Saunders B, Inzlicht. The end of empathy: constructing empathy from a value-based choice. https://doi.org/10.17605/OSF.IO/SM9EC. 2018.
15. Hirshfield LE, Underman K. Empathy in medical education: a case for social construction. *Patient Educ Counsel.* 2017;100(4):785–787.
16. Berry DR. *Bridging the empathy gap: effects of brief mindfulness training on helping outgroup members in need.* Virginia Commonwealth University; https://scholarscompass.vcu.edu/etd. 2017.

12

REFLECTIONS ON AN URBAN THOREAU
A PEACEFUL ENDING TO THE LIFE OF COWBOY

David Wendell Moller

A Special Observation

The best of our human potential is revealed in Cowboy's end-of-life story as the compassion, dedication, and skill of his palliative care team facilitated a death that was full of love, peace, and dignity—in spite of the expected and unavoidable chaos that surrounded it.

Take-Home Lesson

There was something quite exceptional about Cowboy's death. The grim things that darkened and injured him from birth were relieved by the caring embraces of a team of professionals who committed themselves to "loving him until he died." In dying, he found a sense of peace that eluded him throughout life. He opened his heart and even reveled in the empathic attention he received. Most importantly, he was understood and respected in ways that he had never previously been. For this reason, it is fair to say that those horrible features of American unexceptionalism, which harmed him throughout life, were redeemed by the exceptional activities of the palliative care team. Something wonderful literally transpired while he was dying: despite the sadness and chaos of his final months, a transcendence of the injurious consequences of racism and poverty was achieved by mindful presence and the human potential to love one another.

CONCLUSION TO A UNIQUE STORY OF AN AMERICAN LIFE

The great 20th century philosopher Yogi Berra once said, "It ain't over 'til it's over." Yogi's wisdom applies to many situations, whether it is a ball game, life itself, or the story of a person's life. I would thus be remiss if I did not complete the narrative that describes the end-of-life experience of Cowboy. As I noted earlier, there was much in his life that was grim: poverty, racism, mental illness, and estrangement from his family. As I will show, there was much about the end of his life that was wonderful: support, good medical care, gratitude, and reconciliation.

As you will remember, he was getting sicker and winter was rapidly approaching at the point where I interrupted the narrative. Terry Altilio had offered insights into his life and struggles, through a compassionately-crafted dialogue with him, and identified the unique challenges that caring for him posed. So, let us pick up from that point.

Despite the fact that Cowboy had remained brazen in his attitude, his body was betraying him, and he was starting to succumb to his illness. In addition, living in "the cave" was beginning to become unmanageable and even dangerous. For example, one night he suffered chest pains and was short of breath. Trying to get out of bed, he stumbled to the ground. In the dark, on hands and knees, he crawled the full length of the cave to and through the plastic tarp that served as its entrance and exit. He continued crawling up the hill and across the street to a public phone. He called 911 and collapsed onto the sidewalk. The medics arrived promptly, and within 10 minutes or so, Cowboy was at the emergency room of County Hospital, having had a heart attack. Although tests revealed that he had not suffered major damage to his heart, everyone was concerned about his going back home to live under the bridge, alone, in the dark, and with the weather turning cold. Therefore, Linda, still deeply committed to his care, was trying to find a place for him to live after he was discharged. With the assistance of a street minister, who dedicated his ministry to the service of homeless men who were facing serious illness, she was able to arrange for a room at a YMCA for two weeks. There he would be warm in the winter cold and safe. Grateful for her effort, Cowboy went there to stay after being discharged from the hospital. It was situated about a mile from the cave, and he would go there each day to check on his puppy, Cowgirl, and enjoy the familiarity of his home.

The room's being close to the campus enabled Linda to pick him up and drive him to his medical appointments. Most of the time, he would be waiting for her arrival to take him to an appointment, but there were a few occasions when he did not show up. Frankly, Cowboy was always happiest when immersed in street life. Thus, if the spirit moved him or if a "better offer" presented itself, he would go off to gamble, see friends, or return to the cave. Linda would wait for him, agitated and often thinking, "What are we going to do with this guy?" At first when this would happen, she felt not only frustrated, but also disrespected. As she was discovering, her relationship with Cowboy was complicated and challenged her both professionally and personally. The palliative care medical director answered her question directly: "We will love him until he dies." Despite his occasional irresponsibility, that was exactly what she committed to do. However, loving Cowboy was no small challenge. Made difficult not only by his long-term inability to receive or give love but by his unstable mental state as well, caring for this man required special patience. It was energy- and time-consuming, and often put her to the test. "We would constantly do this dance together where he would push me away and then seek me out," she said. Cowboy could not allow her to get too close. Yet he deeply needed and depended upon her. His capacity for intimacy and closeness had been damaged a long time ago in Mississippi, but the human need to be cared about during this difficult time persevered.

"We would constantly do this dance together where he would push me away and then seek me out. . . ."

The first week at the Y went smoothly. Cowboy continued to visit the cave regularly by bus or bicycle. On Thursday afternoons, I would pick him up with a group of medical students, and we would go there together for a "home visit." These visits were always appreciated. He praised the students for their dedication and commitment to becoming physicians. He told jokes, and invariably, when he described how he sometimes shined shoes for a living, he would look down at someone's feet and say, "It looks like those could use a little work." As he was still persuasive and forceful in his personality, a befuddled intern or medical student would have little choice but to remove a shoe. Cowboy would shine it with "spit and polish" while continuing to share the story of his life. He took great pride in this work, and to everyone's surprise, the shoeshine would be really good. Despite the weakening of his body, he was still full of piss and vinegar, especially when presenting his views on racial matters. His rage and anger at his family, including his children, seemed little affected by the toll the disease was taking on his body. During my relationship with him, I had come to learn that Cowboy, in many ways, needed to be angry. Because he had been so deeply injured as a child, anger was one way of responding to the cruelty he endured. For the students not used to such outbursts, these visits were eye-opening. For most of their training, they saw patients in a very narrow, clinical way and seldom in their own environments, and few patients in that setting were so expressive about profoundly personal matters. John, a first-year intern, perhaps put it best when he said, "Thank you for the privilege of getting to meet and know this man." Just as important, the benefits of these visits were mutual. They were valuable for Cowboy in letting him know he mattered. They showed him that there were people who cared enough to visit him in his world and listen to his life story.

During this time, Cowgirl remained faithfully at the cave awaiting his return each day. I checked on her regularly to ensure that she had enough food and water. Ironically, despite prolonged periods of being empty, the cave and its contents remained undisturbed. How unlikely, I thought, that its contents had not been stolen or vandalized.

Unfortunately, despite the good things that were happening, Cowboy's living situation was becoming problematic. He was often unable and unwilling to follow the house rules at the Y. The problem peaked one day when he decided that he did not like the stained white walls of his room, so he went out, got some paint, and began redecorating. A room inspection revealed that the walls and radiator had been spray-painted bright red. Cowboy was to be evicted. He seemed not to care. He would just go back to the cave, but Linda worried that if he returned there, he would be in real trouble. He was continuing to fail physically, and the temperature was dropping into the single digits at night. By pleading with the manager, she was able to convince him to let Cowboy stay one more night. In the meantime, she tried to find somewhere else for him to stay. Essentially unperturbed by the situation, Cowboy told her not to worry and that he would be fine. Having come to love him as she did, she did worry. Once again she went to work on finding a place for him, but he kept insisting that "You can't worry about these things more than I do."

Sometimes good news emerges from misfortune. The next day, before the hour of eviction, Cowboy's breathing difficulties worsened. He was rushed to the emergency room. His pain had intensified, his bowels were failing, and he was in acute respiratory distress. The bad news was that he needed to be admitted to the hospital. That, however, was also the good news, because Linda, despite diligent efforts, had not been able to locate a place for him to stay. His admission provided her with more time. The other part of the good news was that the medical interns who had gotten to know him through their home visits were now back working on the wards at County. Having grown intrigued by and fond of this man, they were all exceptionally dedicated to his care. Thus, under the direction of Dr. G. and Jodi, Cowboy received exemplary medical care. A private room had been arranged. He was settling down, becoming more comfortable, and regaining some strength. It was at this point that I sensed a major transformation in both his attitude and spirit. His seemingly intractable veneer of anger was starting to soften. For the first time, he seemed to be capable of allowing others to take care of him without resisting. Slowly, he was becoming less suspicious and more trusting as his heart was opening just a bit.

I jokingly refer to Linda as the World Wrestling Federation social worker. Seemingly, there is never a problem, no matter how unusual or complicated, that she cannot grasp hold of and "body slam" with resolution for patients and families. While Cowboy was in the hospital, she had been hard at work to find a new place for him to live. It paid off. She was able to locate a small apartment that rented for $250 a month. It was a run-down, roach-infested walk-up in the heart of an inner-city neighborhood known for drugs, gangs, and violence. Even so, it was warm, and there he would be safe. Grateful and glad to be there, Cowboy felt comfortably at home in his new place. He immediately went to work on attacking the roach problem by devising traps made of bleach and water, and would proudly describe how he had solved the problem. His spirit was strong. Cowgirl was with him, having been brought from the cave on the day he was discharged. Thursday afternoon visits with medical students continued, and although his body was being weakened by disease, he remained independent and joyful.

Unfortunately, this new living situation did not last long. Cowboy and Linda had met with the landlady's son to make arrangements for the apartment. He paid, with Linda as a witness, $250 for a security deposit and another $250 for the first month's rent. This person, who was a drug abuser and dealer, absconded with the money. (Subsequently, he disappeared entirely and was thought to have been murdered. The detectives assigned to the case recently gave this news to his mother.) Having received neither rent money nor security deposit, the landlady decided to evict Cowboy. Linda tried to intervene. She assured her that Cowboy had paid the money in full to her son, but the landlady would not be persuaded. Pursuing the matter, Linda pleaded with her to let him stay. However, she remained steadfast in her decision, stating that it was not only about the money, but that "He's going to die, and I don't want him lying dead on the floor above me." So, once again, Cowboy was without a place to stay.

Linda was becoming frustrated at how time-consuming her relationship with Cowboy had become. Expressing this frustration to Dr. G., she vented, "I just don't know what to do for him anymore." Dr. G. repeated what was now becoming a driving mantra of the team's involvement with Cowboy: "We are going to love him until he dies."

> "I just don't know what to do for him anymore." Dr. G. repeated what was now becoming a driving mantra of the team's involvement with Cowboy: "We are going to love him until he dies."

Loving him remained difficult. In fact, Linda had already been criticized by medical students who had been involved in the home-visit program for allowing Cowboy to manipulate and exploit her. At this point she had already invested more than 100 hours in his care. Nonetheless, having grown to love this man as a unique person, she was not about to abandon him, regardless of the demands placed on her. So once again, driven by compassion and the duty to serve, she went to work on finding Cowboy suitable housing. She was able to secure placement in a transitional residence for homeless men discharged from the hospital. Cowboy would be allowed to stay for 30 days, providing he obeyed the house rules. He got off to a reasonably good start, but problems emerged. It is not difficult to understand that obeying rules was not Cowboy's forte, nor would it ever be. His transgressions were not egregious enough to get him evicted this time. Rather, he pushed the envelope sufficiently to become "beloved but difficult," in the words of the house director. He would play his music too loud on occasion, would be late for curfew, and would not always follow the protocol for kitchen behavior. Clearly, he was violating house rules, but the staff felt that they would be able to work productively with him and be successful in nudging him toward greater compliance. However, while Cowboy seemed to be successfully walking the tightrope of acceptable behavior, misfortune once again struck. The spread of his disease was beginning to compromise his bowels. Almost overnight Cowboy became incontinent, and house rules prohibited anyone who was incontinent from being in residence. So, he was evicted, immediately disappeared, and was nowhere to be found. Later we discovered that he had spent some time with a lady friend, spent a night in the back of a car, and stayed with friends at a local underground gambling establishment known as the Pea Shake House. During his shuffle from place to place, Cowgirl disappeared and we had no idea where she was.

We saw him for the first time two weeks later. Cowboy was brought to the emergency room; his pain was elevated, his bowels were not functioning, and he was in respiratory distress. Again he was admitted to the hospital, making this the tenth hospitalization in three months. The pain in his back was intense and made it difficult for him to lie in bed. He spent much of his time sitting, heavily sedated by morphine. He drifted off to sleep regularly and often seemed in danger of falling out of the chair. He knew he was getting sicker and that the end of his life was nearing. He respectfully spoke about God and welcomed the spiritual ministry of the palliative care team chaplain. Medical residents and students continued to look in on him. He remained grateful for their visits. His anger was continuing to dissipate, and he was experiencing an unfamiliar but well-deserved sense of peace and equanimity.

As the days passed, his body continued to be ravaged by disease. Nonetheless, because his medical care remained exemplary, the physical discomfort was minimized. Additionally, perhaps for the only time in his life, he was being nourished and sustained by love. How strange, I thought, that in dying Cowboy was finally finding a sense of comfort that had eluded him throughout life. His major regret at this point was that he feared that Cowgirl was dead. "I think I've lost Cowgirl," he pined with tears welling in his eyes. He went on to remark while gesturing toward the sky, "That's okay, because we will see each other again one day." He was referring to the two of them meeting in heaven.

On one morning after Christmas, I called Cowboy in his hospital room. I began the conversation by saying, "Cowboy, there is someone I want to bring by to see you." "Who is it?" he asked. "Fannie," I said. "Aunt Fannie?" he queried. As it turned out, Linda, during one of her many efforts on his behalf, had stumbled across an aunt who raised Milton for three years in Mississippi. As we were about to learn, before sending him away permanently when he was 13, Milton's mother moved from the plantation for three years and left her son behind with her sister. Aunt Fannie raised him from years five through eight. Although they were mostly estranged throughout his adult life, Fannie had made her way to the urban Midwest, as had her nephew. Coincidentally, she was living less than a mile from the cave.

His response seemed like an epiphany in progress. "Okay. I trust you," he answered. I was particularly amused when he went on to add, "Don't worry, I'll behave myself!" Finally, Cowboy's soul was beginning to find some peace, and his agitation and anger were waning. In the process of dying, he was opening to the possibilities of reconciliation, forgiveness, and fellowship. Vitriol and anger were being left behind almost as if he knew they would be intolerable baggage in the place that lay ahead for him after his life on this earth came to an end.

So later that day, Linda and I brought Fannie, now 80 years old, to see her nephew. There was no antagonism or tension in sight as they reminisced about their lives and relationship. Things were off to a good start, and after five minutes, I seized the opportunity to push the matter further, saying, "Cowboy, with your permission, I'd like to see if we can arrange something else." "What's that?" he replied. "I think it's time to see your children." It was as if he had been anticipating what I had in mind. Showing neither surprise nor anger, he simply said, "I'd like to see them." The communication between us had been clear. Linda now had permission to locate the children, and a reunion, perhaps even reconciliation, might take place. Cowboy immediately returned his attention to the conversation that Linda and Fannie were having, and, of course, being the uncontrollable flirt he was, the discussion inevitably drifted toward "the way" he had with the ladies. "Even as a young boy, he was a 'real charmer,' " Fannie confided. The visit lasted 45 minutes and was richly satisfying for both nephew and aunt. As we drove her home after the visit, Fannie said, "Thank you. It was good to see my nephew."

The last time Michael Smith had seen his father was 20 years before. They inadvertently bumped into each other outside a variety store in an inner-city neighborhood. Upon recognizing his son, Cowboy instinctually recoiled and snarled, "I never gave a fuck about you!" His venom in spewing these words was consistent with the psychoemotional damage he suffered as a child. However, even though Cowboy had bolted from his son's life years ago, Michael nevertheless loved his father and felt the sting of those words deeply. For profoundly complex reasons, Cowboy could relate to his children only as he was raised: hurtfully and spitefully. He had been so damaged by his upbringing, and unfortunately he passed that harm onto his children.

Even though I had previously not known the depth of the estrangement between father and son, I understood fully that the rift was bad. For this reason it was indeed shocking that only a few days later, on December 28, hours after having been contacted by Linda, Michael arrived at his father's bedside. A lot had happened in Michael's life. After having graduated from Ohio State University and completing his graduate work at Harvard, he was drawn back to the city streets. Already damaged emotionally and mentally, "It was the only place I knew to go," he confessed. His life for the past 30 years had not been productive from the point of view of prevailing cultural values. He worked infrequently and lived in poverty. A spiritual quest to the city of Touba in Senegal had led him to convert to Islam. No longer Michael, he was now Sheik Ibrahim.

Frankly, the reunion was largely uneventful. There was too much to be said that could not be said. Cowboy was too sick and the issues were too deep. Their interaction went smoothly, if superficially, with Ibrahim internalizing his emotions. While there, he happened to look into the closet in the hospital room and was horrified by the condition of his father's clothes. They were sooty, dingy, and tattered. Perhaps the only proud memory he had was of the way his father dressed and presented himself. You will remember Cowboy had described this as "cash and flash—flash and cash." In fact, when Milton was living in Chicago, he was named Best-Dressed Black Man by a local black organization on two separate occasions. It was on seeing and smelling his father's clothes that Ibrahim came to learn that he had lived for the past three years under a bridge. He was upset by how poverty and mental illness had shattered the one memory of his father he could recall without regret. At that moment in the hospital room, Ibrahim was gripped by fear and revulsion. He quickly told his father he needed to leave but would be back to see him soon.

Perhaps there is no more awful death than to die with regret, feeling that one's life has been wasted. Perhaps there can be no greater sentence imposed on one's future than to witness the death of a loved one when there is grave and irreconcilable emotional disrepair.

In this regard, Cowboy did not see death as something horrible. His faith in God gave him strength, and in an ironic way he felt satisfied with his life. For better or for worse, despite unimaginable youthful injuries, he had lived life on his own terms. Although he suffered greatly and passed his pain on to his children, he was able to maintain his own style and individuality throughout his life. He had lived with passion, enjoying women, music, work, and fashion. He often impressed others with his zest for life. "I will remember Milton as a man of charm, wit, intelligence, and one who appreciated fashion and complemented style," remarked Barbara, the palliative care team chaplain. Death seemed not so horrible a fate to Cowboy because he had found ways to live without regret and had embraced the possibilities of the life he had been granted.

Maybe most impressive is the fact that at age 65 he had received his General Educational Development (GED) certificate. Throughout his life, he had been resentful of being deprived of an education. As you will recall, he was told he was "too stupid to learn" when he expressed interest in going to school. Cowboy took pride in his vocabulary and his ability to enunciate difficult words and displayed an enthusiasm for learning. Thus, as he spoke about this accomplishment, I sensed that it was almost as if to thumb his nose at his family that he had gotten his high school equivalency diploma. He took delight in the achievement in its own right, certainly, but he also enjoyed "sticking it in their faces." Additionally, Cowboy was always well respected by his peers, who saw him as honest, intelligent, and witty. On the streets he was known as "the mayor," a title bestowed precisely because of these qualities. This helped to explain why the cave would not be ransacked during his myriad absences. In short, as his anger and excitability were

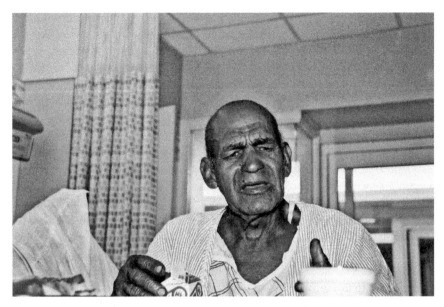

FIGURE 12.1 Peace and gratitude become Cowboy's new normal.

waning in the nurturing arms of a caring group of professionals, Cowboy was at a place where he could review his life with minimum regret and begin to feel a sense of peace (Figure 12.1).

The challenge before Ibrahim, however, was quite different. There was nothing peaceful about being reunited with his dying father. It rekindled painful thoughts about his neglect and abuse. Not only had Cowboy affected his life in hurtful ways, but his death would eliminate any possibility of reconciliation. There may be no greater expression of the pain Ibrahim felt throughout his life than the words of a poem he wrote in 1982, pain brought about by being poor in a culture of affluence and black in a racist society, the injuries of which were exacerbated through abandonment and rejection by his father.

> What about the rape of our body,
> What about the rape of our mind,
> What about the rape of our time,
> What about the rape of our dream,
> What about the rape of our love.

In 1998, while estranged from Cowboy, Ibrahim had self-published a collection of poetry entitled *Invocation for the Mentally Insane, Excerpt Poems for the Lost and Found*. Despite the fact he had not seen his father for 17 years, he wrote the following words of special thanks in the acknowledgment section: "To My Father, (A Surviving King)." Throughout the years of exile from his father, Ibrahim yearned for connection. His heart remained conflicted between rage and anger toward him and the need to love and forgive. Tension between those emotions would never be more pressing than at this particular point in his life.

Ibrahim remained true to his word and returned to see his father the following day. He brought with him a newly-purchased shirt and pair of shoes. "I just cannot bear the thought of my father wearing those clothes," he remarked. Although he seemed to understand that Cowboy would never be well enough to wear his new outfit, "at least he would have something decent to be buried in," Ibrahim stated. At this point, he was unaware that months before Cowboy had decided against a funeral for several reasons, one of which was the belief that "No one would come," and that "If people are interested in seeing me, let them do it while I'm alive."

During this period, Dwight, Cowboy's other son, also came to visit. Having worked for a local affiliate of CBS, he was now a pastor in Dayton, Ohio. Dwight had been estranged from Cowboy off and on for most of his life. They had had a major falling out many years ago and had not seen each other since. Dwight had sought to contact him just the previous year, but their paths unfortunately never crossed. When first contacted by Linda, Dwight was in shock. He had come to think his father was probably dead. Hearing that he was still alive was startling and opened a floodgate of conflicting emotions, anger, and confusion. Nonetheless, true to his ministry as a Christian pastor, and driven by a personal need to find reconciliation, he arrived at Cowboy's bedside also on December 28. He came alone and in secret. The situation was so bad that he could not even tell his mother what he was up to, as this ex-wife and Cowboy were bitterly estranged. As he walked into the room on the sixth floor and saw his now-dying father for the first time in years, the experience was overwhelming: wounds were reopened, and a painful intensity ensued. However, despite this background and these issues, their conversation was amicable. The past was not brought up, and Cowboy was pleased to see his son. Dwight stayed for about an hour and then left to travel back to Ohio. He drove in deep reflection about the anticipated loss of his presumed-dead father and their embittered relationship.

Cowboy was in a different state of mind. Having gotten to a peaceful place in his life, seeing his sons did not have a significant emotional impact on him. He simply enjoyed their visits. On the other hand, for Ibrahim and Dwight, the emotional consequence was huge. Feelings that had been deeply buried were stirred. As a result, they were shaken by their encounters with him. In response, they individually retreated to their private lives: Dwight to his ministry in Dayton and Ibrahim to the solitude of the reclusive spiritual journey he had been on for the past two years. They would not see their father again for 17 days. Unfortunately, Linda was unable to locate Cowboy's daughter, who was reportedly living in Chicago at this point, so a reunion between Shirlene and her father did not take place.

In the meantime, insurance regulations required that Cowboy be discharged from the hospital. The residents had already delayed discharging him because they knew he had nowhere to go. Unable to justify hospitalization any longer, they transferred Cowboy to the nursing home. Deerfield Village would become his final residence before death. He knew he was dying. Be that as it may, thanks to good control of pain and other symptoms, he was still able to enjoy life. He paid off all his debts, most of which were from money borrowed from friends or gambling associates. He reveled in the love displayed by the palliative care team. He quickly became a favorite of the health service professionals who worked on his floor at Deerfield. He was not bothered by the fact that his sons had not returned to visit nor bothered to call. Instead, he focused on positive things: his love of women (especially Linda), his favorite music, and his unwavering belief in God. In a strange way, this was a good time for both Cowboy and those who cared for him.

Over the next three weeks, things remained pretty much the same. Cowboy enjoyed being the center of attention at Deerfield. Although they had not known him long, many of the staff came to care deeply about this "interesting" and "cool" man. None of his children was involved. We still had not been able to track down his daughter, and his sons had not returned. Cowboy gave this no thought whatsoever. Friends from the neighborhood would visit, including Dr. Ralph of the federally funded Homeless Initiative Program. "I'd visit and we'd talk about music. Cowboy loved jazz," Ralph said.

Occasionally, if he were feeling up to it, someone would take him out for a while, back to the streets where he felt most at home: to look for Cowgirl, to say hello to friends, perhaps to stop at Burger King for a cup of coffee. During these weeks, there were two constants in his life: the progression of his disease and the abiding love of those at County whose lives he'd touched. Cowboy, often alone in life, was now befriended in dying.

On Thursday, January 10, Linda and I were riding back to campus after having participated in a community presentation about caring for the dying poor at County. After our talk, at which we told a bit of the story of Cowboy, the first question asked was, "What happened to the dog?" We explained that she had been missing then for six weeks and was feared dead. Multiple attempts to find her at the pound and in the neighborhoods had been unsuccessful. We mentioned that Cowboy grieved and cried over her loss but felt confident that they would "see each other again one day." Later, as Linda and I continued talking about the enthusiastic response of the audience, an idea occurred.

"We don't have to rush back. Let's take one more drive through the neighborhood," I said. So we drove to the cave and then up Martin Luther King, Jr. Street to the apartment where Cowboy had briefly lived before being evicted. We were looking for Cowgirl as we circled the streets. Not surprisingly, she could not be found, but maybe Yogi knew what he was talking about after all, and it would not be over until it was over. As we searched, one final thought occurred. "Let's check with the landlady about the dog," I suggested.

Linda, a bit concerned, asked, "Do you think she'll talk to us?"

"All she can say is no."

"Let's do it," she decided.

We rang the bell and were graciously received by Mrs. M. She talked painfully about how her son was missing and presumed dead. She elaborated on her faith and reliance on God throughout this difficult time. We hesitated to inquire about Cowgirl, as her disappearance paled in comparison to this mother's grief. Nonetheless, we asked and she responded, "Oh yes, I see her every day at 5:30."

"At night?" we queried.

"No, I feed her every morning at 5:30, and then she goes off."

Unbelievable, we thought. Cowgirl is alive! As it turned out, day after day she sat outside the door waiting for Cowboy to return after his eviction. Mrs. M. began feeding her at that point. When the apartment was rented shortly thereafter, the new tenant did not like the dog hanging around, and he kicked her, injuring a hip. As a result, Cowgirl would come to the house to be fed early in the morning but would wander off soon thereafter to avoid further abuse. Stunned by the news that she was still alive, we knew we had one more challenge in front of us. We needed to find and retrieve Cowgirl.

On Sunday, January 13, we went back to the neighborhood and began our search. As if it were supposed to happen, we found Cowgirl almost immediately. She appeared bigger, having grown, and her fur was thickened by the winter weather. She was also frightened and hurt. We were able to corral her in a backyard. She was trepidatious but not aggressive. Cowboy had once told me, "She doesn't like most people, but now that she knows you, she'll never hurt you. Nope, she won't." Talking gently to her, I tried to approach slowly. It took an hour and 45 minutes before I was able to get a leash around her. Getting her into a car was just as difficult, but we persisted and finally succeeded.

Joining us in trying to capture Cowgirl were Peggy, a respiratory therapist at Deerfield Village, and her husband, Tom. When Peggy, who is an animal rescuer, learned that Cowgirl was alive, she offered to take her in and find her a foster home. During the effort to get Cowgirl into Peggy's truck, a nurse at Deerfield paged Linda. Cowboy had taken a dramatic turn for the worse, and it seemed that death would not be far away. Linda went on to the nursing home to be with him. Peggy, Tom, and I continued our struggle with Cowgirl.

Once we got her inside the truck, we drove straight to the nursing home. Cowgirl was resistant but not aggressive as we dragged her into the building, onto the elevator, and down the fourth-floor hallway into Cowboy's room. As soon as she saw him, she sprang to life. She rushed to him, climbed onto the bed, and lay across his chest. Licking his face and hands, she aroused Cowboy. Weakly opening his eyes, he smiled and put his arm around her, saying ever so faintly, "Cowgirl's here!"

> Weakly opening his eyes, he smiled and put his arm around her, saying ever so faintly, "Cowgirl's here!"

Over the next two hours, many of the staff roamed into the room. News of this event had even spread to other floors, and people wanted to have a look. The general sentiment was perhaps best expressed by a nurse who said, "Amazing. Just amazing." Dr. Ralph stopped in to say goodbye to his friend. Barbara came as well to offer spiritual support. I went to pick up Fannie, who sat quietly by his side throughout the afternoon. Before leaving she bent over, kissed him, and said, "I love you, Milton." Tears were streaming down her cheeks. There was a real gathering of community at Milton's bedside, a tribute to the capacity of this man to touch our lives. Around 5:00 that Sunday afternoon, Peggy left with Cowgirl, who eagerly went with her following the smell of Cowboy's slippers and pajamas. Linda and I kissed him and promised to return in the morning (Figure 12.2).

We arrived around 8:00 A.M. the next day. Dr. G. was already there, having brought a cup of coffee. Cowboy was able to take a few sips, and the nurse practitioner sighed, "It's all about pleasure at this point." Barbara came to pray. All of his physical needs, especially relief from respiratory distress and pain, were well attended to by the nursing staff. Death was imminent, but given the extent of his physical decline, he was remarkably peaceful. Around noon, Linda and I needed to leave. I kissed him on the forehead, saying, "Thank

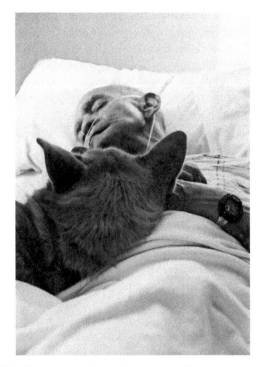

FIGURE 12.2 Best friends sleeping together before saying goodbye.

you for being my friend, Cowboy." He managed a smile. It was now time for Linda to say goodbye to her dear friend. "Milton, I have something for you," she said, arousing him. "It's what you always wanted." With grace and ease, she leaned over and kissed him on the lips. Their eyes met briefly, and he uttered what were to be his final words: "Thank you. I loved that."

We knew that Cowboy would soon be dead, and Linda went off to call Dwight and Ibrahim. She informed them that if they wanted to see their father before he died, they had best come immediately. They did, returning for the first time since the initial re-union. Cowboy was unconscious by then, and he never knew that they spent several hours with him that night.

The next day I went to see Cowboy around 6:45 A.M. There was a group of people milling around the nurses station, and as soon as I got off the elevator I knew something was up. Cowboy had died in his sleep at 1:55 A.M. on Tuesday, January 15. I called Linda to tell her the news. The nurses, other staff, and I lingered together for a while. They offered their remembrances, and I shared with them pictures of the reunion with Cowgirl that had taken place on Sunday. After 10 minutes, they scurried off to their respective duties. I went down to his now-empty room with a reporter I had brought to meet him. Together we sat in the dark, and I reminisced about our relationship, offering suggestions as to why so many people were drawn to him. Despite great sadness, I felt joy in being a part of this uncommon experience, and I felt pride in how Cowboy had been so well served by the professionals at County.

I can only imagine that as he climbed the stairway to heaven, he was greeted by St. Peter, who applauded, saying, "Hey, Cowboy! Great death!" Perhaps St. Peter followed up with, "Now it's time to talk a bit about your life, before you are getting through here!"

Linda had notified Ibrahim and Dwight of their father's death, and the four of us were scheduled to meet at 2:00 that afternoon. Their dominant feelings at this point were gratitude and confusion. They were thankful for the good care that Cowboy had received at County, especially finding comfort that so many different individuals had taken an interest in their father. Their confusion was essentially overwhelming, however. Theirs was a unique and especially burdensome grief, and they felt the sting of a tidal wave of painful emotions that swept over them. They were suffering the loss of their father, a father they never really knew. Moreover, they were remembering instances of neglect and abusive treatment, and they were glaringly reminded of how they suffered all those years. Their struggle was to grieve the death of a father who was never capable of loving them but whose love they so desperately needed.

Dwight began. "My father grew up in the South?" I was shocked. I never imagined the separation between father and children had been so severe that they did not even know his birthplace. "Yes," I replied, "in Mississippi." I went on to describe his experiences as a boy and the recent circumstances of his life in the cave. All the while I was thinking to myself that Linda and I knew Cowboy far better than they did. How sad.

Both Ibrahim and Dwight were hungry for information and details. Any bit of knowledge that would help them make a connection with their father was appreciated. They hung on every word with anticipation that something might be revealed that would provide understanding and meaning. We showed pictures, which they passed back and forth as if they were sacred objects. Ibrahim seemed especially frightened. "I worry that I am going to wind up like this myself one day." A few tearful moments later it was as if a light bulb had turned on. "You know, there's a man at Harvard who went off and lived in isolation. His name was Henry David Thoreau. What I see here in my father is Thoreau." "An urban Thoreau?" I inquired. "Exactly. Except that Henry David would leave Harvard and go to Walden Pond by choice. My father never had a choice. He never had the opportunity to attend Harvard as I did, and the circumstances of his life led him to live like this." Ibrahim was carving out a strategy for coping with the tragedy of Cowboy's life and death. In doing so he would filter his suffering through the image of his father as a creative and irrepressible rebel who lived his life as a form of protest.

Dwight, on the other hand, was struggling to comprehend the loss and pain as a Christian minister. He indicated that just the past Sunday he had given a sermon entitled "Dancing with Broken Bones." He turned directly to Ibrahim and spoke to him about how their father lived and danced with broken bones. Tears streamed down his cheeks. In this conversation he was trying to cope with his father's transgressions by forgiveness and understanding, an understanding based on coming to recognize for the first time that much of Milton's irresponsibility as a father had been produced by the injuries he suffered as a boy. To this day, Dwight is still working on forgiveness.

After four-emotionally draining hours, Ibrahim asked where Cowboy's body was and if he could see it. Linda made a phone call and alerted the morgue that we were coming. Dwight wanted to walk with us but waited outside while Linda, Ibrahim, and I went inside. Reverently, Ibrahim knelt beside his father's body. He began. "Father, I know you can hear me." He then proceeded to talk to and pray for him in both English and Arabic. All the while he was gently touching his father, as if to hold on to a connection that had never existed. After 10 minutes, he kissed Cowboy on the forehead and gently zipped up the body bag. The three of us went outside to rejoin Dwight. Dwight and Ibrahim left the hospital to return to their respective homes. Linda and I hugged goodbye, each of us going off to reflect on the impact Cowboy had made on our lives.

> Their eyes met briefly, and he uttered what were to be his final words: "Thank you. I loved that."

The first of two memorial services was held at noon on Wednesday. Staff from the Homeless Initiative Project and Deerfield Village gathered at the cave for a 20-minute ceremony. There were several police officers in attendance, cops who were fond of Cowboy and had protected him. Two of them had tears in their eyes as they told about their relationship. "He was a remarkable man," Officer Terri noted. "We always would keep an eye out for him." I finally understood why the cave would remain undisturbed when Cowboy was absent. The word on the street was not to mess with it, and the cops really did look after him. In fact, they visited almost every day, making the cave a "protected site." Thinking about how Cowboy had formed and creatively used these relationships to secure his survival brought a quiet smile to my face. All those years ago in Mississippi, he had learned how to survive by cultivating relationships with those who could help him. That very ability, which he developed as a boy, continued to serve him until the very end.

A local TV station had gotten wind of Cowboy's story and decided to cover the memorial service. In fact, as the news spread, the media became quite interested in this uncommon life story. Five television spots, two of which were the lead story, and two newspaper columns appeared over the next five days. How ironic. Cowboy, so invisible in life as thousands of people drove over and past his home every day without regard for him, was becoming a celebrity of sorts in death. Too bad he wasn't there to see the outpouring of interest in the community. Frankly, he would have loved it.

The next day I took Terrence, the first-year medical student who regularly saw Cowboy, on a bereavement visit to see Ibrahim. We picked Cowboy's son up at his home on the east side of the city. Because Ibrahim wanted to see where his father had lived, we headed downtown to the cave. A television reporter and camera crew were scheduled to meet us there at 3:00 P.M. Ibrahim entered the car in a somber mood. After exchanging hellos, he quickly began talking about Thoreau. Opening a portfolio filled with papers, he proceeded to read a passage from Thoreau's book *Civil Disobedience*. His voice trembled with anger as he continued reading. "This is my father. This is my father," he fumed, referring to the dehumanizing impact of the state and political economy to which he believed his father had fallen victim. Ibrahim's mind was whirling in the heavens and stars with ideas that legitimized his father's suffering and lifestyle. In this journey he was struggling to explain his father's life and searching for meaning to his own emotional pain. "My father's soul is not at peace," he lamented. "We are going to have to set it free." Terrence and I listened carefully, assuring him that Cowboy had been wonderfully cared for in the preceding months. In addition, we assured him that we had both noticed that a transformation had occurred. For the first time in his life, Cowboy had been able to

acknowledge love. I went on to add that I believed that Cowboy's soul was at peace because of the warming fires of fellowship that saw him into his death. Ibrahim, still agitated, was not convinced.

We arrived at the cave, and the news crew was waiting. I told Ibrahim about the first
time I had met Cowboy and how he had brought gifts out to Linda and me on the hill.
I joked about how he was cleanly shaven and sporting a nice-smelling cologne, and how
I came to realize later on, after witnessing his relentless flirtations with her, how that was
clearly for her benefit, not mine. Slowly, we went down the hill and entered through the
plastic tarp. Ibrahim seemed mesmerized by the sight. Slowly, he walked from place to
place, gently touching items at random. He was overwhelmed by what he saw, and the
feelings engendered were shaking him visibly. Still struggling to make sense of his father's
life, he announced to the reporter that on January 22, which would have been Cowboy's
74th birthday, he would begin a hunger fast to bring attention to the predicament of the
homeless in America. It would be in four parts: 10 days of fruit, then 10 days of juice,
10 days of water, and the last 10 days he would consume nothing but air. He invited the
reporter to cover the fast. Shana said she would think about it.

The second memorial service was held on Saturday. About 60 people were in attendance, including Cowboy's daughter who was finally located by Linda, and Ibrahim's
mother. The palliative care team was there, as were some students and friends of Cowboy
from the community. Some who had never even met him came. They had been moved
to attend by the stories in the media. Linda and I gave eulogies, and Dr. G. read from the
scripture. As I spoke about Cowboy, I lit a black candle in front of the memorial board
to symbolize the dark side of his life: poverty, racism, emotional damage, alienation, and
mental illness. I concluded by asking Linda to join me and we all listened to the song
"Cowboy, Take Me Away." We stood, arms around each other, listening to the words and
saying goodbye to a dear friend.

Dwight spoke next and focused on the value of forgiveness. Then Ibrahim eulogized
his father for nearly an hour, reading from the Koran and the Bible and sometimes
speaking in Arabic and translating back into English. His theme was based on a sermon
his brother had given the previous Sunday: "Dancing with Broken Bones." "My father
danced with broken bones," he said gravely and often throughout his brilliant and impas-
sioned "performance." At the end of the service, the black candle was extinguished and
we proceeded to the cave for a final farewell.

The television crew was waiting for us. On arrival we assembled in the "lounge area,"
where Linda lit a white candle that symbolized the reconciliation, forgiveness, and transcendence that had transformed Cowboy's life during his end-of-life experience. Sadly,
I noticed that the cave had already been ransacked and trashed. Broken liquor bottles
were strewn about, and Cowboy's possessions had been pilfered. News about his death
had spread throughout the streets, and "crack heads have moved in," reported Dr. Ralph.
A few prayers were offered, along with remembrances of Cowboy. I offered the final
prayer, concluding with the words, "Cowboy is no longer dancing with broken bones."
I prayed silently that his soul had found peace, for secretly I agreed with Ibrahim. After
the service, Dwight went back to Ohio; his daughter to Chicago; and Ibrahim went to his

inner-city mosque. Linda and I, with friends who were in attendance at the service, went for a glass of wine and commiserated about the joys of having known Cowboy.

Ibrahim successfully completed his hunger strike 40 days from its beginning. The day he broke it, a rally was held and a march organized from the cave to the state house. One of the police officers who regularly visited Cowboy at the cave provided a police escort for the group of 30 or so people who were participating. Ibrahim walked with a sandwich board over him that stated:

40-DAY FAST FOR
THE HOMELESS
THIS IS DAY
40
ONE GOD
ONE PLANET
ONE
HUMANITY

About midway on the walk from the cave to the state house, the procession passed a fire hydrant. On it were written the following words, "Piss here nigger." As we walked away, I thought how bitterly appropriate the words seemed, given the legacy of racism that fractured Milton as a boy. I also imagined God shedding a tear in His heaven at this precise moment, lamenting how easily and pervasively humans can hate and harm each other, and how Cowboy's story reflected that fact about the human condition. I also imagine God's spirit being buoyed by His observance of the love and mindful presence that was bestowed upon Cowboy, and how that represented all that is right and good about the human potential. Cowboy is gone, but his story is alive and well, its lessons providing a map of the human condition. They show that the American institution of slavery and our societal history of racism are relevant in the 21st century. The evil of hatred and potential for cruelty that seem all too much a part of our humanity are shown to have had a fracturing impact on this man's mind and soul. They demonstrate the injurious consequences of poverty as well. On the other hand, they reveal Cowboy's creativity and love of life, and how he demonstrated a remarkable sense of resilience and inner strength. Perhaps most important of all, the lessons of Cowboy's story declare the redemptive power of love and illuminate the healing and transforming impact of "mindful presence" in the lives of the most vulnerable among us.

In gratitude for the care he received and for the attention of the students who became his friends, Cowboy left his body to the medical school so that even after death he might continue to teach the next generation of doctors. All I can do at this point is to hope and pray that, like Mrs. Angel, Cowboy will find rest, real rest, and peace, real peace. And that his narrative, along with those reflected in the other stories in *Dancing with Broken Bones*, will be heard and honored so that the sufferings of those who live and die at the margins may be healed.

WHAT HAPPENED TO COWGIRL?

Animals often evoke a strong emotional reaction in us. For many people they are not just pets, but beloved members of the family. They elicit joy upon their arrival and generate an authentic sense of loss and grief upon their departure. They stimulate sadness when they suffer and bring delight through their friendship and playful presence in our lives. These feelings reflect the strong bond and sense of relationship that can develop between humans and animals.

The bond that developed between Cowboy and Cowgirl was especially strong. Unlike many throughout his life, she accepted him for who he was. She judged him not for his lifestyle, personal qualities, or racial heritage. And for this reason, in late life, Cowgirl became his best friend, serving as his companion-in-residence at the cave. It is only fitting that these best friends were reunited after her disappearance and shortly before his death. As she left the nursing home that day, following the scent of Cowboy's slippers, she was taken home by Peggy, who as you will recall was a respiratory therapist at Deerfield Village. Peggy successfully fostered her adoption, and Cowgirl, fully healed from her injury, went to live on a spacious farm that is far removed from the inner-city intersection where she would patiently wait for the return of Cowboy. It remains to be seen, however, if Cowboy was right in his assertion that they would meet up again, joining him in heaven, after her life on this earth is finished.

13

COWBOY'S LEGACY
REFLECTIONS ON END-OF-LIFE
CARE OF THE URBAN POOR

Shirley Otis-Green

The dying need the community, its help, fellowship, care and attention, which will quiet their distress and fears and enable them to go peacefully. The community needs the dying to make it think of eternal issues and to make it listen and give to others.
—Dame Cicely Saunders

Cowboy's narrative in David Moller's *Dancing with Broken Bones: Poverty, Race, and Spirit-filled Dying in the Inner City* (2012)[1] describes a life lived through a prism of poverty and racism. The marginalization and stigmatization of the disenfranchised blind us to (and shield us from) the myriad ways that these social realities increase the suffering of the dying urban poor. Moller recognized that, for the economic statistics surrounding the numbers of homeless persons facing end of life to have meaning, they must first have a face. Cowboy's story provides the framework in which we can consider the impact of a lifetime of racism, violence, abuse, and poverty.

MARGINALIZATION

Cowboy was born into a world of poverty and racism in the rural South of Depression-era America. His extended family ostracized both him and his young mother, leaving an indelible imprint that continued into the next generation. Cowboy found that his biracial heritage closed doors for him wherever he traveled and became the foundation for his marginalized existence. Limited education, skills, and social support compounded the wounds of his violent past and magnified the barriers that he faced in attempts to escape a life of poverty. Although resilient and "street savvy" and often able to charm his way into the hearts of others, he experienced a lifetime of brief serial relationships. Over time, he alienated his family and took up residence under a bridge, with his dog, Cowgirl, his closest companion.

Cowboy, like many who live in poverty, was forced to make critical decisions daily regarding how to use his limited resources so as to survive and get along. These "forced choices" required minute-by-minute compromises that may seem contradictory to his longer-term best interests (for example, the decision to use limited resources to buy cigarettes). Living on the street requires decisions about what items can be transported with you (and which will have to be left behind) and which "found" items are worth carrying "home" (and again, which, though potentially useful in the future, will have to be left behind).

The cumulative consequences of living a life with thousands of such choices multiplies the risk that decision fatigue will set in, resulting in less psychic energy being available for "higher level" decision-making.[2] An appreciation for the implications of living with chronic decision fatigue contributes to our understanding of how the stress associated with an overwhelming number of such daily decisions contributes to a pattern of compromised capacity for long-term decision-making.

The diagnosis of lung cancer in his 70s brings Cowboy face to face with a regimented and impersonal medical system, one which was poorly adapted to the unique needs of the "homeless" or "mentally ill."[3] Although still charismatic and often congenial, Cowboy remained alienated and outside the social "safety net," challenging his caregivers to craft a personalized care plan, one that would require them to extend themselves beyond the normative boundaries of the safety-net system, in order to address his complex needs not only for medical care but for shelter. Caring for Cowboy in the midst of the chaos and complexity that surrounded him increased their risk for moral distress and burnout. Cowboy's experience, while unique, is not atypical. The poor face limited options regarding care and find themselves dependent upon a deeply fragmented healthcare "system" that is ill-designed to meet their multidimensional needs.[4,5] The lack of an integrated system of care contributed immeasurably to the further marginalization of Cowboy and presented nearly insurmountable challenges for his healthcare providers.

As Cowboy's disease progressed, he responded with increased anxiety as hospitalization and its associated "institutionalization" threatened his identity and self-worth. Hospital discharges resulted in further disenfranchisement and demoralization when he was evicted from the shelters that had reluctantly accepted him. The aspects of his life that most contributed to his sense of meaning and purpose were stripped from him as he found himself "placed" in various "homes." Losing the ability to care for and be with his beloved Cowgirl compounded the impact of his grief and further compromised his ability to "manage" his disease. As Cowboy's vulnerability intensified, he relied increasingly upon the palliative care team who had committed themselves to assisting him improve his well-being.

PROFESSIONALISM AND ETHICAL PRACTICE

The palliative care team's commitment to care for Cowboy came at a tremendous personal and professional price. Cowboy's needs for comprehensive, person-centered care transcended the scope of what the US healthcare system is currently designed to supply. His caregivers were caught in an ethical trap. Truly caring for Cowboy required that his care providers either work outside the boundaries of conventional medical practice, or ignore major aspects of his suffering. Neither strategy was ultimately sustainable. Cowboy's situation was an uncomfortable reminder that our current healthcare "system" is not only untenable, but ultimately unconscionable for all involved, and poorly designed to address the social determinants of health that magnified his suffering.

Professional healthcare providers are taught to work within the limits of their "scope of practice" and are reminded to develop "healthy boundaries" to "protect" themselves as they encounter the suffering of others. The challenge is that we are each responsible to determine where our professional boundaries will be for any given situation. The lack of mentorship and support leaves us vulnerable and at risk for ethical and moral distress and burnout.[6]

ETHICAL AND MORAL DISTRESS

Ethical and moral distress occurs when we finds ourselves in the unenviable situation of being thwarted in being able to do what we believe needs to be done. The contradiction between what we feel needs to be done and what we are expected to do (or what we are allowed to do) results in ethical and moral distress and is a significant contributing factor in the decision of many providers to prematurely leave the field of health care.[7] Palliative care professionals are especially vulnerable to this stress due to our exposure to intense and often unrelieved suffering.[8] We must each find a way to reconcile this paradox if we are to maintain our ability to compassionately do this work. Finding mentors who can offer guidance regarding this complex negotiation is crucial. New members of the team are particularly vulnerable to this ethical and moral distress and are particularly in need of mentorship and support to guide them.[9]

Linda, his palliative social worker, responded to Cowboy's non-medical concerns with unmatched empathy and dedication and committed herself to his care regardless of personal cost and professional criticism. Awareness that Cowboy's needs received more attention than did others' (who were perhaps equally needy and equally deserving) created an ethical challenge for the reflective practitioner. How do we reconcile ourselves with the uncomfortable reality that we "can't be all things to all people?" As Cowboy's needs continued to escalate, this intensive level of care became increasingly difficult to sustain and took an ever-increasing toll on this dedicated social worker's well-being. We can speculate that as a palliative social worker, she was deeply motivated to redress some of the social injustices that Cowboy had experienced throughout his tumultuous life, yet her professional role offered only limited "authority" to respond to these overwhelming needs.[10]

As a social worker, Linda was trained to think in terms of systems and to recognize the benefits of enhancing Cowboy's network of social support.[11] No doubt, in her career at this safety-net urban hospital, she had encountered numerous socially-isolated individuals who, upon death, became "unclaimed bodies" within the county morgue system. As Cowboy's illness escalated, her motivation to assist him in reconciliation with his children intensified, perhaps in hope of preventing this scenario for Cowboy.

> His caregivers are caught in an ethical trap. Truly caring for Cowboy requires that his care providers either work outside the boundaries of conventional medical practice or ignore major aspects of his suffering.

Yet even Cowboy recognized the inherent futility and tremendous burden that was imposed on the team members that resulted when his care providers seemed to be more concerned than he was regarding specific health outcomes. "You can't worry about these things more than I do, he instructed them."[12] Being in such untenable situations increases the palliative care team's risk for moral distress and burnout, along with feelings of helplessness.

Palliative care professionals are asked to sit with the suffering of others and to do so in a system that is poorly designed to support us in this task. Not surprisingly, then, we may find ourselves becoming numb to the pain of others in an attempt to protect ourselves. Consistent exposure to physical, psychological, social, spiritual, and existential suffering impacts all care providers, who often lack appropriate self-care strategies.[13] Failure to care for ourselves may result in a tendency to distance ourselves from the very people most in need of our caring and support. Reflective practice can help us to identify the early signs of burnout so that we might implement robust strategies to address these concerns and remain committed and compassionate care providers.[14,15]

> Cowboy's story reminds us that the care of the dying is best done in the community.

Despite the very real challenges inherent in working with this population, palliative care providers are also privileged to be witnesses to moments of incredible grace and healing. Walking with Cowboy through his struggles was a transformative experience for all involved. His humanity, resilience, generosity, humor, and spirit left a powerful legacy for his care providers, his family after they were reconciled, and his community. His courage in facing his dying and his willingness to invite others to learn from his experiences profoundly changed the way "his students" practice medicine. Confidence that one's work is meaningfully making a difference in the lives of others is a powerful antidote to burnout

THE NEXT GENERATION OF PALLIATIVE CARE: INTEGRATING ADVOCACY AND LEADERSHIP IN THE TRANSFORMATION OF HEALTH CARE

Advocacy and leadership are essential elements of professionalism. The "Cowboys" of our world remind us of our need to be advocates for a system where competent and compassionate care is reliably and humanely delivered for all. Healthcare professionals have an ethical obligation to be advocates for a reformation in the delivery of care.[16] We understand the brokenness of the system. We see the unmet needs of the underserved and experience the personal and professional impact of misaligned incentives in a bureaucracy that too often harms those it is meant to heal. We are the ones who realize the urgency to transform our current "non-system" of healthcare into one that recognizes the inherent dignity and worth of each individual and is committed to providing an environment where the search for meaning and purpose are of as much attention as lab values and blood draws.[17,18] (Figure 13.1).

The next generation of palliative care professionals is needed to continue the field's pioneering efforts to build a more-humane healthcare system where culturally-appropriate

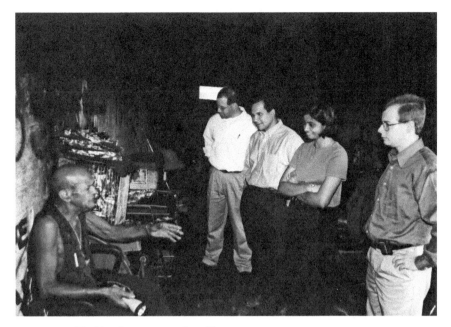

FIGURE 13.1 Teaching the next generation of doctors.

care is delivered in a comprehensive, community-based environment.[19,20] This new system will emphasize the importance of personalized communication to identify truly person-centered and family-focused goals of care. Patients' pain and symptom management needs will be reliably addressed by an interprofessional team of skilled professionals who can competently address the complex and multidimensional concerns of those with a history of mental illness or substance abuse.[21] Committed and compassionate leaders are needed to ensure that health care can be sustainably delivered and will be reliably accessible to diverse populations without regard to social status or economic class.[11,22]

> We understand the brokenness of the system. We see the unmet needs of the underserved and experience the personal and professional impact of misaligned incentives in a bureaucracy that too often harms those it is meant to heal.

SUMMARY: COWBOY'S LEGACY

Cowboy's story reminds us that the care of the dying is best done in community. His increasing vulnerability is an uncomfortable reminder that we, too, may someday be dependent upon others to meet our needs. Despite our attempts to distance ourselves from the dying, we each may all too soon find ourselves alienated and marginalized in the very institutional "system" that at present so poorly cares for others. Cowboy is a reminder that we may also one day have to rely upon others for compassionate and competent care that is reliably delivered. Cowboy's story calls us to action, for in designing a system that will reliably meet his needs, we are also taking steps to better assure that our own needs will be met when our time comes.

REFERENCES

1. Moller D. *Dancing with Broken Bones: Poverty, Race, and Spirit-filled Dying in the Inner City.* New York: Oxford University Press; 2012.
2. Vohs KD, Baumeister RF, Schmeichel BJ, Twenge JM, Nelson NM, Tice DM. Making choices impairs subsequent self-control: a limited-resource account of decision making, self-regulation, and active initiative. *J Pers Soc Psychol.* 2008;94(5):883–898.
3. Otis-Green S, Rutland C. Marginalization at the end of life. In: Berzoff, Silverman (Eds.). *Living with dying: a handbook for end-of-life healthcare practitioners.* New York: Columbia University Press; 2004:310–324.
4. Lewis JM, DiGiacomo M, Currow DC, Davidson PM. Dying in the margins: understanding palliative care and socioeconomic deprivation in the developed world. *J Pain Sympt Manag.* 2011;42(1):105–118.
5. Colon Y. Working with sociocultural and economic diversity. In: Christ G, Messner C, Behar L (Eds.). *Handbook of Oncology Social Work.* New York: Oxford University Press; 2015:263–267.
6. Otis-Green S. Embracing the existential invitation to examine care at the end of life. In: Qualls SH, Kasl-Godley J (Eds.). *The Wiley series in clinical geropsychology: end-of-life issues, grief and bereavement: what clinicians need to know.* Hoboken: NJ: John Wiley and Sons; 2011:462–481.
7. Sardiwalla N, VandenBerg H, Esterhuyse KGF. The role of stressors and coping strategies in the burnout experienced by hospice workers. *Cancer Nurs.* 2007;30(6):488–497.
8. Kamal AH, Bull JH, Wolf SP, et al. Prevalence and predictors of burnout among hospice and palliative care clinicians in the U.S. *J Pain Sympt Manag.* 2016;51(4): 690–696.
9. Kearney MK, Weininger RB, Vachon, MLS, Harrison RL, Mount BM. Self-care of physicians caring for patients at the end of life: being connected . . . a key to my survival. *JAMA.* 2009;301(11):1155–1164.
10. Smullens S. *Burnout and self-care in social work.* Washington, DC: NASW Press; 2015.
11. Altilio T, Otis-Green S (Eds.). *Oxford textbook of palliative social work.* New York: Oxford University Press; 2011.
12. Moller DW. *Dancing with Broken Bones: Portraits of Death and Dying Among Inner-City Poor..* New York: Oxford University Press; 2004:66.
13. Sinclair S. Impact of death and dying on the personal lives and practices of palliative and hospice care professionals. *CMAJ.* 2011;183(2):180–187.
14. Perry B. Why exemplary oncology nurses seem to avoid compassion fatigue. *Can Oncol Nurs J.* 2008;18(2):87–99.
15. Showalter SE. Compassion fatigue: What is it? Why does it matter? Recognizing the symptoms, acknowledging the impact, developing the tools to prevent compassion fatigue, and strengthen the professional already suffering from the effects. *Am J Hospice Palliat Med.* 2010;27(4):239–242.
16. Otis-Green S. Legacy building: implications for reflective practice. In: Altilio T, Otis-Green S (Eds.). *Oxford textbook of palliative social work.* New York: Oxford University Press; 2011-A:779–783.
17. Borneman T, Brown-Saltzman K. Meaning in illness. In: Ferrell BR, Coyle N, Paice JA (Eds.). *Oxford textbook of palliative nursing, third edition.* New York: Oxford University Press; 2010:554–563.
18. Chochinov HM. Dignity-conserving care: a new model for palliative care. *JAMA.* 2002;287(17):2253–2260.

19. Ferrell BR. Humanizing the experience of pain and illness. In: Ferrell BR (Ed.). *Suffering.* Sudbury, MA: Jones and Bartlett Publishers; 1996:3–27.

20. Lynn J, Schuster JL, Kabcenell A. *Improving care for the end of life: a sourcebook for health care managers and clinicians.* New York: Oxford University Press; 2000.

21. Altilio T, Otis-Green S, Hedlund S, Cohen Fineberg I. Pain management and palliative care. In: Gehlert S, Arthur Browne T (Eds.). *Handbook of health social work, second edition.* Hoboken, NJ: John Wiley and Sons; 2012:590–626.

22. Otis-Green S, Rutland C. Marginalization at the end of life. In: Berzoff P, Silverman J (Eds.). *Living with dying: a handbook for end-of-life healthcare practitioners.* New York: Columbia University Press; 2004:310–324.

EPILOGUE
A CALL TO ACTION: CARING AT THE MARGINS

Diane Meier and Stacie Sinclair

Dancing with Broken Bones gives readers the privilege of meeting those who are forgotten or ignored in our society, often from the moment they are born until they draw their last breath. Each story—Cowboy, Mr. Green, the Wheelers, and the Whites—is important because these people existed. Because they mattered. Because they were courageous enough to share their most vulnerable moments with an audience that their experiences should have taught them to mistrust. The best way to honor their generosity is by absorbing their unique stories and integrating their lessons as we encounter new people throughout our lives.

Yet from the collection of these patients' experiences, there is another story to be told. Their lives and deaths tell of a failure in public policy to protect people living on the margins of our society. Every new administration and Congress grapples with decisions on what role federal and state governments should play in caring for low-income and homeless populations, which programs will be most effective, and how much of the budget can be "sacrificed" to these line items. Ideology plays a prominent role, as does economic context, and we have seen the public safety net expand and contract with almost every transition of power. Yet even in the most generous of administrations, the piecemeal nature of this country's social welfare programs leaves ample room for underserved populations to fall through the cracks. By considering what healthcare—and to a lesser extent, welfare—policies were in place when this book was written, what has changed since that time, and what policies the current administration has proposed, readers will be better equipped to advocate for those who are too sick and too poor to do so for themselves.

HEALTHCARE AND THE SAFETY NET OVER THE PAST THREE ADMINISTRATIONS

Much has changed since the initial publication of *Dancing with Broken Bones* in 2004. As Dr. Moller was caring for and collecting stories from his patients, there was relative economic prosperity in the Clinton and early Bush administrations. This would eventually give way to the largest recession since the Great Depression under the late Bush/early Obama administrations, increasing the percentage of the population in poverty from a low of 11.3% in 2000 to a high of 15.1% in 2010 before leveling off (see Box 14.1).[1] Each

Box 14.1 The Federal Poverty Level

A critical element of determining eligibility for government safety net programs has been operationally defining "poverty." Over time, the federal government and other stakeholders have developed multiple methodologies for calculating poverty,[1] but eligibility for many of today's programs is grounded in the work done by Social Security Administration economist Mollie Orshansky in 1963–1964. Originally based on US Department of Agriculture estimates that families spent approximately one-third of their after-tax money on food, her formula essentially multiplied the estimated value of the economy (i.e., bare minimum) food plan times three. Although not developed to be a new measure of poverty—historians paraphrased Ms. Orshansky saying that the thresholds would be better considered "as a measure of income **inadequacy**, not of income adequacy"—the formula was officially adopted to calculate the Federal Poverty Level (FPL) guidelines in 1969 and has since remained largely unchanged.

While eligibility for some means-tested government programs can be based on slightly higher income levels (e.g., the Children's Health Insurance Program [CHIP] provides health insurance to children in families making up to 138%), many more programs are limited to those earning less than or equal to 100% of the FPL. This is problematic as the guidelines are very low (see Table 14.1), and with the exception of Alaska and Hawaii, do not vary by region. And it is worth noting that there is tremendous inequality, with approximately more black (24%) and Hispanic (21%) households living in poverty than white (9%) households.[53]

Table 14.1 Federal Poverty Level (FPL) Guidelines

Persons in Family/ Household	2000	2010	2017
1	$8,350	$10,830	$12,060
2	$11,250	$14,570	$16,240
3	$14,150	$18,310	$20,420
4	$17,050	$22,050	$24,600
8	$28,650	$37,010	$41,320
Each additional person	$2,900	$3,740	$4,180

Source: Office of the Assistant Secretary for Planning and Evaluation

Note: FPL amounts are higher in Alaska and Hawaii

administration made changes to health and/or welfare policies, either while executing its own priorities or in response to external crises. What follows is a discussion of selected policies and programs that had implications for the dying poor, either in terms of direct support or general attitudes toward those who are considered "deserving" and those considered "undeserving" (Box 14.1).

CLINTON EFFORTS TO "END WELFARE AS WE KNOW IT" AND ESTABLISH UNIVERSAL HEALTHCARE

During the Clinton administration, the economy performed well in several key indicators—unemployment (below 4% by 2001), labor force participation (67.2%), gross domestic product (GDP) growth (3.8%), and wage growth (increase from $661/week to $700/week for the median household).[2-4] Although income inequality began to rise more rapidly than it had in previous generations, particularly for the top 10%,[5] the country's relative prosperity probably made the idea of welfare reform more palatable to the populace. In 1996, President Bill Clinton signed into law the Personal Responsibility and Work Opportunity Reconciliation Act (PRWORA). Its most notable provision was the termination of the Aid to Families with Dependent Children (AFDC) program, which was replaced by the Temporary Assistance for Needy Families (TANF) program. The former program provided cash assistance payments based on need as defined by the state, while the latter created a block grant that effectively capped federal contributions.[6] TANF eliminated the "entitlement" status of welfare since program eligibility did not necessarily ensure receipt of support if funds were already fully expended; indeed, by 2002, only 48% of households that were eligible for TANF received it (down from 82% in 1992).[7] It also increased work participation requirements, imposed a lifetime limit on the amount of time a family could receive federal assistance, and gave states latitude to transfer up to 30% of the federal funds to other programs. While these changes might not have had a significant impact on low-income childless adults such as Cowboy or Mr. Green, who were generally ineligible to receive payments under either AFDC or TANF, they signaled a paradigm shift toward more restrictive policies for impoverished populations and were met with some controversy.[8] Subsequent evaluations showed that welfare reform did not have any statistically significant effects on poverty or deep poverty,[9] nor did it reduce the intergenerational transmission of poverty (Box 14.2).[10]

In addition to welfare, reforming the healthcare system was an early priority of the Clinton administration; however, despite much effort, the President and Congress were unable to pass national health insurance legislation.[11] Absent comprehensive health reform, President Clinton made a few changes at the margins. For example, his administration established Programs of All-inclusive Care for the Elderly (PACE) as a permanent Medicare benefit and an optional Medicaid benefit under the Balanced Budget Act of 1997 (BBA).[12] This program allows eligible beneficiaries to remain in the community while receiving comprehensive services from an interdisciplinary team. PACE is effective in meeting the needs of low-income, aging patients, a significant percentage of whom will live for several years with multiple chronic conditions, functional and cognitive limitations, and high healthcare utilization. President Clinton also established the State Children's Health Insurance Program (SCHIP, now more commonly referred to as CHIP), a federal–state partnership that provides health coverage to children whose family income is above the Medicaid eligibility threshold but is still low enough to make accessing insurance difficult. Evaluations of this program demonstrated success in reducing uninsurance rates among children and improvements in access to care, including preventive services.[13] There is also some evidence to suggest that CHIP has contributed to a reduction in avoidable hospitalizations and mortality among low-income children, although results are variable.[14]

Box 14.2   US Spending on Healthcare Versus Social Supports

Experts note that despite spending more on healthcare per capita than all other developed countries in the world (estimated average of $10,350 in 2016,[54] with the top 5% averaging $47,498[55]), the United States fares worse on many key health indicators such as life expectancy and multimorbidity. Meanwhile, the United States spends a far smaller share (approximately 9%) of its GDP on social services such as housing, nutrition, and income supports. This is notable, as recent models point to the fact that medical care only accounts for 10% of overall health, with social circumstances and environmental factors contributing at least 20% (Figure 14.1).

   Spending on social supports and services such as housing, nutrition, and income support can have a positive impact on health outcomes and healthcare costs.[57] One study found that higher spending on social supports as compared to spending on healthcare in states was positively correlated with better health outcomes. Spending (or lack thereof) on social supports also manifests in disparate health outcomes for underserved and diverse communities. As policymakers continue searching for solutions to contain healthcare spending as a percentage of GDP, only proposals that include addressing upstream social determinants of health will be effective in the long run.

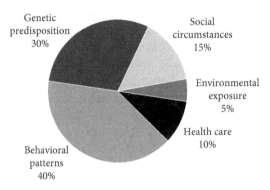

FIGURE 14.1 Determinants of health.
Source: Schroeder SA, *N Engl J Med*, September 2007; adapted from McGinnis JM, Russo PG, Knickman JR, *Health Aff*, April 2002.

BUSH-ERA POLICIES AND THE START OF THE GREAT RECESSION

Early in President George W. Bush's campaign, he described himself as a "compassionate conservative." This philosophy appeared to manifest itself in policies that demonstrated some level of commitment to the needy but also a desire to reduce individual dependence on the government. His reauthorization of TANF as part of the Deficit Reduction Omnibus Reconciliation Act of 2006 included even more stringent work requirements and minimum benchmarks that recipients had to meet, increased pressure on states to reduce their caseload, and provided states with more authority to limit assistance.[7]

Furthermore, it shifted the program away from welfare checks (fungible payments) to non-cash assistance such as short-term childcare, job search assistance, and substance-use disorder treatment. Perspectives on cash versus non-cash assistance are mixed: while some argue that cash benefits create a disincentive to work and can be used inappropriately, others think that specific support services can be complicated for states to administer, may be difficult for beneficiaries to access, and do not address all of the underlying causes of the need for assistance.

In the meantime, as TANF benefits declined, the Earned Income Tax Credit (EITC) began to provide a larger share of cash assistance to low-wage families. Designed as a refundable tax credit, the EITC was found to be relatively effective in lifting certain populations out of poverty[15] and perhaps could have benefited someone like Mr. White who had a wife and four children and consistently worked full time for 25 years. That being said, there were important gaps in the benefit design, including the calculation of phase-in and phase-out rates that maximized the credit amount to those whose income was closest to the Federal Poverty Level (FPL), very low credits to low-wage childless workers, and no assistance for those not working.

The Bush administration's most significant domestic contribution to improving healthcare access for low-income and seriously ill populations was its investment in Federally Qualified Health Centers (FQHCs). In many communities, FQHCs are the primary point of care, and because of their mandate to provide services regardless of ability to pay, they serve a disproportionate share of Medicaid and low-income patients (roughly two out of every three patients living in poverty).[16] President Bush's Health Center Growth Initiative (HCGI) sought to add new or expand existing health centers over five years by distributing grants for expanded medical capacity (EMC) and new access points (NAPs).[17] By the end of the initial project period, there were more than 1,200 new and expanded access points in medically underserved areas. Centers that received both NAP and EMC funding saw significant growth in the number of patients they were able to see, compared to those who received no funding (58% increase compared to 10% increase, respectively), and much of the increased volume was composed of Medicaid beneficiaries and those with incomes of less than 200% of the FPL. The HCGI was followed by the passage of the Health Care Safety Net Act of 2008, which reauthorized appropriations to continue funding the health centers program. The Obama administration would build on these efforts in the following years. Despite the positive trend in community health center expansion, however, stakeholders expressed concern that an estimated 56 million people in the country still had inadequate access to primary care by the end of 2008.[18]

Other notable Bush-era health policies included the Health Insurance Flexibility and Accountability (HIFA) demonstrations and the Medicare Prescription Drug, Improvement, and Modernization Act (MMA). The HIFA demonstrations provided states with more flexibility in their Medicaid and SCHIP programs through a Section 1115 waiver, in an effort to test strategies for expanding coverage.[19] Although state budget shortages and low enrollment among participants presented challenges, an early examination of ten state HIFA waivers showed enthusiasm for the benefit and cost-sharing flexibility, as well as "a particular interest in expanding coverage to groups that historically have been excluded from publicly-sponsored coverage, such as childless adults, higher-income parents, and the working poor."[20] Meanwhile, the MMA significantly expanded

Medicare through a number of programs and changes, including the establishment of Health Savings Accounts and their associated high-deductible health plans, and the transition from Medicare+Choice to Medicare Advantage. The establishment of the Medicare Prescription Drug Benefit (Part D) probably helped low-income patients with serious illness; an early evaluation showed that it reduced the percentage of older Americans who lacked drug coverage and led to significant increases in filled prescriptions and decreased drug costs,[21] and as of September 2016, nearly 41 million Medicare beneficiaries were enrolled in Part D plans.[22]

Altogether, President Bush's policies indicated high-level concern for vulnerable populations and took steps to strengthen certain elements of the safety net. However, these new programs fell short of the comprehensive reform needed to ensure access for low-income and seriously ill persons, leaving gaps in healthcare coverage and essential services and supports. The Great Recession exposed these gaps as people began losing their jobs and, by extension, their employer-sponsored health insurance. The official poverty rate increased by 2.5% between 2007 and 2011,[23] while the uninsurance rate among 18- to 64-year-olds peaked at 18.2% in 2010.[24] The consequences of the Great Recession were also felt more deeply among communities of color, with African Americans and Hispanic families experiencing significantly larger losses in wealth than white families.[25]

OBAMA'S ECONOMIC RECOVERY AND THE AFFORDABLE CARE ACT

Within the first month of his administration, President Obama passed the American Recovery and Reinvestment Act of 2009 (ARRA), an $831 billion stimulus package developed to cushion the impact of the Great Recession and accelerate economic recovery. At a high level, it provided tax incentives for individuals (including a $4.7 billion expansion to the EITC for families with children); invested in healthcare (including $86.8 billion to Medicaid, and $25.8 billion to promote adoption of health information technology), education, energy, infrastructure, housing, and scientific research; and infused $82.2 billion into means-tested and social insurance safety net programs, including Social Security, Supplemental Security Income (SSI), Meals on Wheels, food stamps, and TANF payments.[26] While there are many conflicting opinions on whether the ARRA was the most effective approach to recovery, evidence suggests that investments in the safety net were beneficial, with funding being distributed across multiple demographic groups.[23] It is likely that every patient described in *Dying at the Margins* could have benefited from several of these expanded programs.

As important as the stimulus package was, health policy was a cornerstone of the Obama administration. President Obama passed several pieces of healthcare legislation, including the CHIP Reauthorization Act of 2009, which expanded the program to an additional 4 million children as well as pregnant women,[27] and the bipartisan Medicare Access and CHIP Reauthorization Act of 2015 (MACRA), which—in addition to renewing CHIP for two years—accelerated the transition to value-based payment for clinicians caring for Medicare Part B beneficiaries. However, much of Obama's legacy will be linked to the Patient Protection and Affordable Care Act (PPACA, or ACA), which brought dramatic changes to almost every part of the healthcare system. The following sections discuss some of the provisions that had the most impact on low-income and seriously ill populations.

Medicaid Expansion

The ACA expanded the eligibility criteria for Medicaid so that parents and childless adults with incomes between 100% and 138% of the FPL (approximately $33,465 for a family of four in 2016) could enroll in the program. The expansion was designed in such a way that the federal government would fund 100% of the expansion costs for the first three years starting in 2014, and then gradually taper down to a 90/10 split with the states. Medicaid expansion was originally intended to cover all US adults in this income bracket; however, the Supreme Court's 2012 ruling effectively made it optional. As of publication, 31 states and the District of Columbia had chosen to expand Medicaid, resulting an increase of approximately 14.5 million adults to the program.[*],[28] Evaluations on the impact of expansion on access to care and health outcomes have shown an increase in the percentage of patients having annual wellness visits and preventive services (e.g., blood pressure screenings, flu shots),[29] increased prescription utilization,[30] and lower out-of-pocket spending for patients with chronic conditions.[31,32]

Health Insurance Exchanges and Subsidies

The ACA established "exchanges" (a.k.a. "marketplaces") wherein individuals who did not have employer-sponsored insurance could purchase a health plan. All states had the option of establishing their own exchanges, but many chose to partner either with other states or with the federal government, with 28 states electing to simply use the federally facilitated marketplaces.[33] At the same time, the ACA provided federal subsidies and cost-sharing reductions to purchase coverage on the individual market for those with incomes between 138% and 400% of the FPL (or more than 100% of the FPL for those in states that did not expand Medicaid). From 2013 to 2014, the share of low-income workers who purchased health insurance in the individual market rose from 6% to 10%.[34] One analysis of the individual marketplaces showed a significant drop in the uninsured rates for those with family incomes of less than $48,500, with respondents reporting greater ease in finding affordable health plans and an increased ability to obtain needed care.[35]

Other relevant provisions related to individual coverage include "guaranteed issue," meaning insurers cannot deny coverage due to preexisting conditions; a ban on annual and lifetime coverage limits; protection from losing insurance in the event of illness; and an annual limit on out-of-pocket expenses for individuals and families. All plans were also required to cover 10 "Essential Health Benefits," which include:

1. Ambulatory patient services
2. Emergency services

---

* This total is split into two groups—those who were newly eligible for Medicaid under expansion rules (approximately 11.2 million people) and those who had been eligible prior to the expansion but for some reason had not previously enrolled (approximately 3.3 million).

3. Hospitalization
4. Maternity and newborn care
5. Mental health and substance use disorder services, including behavioral health treatment
6. Prescription drugs
7. Rehabilitative and habilitative services and devices
8. Laboratory services
9. Preventive and wellness services and chronic disease management
10. Pediatric services

Community Health Centers Expansion

Building on the FQHC expansion under the Bush administration, the ACA included several billion dollars to increase the number of new centers and update existing ones.[36] There are several different kinds of FQHCs across the United States in addition to the standard ones that serve a variety of underserved populations or areas, including health centers that provide care to migrant and seasonal agricultural workers and their families; healthcare for the homeless programs that provide care to homeless individuals, including substance abuse and mental health services; and public housing primary care programs that provide care to public housing residents, often on or near public housing premises. The increased ACA funding, along with the growing proportion of patients who had coverage through Medicaid expansion or the individual markets, helped stabilize the centers' budgets and increase their capacity (e.g., higher staff-to-patient ratios). Thus, more patients have been able to access preventive services sooner, improving overall health and allowing patients who might have serious illnesses to detect problems sooner. Despite these benefits, it is worth noting that the centers continue to see a disproportionate share of low-income patients who are unable to pay deductibles and cost-sharing (particularly in non-expansion states) and tend to be in poorer health.

Alternative Payment Models and Other Demonstration Projects

The ACA expanded programs and demonstrations designed to accelerate the transition from a healthcare system that pays for volume to one that pays for value. The Centers for Medicare and Medicaid Services (CMS) managed much of this activity, overseeing various quality-reporting programs as well as the newly established Center for Medicare and Medicaid Innovation (CMMI). CMMI was charged with testing innovative payment and delivery models that could improve the care provided, improve health outcomes, and reduce overall cost to the healthcare system. Several models focused on low-income populations in both Medicaid and Medicare, improvements in the care of serious illness (e.g., the Oncology Care Model), and at least one model targeted care at the end of life (Medicare Care Choices Model). Several palliative care models were tested through the Health Care Innovation Awards. And the recent announcement of the Accountable Health Communities model provided formal acknowledgment of the need to support health-related social needs (e.g., food insecurity, unstable housing), as these have been shown to play an outsized role in health outcomes—even more than medical care itself.

The ACA also supported the transition to "whole-person" care through the creation of Accountable Care Organizations (ACOs). Groups of physicians, hospitals, and other providers could establish networks that allowed for greater coordination of care for an assigned population and, in some cases, increased flexibility to pay for services that may not be allowed under traditional Medicare, including care navigation and linkages to community-based organizations, social service agencies, and public health resources. In exchange, ACOs agreed to be accountable for the outcomes of their patients—as well as the overall cost of care—and could receive incentive payments and/or shared savings, depending on the arrangement, the level of risk accepted, and the amount of money saved.

Approximately 20 million people gained coverage under the ACA, the uninsurance rate dropped to 12.4% from 18.2% in 2016,[37] and health spending slowed considerably after the law's passage.[38] The ACA benefited low-income and homeless persons by making health coverage more accessible and affordable for a portion of this population, covering treatment for issues that disproportionately affect them, and moving toward a more person-centered system of care that rewards high-value services. Providers such as those working in Health Care for the Homeless projects observed double-digit increases in health coverage in Medicaid expansion states between 2012 and 2014; this contributed to larger revenue gains, which in turn increased the projects' financial stability.[39]

Yet the ACA had many shortcomings as well. Approximately 27 million non-elderly individuals remained uninsured by the end of 2016; the health insurance exchanges in several states struggled to retain insurers and keep premiums affordable; and, in some areas, access to coverage did not necessarily translate into access to care. It is beyond the scope of this epilogue to discuss the politics surrounding the ACA's passage and rollout, but one of the Obama administration's greatest failures was its inability to clearly communicate to the public what the law did. This created ample opportunity for opponents to undermine the ACA's implementation (e.g., failing to approve risk-corridor payments to insurers that agreed to cover high-need, high-risk patients) and mount a campaign that eventually gained enough traction to threaten the law's survival.

SIGNALS FROM THE TRUMP ADMINISTRATION
ON SUPPORT FOR THE DYING POOR

On January 20, 2016, Donald Trump was sworn in as the 45th President of the United States. Bolstered by a Republican majority in both the House and Senate, one of the new administration's first priorities was to honor its campaign pledge for the swift repeal and replacement of the ACA. Leadership began working to coalesce around solutions that would undo the "regulatory burdens" and "executive overreach" of the healthcare law while maintaining popular patient protections and coverage gains (at least in the short run). However, proposals such as the "American Health Care Act," then-Representative Tom Price's "Empowering Patient First Act," and House Speaker Paul Ryan's "A Better Way" provide insight into some of the strategies favored to accomplish this administration's goals.[40] It is worth noting that not all the proposals are inherently bad; like everything, the impact will depend on the details. However, there are several proposals that could negatively impact low-income, seriously ill populations, including:

- Sunsetting or fully repealing Medicaid expansion, which would rapidly undo the coverage gains made under the ACA;
- Implementing Medicaid work requirements, which fail to acknowledge that most low-income persons and Medicaid recipients who can work already do so, and if they don't, it may be due to other systemic barriers;[41]
- Converting Medicare to a premium support system, which, if not implemented carefully, will limit choices and access for low-income beneficiaries or make coverage unaffordable;[42]
- Repealing marketplace subsidies and replacing them with fixed tax credits based on age rather than income;
- Imposing a substantial penalty on individuals who fail to maintain continuous coverage;
- Implementing high-risk pools, which, in the past, have failed due to high costs and limited coverage;[43] and
- Converting federal support for Medicaid from a calculated match rate to a per capita allotment or a block grant.

The last proposal is particularly alarming because it would significantly reduce the amount of federal funding provided to states. States would feel the impact most acutely in their care of seriously-ill beneficiaries, including older adults who rely on Medicaid for long-term services and supports and children with life-limiting illness since a per capita cap would not account for higher costs of individuals in these populations. This would put states that are already facing budgetary pressure in the difficult position of having to modify or even eliminate certain benefits (including the "optional" hospice benefit) for vulnerable patients if block grants do not provide enough resources to care for everyone who is entitled to Medicaid coverage. Alternately, it is feasible that block-granting Medicaid could lead to waitlists similar to those seen with TANF, wherein those eligible for benefits could be denied coverage due to lack of funds. This could be catastrophic in the context of serious illness (Figure 14.2).

Absent legislation, the administration can make several substantive changes to ACA implementation through regulation. Early in his tenure, Secretary of Health and Human Services (HHS) Tom Price delayed implementation of several bundled payment models and informed state governors of increased flexibility in setting Medicaid premiums and cost-sharing. Other actions Secretary Price could take include:

1. Ending cost-sharing payments to insurers.
2. Failing to enforce the individual mandate that is designed to keep younger and healthier people in the marketplace risk pool.
3. Reducing reimbursement payments to insurers.
4. Making liberal use of the ACA's state innovation waivers, allowing states to overhaul their markets if they meet certain requirements.

While these actions might not result in what stakeholders would consider full repeal, they could nonetheless threaten the sustainability of several fundamental ACA provisions.

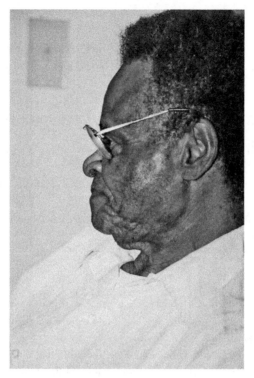

FIGURE 14.2 Their stories attest to a failure in public policy and an unwillingness to address the injustice of disparities in health and wealth.

Beyond healthcare, the Trump administration's first budget blueprint made a strong statement about its commitment to low-income and seriously ill populations. Looking only at discretionary programs, this budget proposed to cut billions of dollars in funding to several of the agencies and programs that care for the most vulnerable populations.[44] For instance, the $6.2 billion cut to the US Department of Housing and Urban Development (HUD) included the elimination of Community Development Block Grants; these grants fund programs such as Meals on Wheels, local improvement and anti-poverty efforts, rental assistance, and affordable housing initiatives. The $15.1 billion cut to HHS included the elimination of $403 million in health professions and nursing training programs, which often include commitments from those who receive assistance to work in health professional shortage areas. The budget also proposed the elimination of several agencies outright, including the Appalachian Regional Commission, which promotes economic development in depressed communities, and the United States Interagency Council on Homeless, which coordinates efforts among 19 federal member agencies to end homelessness in America. While it is unlikely that Congress will execute all the proposed cuts in President Trump's budget blueprint, it sends a powerful message on how this administration will prioritize low-income and homeless populations and those with serious illness over the next four years.

WHAT COMES NEXT

Of the stories contained in this book, almost all the care, services, and supports the patients received were examples of minor policy successes—the funding of the county hospital and affiliated nursing home that provided care to patients despite continuing to operate at a $20 million annual loss; Medicare and Social Security, which provided healthcare coverage and some financial support for those fortunate enough to have an "identity": the well-trained care team that could go out into the community to accompany the patients in their final days. But the successes pale in comparison to the inability of our safety-net system to meet these patients' basic human needs throughout their lives. Ernest, Cowboy, and Mr. Green deserved to grow up in supportive environments where they had food, housing, and protection from abuse. Mr. White and his family deserved health insurance from a job he worked at for more than 25 years. Mr. Noble deserved a disability policy that could keep him out of poverty while he struggled to maintain part-time work. Mrs. Angel and Mr. Wheeler deserved healthcare professionals trained in effective communication, who could provide clear and honest information about their terminal conditions so they could make informed decisions. Mr. and Mrs. White deserved to spend their final months in a nursing home that was adequately staffed. All the patients' families and caretakers deserved assurances that their loved ones would receive treatment that preserved quality of life without simultaneously worrying that this care would bankrupt them. And all the dying poor whose stories were not collected for this book deserve to live in a society where their needs are met and their lives are valued.

In Support of the Public Safety Net

Proposals to cut or overhaul Medicaid, Medicare, and other safety-net programs often stem from concerns that they occupy too much of the federal budget or that the programs in their current form have expanded too far beyond what the original legislators intended. Many people, regardless of political affiliation, also share concerns about whether their tax dollars are being spent effectively and how the country will be able to manage the continued growth of entitlement spending. Leaving aside arguments about the relative efficiency of these programs, or the fact that society absorbs the costs of caring for low-income patients in one way or another (e.g., uncompensated healthcare, lost productivity), it is worth considering the common-sense reasons why the public safety net is necessary.

Payment for medical care changed dramatically in the mid-20th century. Prior to World War II, doctors who treated self-pay patients across income brackets had more flexibility in what they could charge their patients. It was not uncommon to charge financially secure patients more so that the doctors could provide services to low-income patients on a sliding scale. In particularly poor circumstances, the patient could trade goods, or the doctor might simply donate the care. This arrangement was helped by the fact that medicine was not as sophisticated as it is today.[45] There were far fewer treatments and procedures available and, as most care was provided in the home, less overhead for providers. This changed after the Second World War, when private and government insurance entered the market and developed formal fee schedules. As insurers began to systematize prices, doctors were less able to use fees from wealthy patients to compensate for others' care. The invention of new therapies and the gradual shift toward hospital-based care contributed to increased healthcare costs. These trends limited access to care for many people, particularly low-income patients. It could take years for an uninsured patient who required a hospitalization to pay off the bill, and in many instances, people would decide to forgo care. The creation of Medicare and Medicaid helped resolve some of these issues for millions of people.

A healthy contingent of US residents believe that social insurance should be left to philanthropy and voluntarism, as this would give people greater control over how they spend their resources. This is a noble idea, and it should be celebrated that Americans donated more than $370 billion to charity in 2015.[46] Unfortunately, there are several problems with relying on charity to pay for the safety net. First, resources often dwindle in times of greatest need, such as during the most recent recession, and they tend to be unevenly distributed based on geography. Second, people often limit their contributions to a few "pet" issues, and overlook other less attractive or visible causes that may still need support. Third, people tend to donate to organizations that have established infrastructure, as well as power and broad visibility; local charities often do not have a large enough marketing budget to recruit new donors, and philanthropists tend to prefer "bricks and mortar" operations. Finally, charitable giving over the past several decades has increased in total dollar amount, but consistently hovers around 2% of the GDP.[47] Private philanthropy is important but, without a central coordinating body designed to distribute resources across issues based on need rather than personal preference, critical needs will go unmet.

There is certainly room to improve efficiency in public safety-net programs,[48] and if the CMMI demonstrations were any indication, many people would welcome proposals that could improve the quality of services while reducing the overall cost. But with millions of people relying on hundreds of means-tested and social insurance programs to meet their basic needs, proposals to simply slash funding without a considered replacement are unconscionable and should be soundly rejected.

Policies Needed to Support the Dying Poor

Considering the current administration's priorities, the first policy battle is one of preservation. The ACA's role in extending coverage to 14 million low-income people through Medicaid expansion has shown evidence of increasing access to care and improving health outcomes. Stakeholders must also advocate against converting Medicaid to block grants and insist that any proposal to do so be accompanied by extensive evidence supporting that it will not harm beneficiaries. Unfortunately, there has not been the same mobilization around protecting Medicaid as has been the case with Medicare, in large part because Medicaid recipients are among the most vulnerable groups in this country. Yet Medicaid serves almost 20 million more beneficiaries and will continue to be the default payer of long-term services and support for older adults until policymakers develop an alternative.

In addition to maintaining coverage gains, preserving FQHC expansion will remain critical to meeting the needs of low-income populations. The continued presence of well-staffed community health centers will ensure that patients receive the preventive services needed to keep them healthy for as long as possible, allow for early detection should something go wrong, and provide access to pain and symptom management when needed. While the President's budget blueprint referenced supporting direct health services administered in community health centers, it did not specify how much would be dedicated to this effort.

The continued development of alternative payment models focused on caring for seriously ill patients holds great promise for improving health outcomes while reducing costs. Many of these models consider the circumstances of low-income and homeless patients, and have the flexibility to cover social services and supports as needed. PACE and Independence at Home, which have been proven to improve both outcomes and spending, should be expanded.

Finally, there must be a greater investment in ensuring that all patients with serious illness have access to palliative care, regardless of socioeconomic status or setting of care. The Palliative Care and Hospice Education and Training Act takes steps toward achieving this by establishing workforce training programs for clinicians of all types to ensure that they have skills in pain and symptom management, communication, and helping patients negotiate the healthcare system; enhancing research on improving the delivery of palliative care; and creating a national education and awareness campaign to inform patients, families, and health professionals about the benefits of palliative care and available supports and services.

It is individual stories like the ones contained in this book that remind policymakers of their obligation to improve the healthcare system for vulnerable patients and families. Keep doing the good work.

REFERENCES

1. Chaudry A, Wimer C, Macartney S, et al. Poverty in the United States: 50-year trends and safety net impacts. HHS. https://aspe.hhs.gov/system/files/pdf/154286/50YearTrends. pdf. Published March 2016. Accessed March 22, 2017.
2. Matthews D. The Clinton economy, in charts. *Wonkblog.* https://www.washingtonpost. com/news/wonk/wp/2012/09/05/the-clinton-economy-in-charts/?utm_ term=.6bb674dc8d5e. Published September 5, 2012. Accessed March 22, 2017.
3. Casselman B. No, Bill Clinton does not "know how" to fix the economy. *FiveThirtyEight.* https://fivethirtyeight.com/features/no-bill-clinton-does-not-know-how-to-fix-the-economy/. Published May 20, 2016. Accessed March 22, 2017.
4. Mishel L, Gordon C. Real hourly wage growth: The last generation. *Working Economics Blog.* http://www.epi.org/blog/real-hourly-wage-growth-last-generation/. Published October 10, 2012. Accessed March 22, 2017.
5. Andrews EL. Economic inequality grew in the 90's boom, Fed reports. *New York Times.* http:// www.nytimes.com/2003/01/23/business/economic-inequality-grew-in-90-s-boom-fed-reports.html. Published January 23, 2003. Accessed March 22, 2017.

6. Aid to Families with Dependent Children (AFDC) and Temporary Assistance for Needy Families (TANF) overview. https://aspe.hhs.gov/aid-families-dependent-children-afdc-and-temporary-assistance-needy-families-tanf-overview-0. Published November 11, 2009. Accessed March 22, 2017.

7. Allard SW. The changing face of welfare during the Bush Administration. *Publius: The Journal of Federalism*. 2007;37(3):304–332. doi:10.1093/publius/pjm013.

8. Vobejda B. Clinton signs welfare bill amid division. *The Washington Post*. http://www.washingtonpost.com/wp-srv/politics/special/welfare/stories/wf082396.htm. Published August 23, 1996. Accessed April 8, 2017.

9. McKernan S, Ratcliffe C. The effect of specific welfare policies on poverty. The Urban Institute. http://www.urban.org/sites/default/files/publication/50861/411334-The-Effect-of-Specific-Welfare-Policies-on-Poverty.pdf. Published April 2006. Accessed May 2, 2017.

10. Hartley RP, Lamarche C, Ziliak JP. Welfare reform and the intergenerational transmission of dependence. *University of Kentucky Center for Poverty Research Discussion Paper Series, DP2016-01*. http://www.ukcpr.org/sites/www.ukcpr.org/files/documents/DP2016-01_Hartley_et_al.pdf. Published September 2016. Accessed May 2, 2017.

11. Clymer A, Pear R, Toner R. The health care debate: What went wrong? How the health care campaign collapsed, a special report. *New York Times*. http://www.nytimes.com/1994/08/29/us/health-care-debate-what-went-wrong-health-care-campaign-collapsed-special-report.html?pagewanted=all. Published April 29, 1994. Accessed March 29, 2017.

12. The Clinton Presidency: Improving the nation's care. The Clinton-Gore Administration: A Record of Progress. https://clinton5.nara.gov/WH/Accomplishments/eightyears-07.html. N.d. Accessed March 29, 2017.

13. Hoag S, Harrington M, Orfield C, et al. *Children's Health Insurance Program: an evaluation (1997–2010)*. Washington, DC: Office of the Assistant Secretary for Planning and Evaluation; 2011.

14. Paradise J. The impact of the Children's Health Insurance Program (CHIP): what does the research tell us? Kaiser Family Foundation. http://kff.org/medicaid/issue-brief/the-impact-of-the-childrens-health-insurance-program-chip-what-does-the-research-tell-us/. Published July 17, 2014. Accessed March 29, 2017.

15. Center on Budget and Policy Priorities (CBPP). *Policy basics: the Earned Income Tax Credit*. 2016. http://www.cbpp.org/research/federal-tax/policy-basics-the-earned-income-tax-credit. Accessed March 15, 2017.

16. Pound WT. *Community Health Centers: a primer for legislators*. National Conference of State Legislatures; 2011. http://www.ncsl.org/portals/1/documents/health/CHCPrimer811.pdf. Accessed March 14, 2017.

17. Shi L, Lebrun LA, Tsai J. Assessing the impact of the Health Center Growth Initiative on health center patients. *Public Health Rep*. 2010;125(2):258–266.

18. Sack K. Expansion of clinics shapes Bush legacy. *New York Times*. http://www.nytimes.com/2008/12/26/health/policy/26clinics.html. Published December 25, 2008. Accessed March 14, 2017.

19. Engquist G, Burns P. *Health Insurance Flexibility and Accountability Initiative: opportunities and issues for states*. Princeton, NJ: The Robert Wood Johnson Foundation; 2002.

20. Coughlin TA, Long SK, Graves JA, Yemane A. An early look at ten state HIFA Medicaid waivers. *Health Aff*. 2006;25(3):w204–w216. doi:10.1377/hlthaff.25.w204.

21. Briesacher BA, Zhao Y, Madden JM, et al. Medicare Part D and changes in prescription drug use and cost burden: national estimates for the Medicare population, 2000–2007. *Med Care.* 2011;49(9):834–841. doi:10.1097/MLR.0b013e3182162afb.

22. Kaiser Family Foundation (KFF). The Medicare Part D Prescription Drug Benefit. Kaiser Family Foundation; September 2016. http://files.kff.org/attachment/Fact-Sheet-The-Medicare-Part-D-Prescription-Drug-Benefit. Accessed March 15, 2017.

23. Moffitt RA. The great recession and the social safety net. *Ann Am Acad Pol Soc Sci.* 2013;650(1):143–166. doi:10.1177/0002716213499532.

24. Cohen RA, Martinez ME, Zammitti EP. Health insurance coverage: early release of estimates from the National Health Interview Survey, 2015. National Center for Health Statistics. https://www.cdc.gov/nchs/data/nhis/earlyrelease/insur201605.pdf. Published May 2016. Accessed May 2, 2017.

25. McKernan S, Ratcliffe C, Steuerle E, Zhang S. Impact of the Great Recession and beyond: disparities in wealth building by generation and race. Urban Institute. http://www.urban.org/sites/default/files/publication/22551/413102-impact-of-the-great-recession-and-beyond.pdf. Published April 2014. Accessed May 2, 2017.

26. Obey DR. H.R. 1—American Recovery and Reinvestment Act of 2009. Congress.gov. https://www.congress.gov/bill/111th-congress/house-bill/1?r=1. Published January 26, 2009. Accessed March 29, 2017.

27. KFF. Children's Health Insurance Program Reauthorization Act of 2009 (CHIPRA). Kaiser Commission on Key Facts: Medicaid and the Uninsured. https://kaiserfamilyfoundation.files.wordpress.com/2013/01/7863.pdf. Published February 1, 2009. Accessed March 29, 2017.

28. KFF. Medicaid Expansion Enrollment. http://kff.org/health-reform/state-indicator/medicaid-expansion-enrollment/?currentTimeframe=0&sortModel=%7B%22colId%22:%22Location%22,%22sort%22:%22asc%22%7D. Published March 31, 2016. Accessed March 29, 2017.

29. Kirby J, Vistnes J. Access to care improved for people who gained Medicaid or marketplace coverage in 2014. *Health Aff.* 2016;35(10):1830–1834. doi:10.1377/hlthaff.2016.0716.

30. Ghosh A, Simon K, Sommers B. *The effect of state Medicaid expansions on prescription drug use: evidence from the Affordable Care Act.* 2017. http://www.nber.org/papers/w23044?utm_campaign=ntw&utm_medium=email&utm_source=ntw. Accessed March 30, 2017.

31. Pines JM, Zocchi M, Moghtaderi A, et al. Gaining coverage through Medicaid or private insurance increased prescription use and lowered out-of-pocket spending. *Health Aff.* 2016 Sep 1;35(9):1725–1733. doi:10.1377/hlthaff.2016.0091.

32. Antonisse L, Garfield R, Rudowitz R, Artiga S. The effects of Medicaid expansion under the ACA: Updated findings from a literature review. The Kaiser Family Foundation. http://files.kff.org/attachment/Issue-Brief-The-Effects-of-Medicaid-Expansion-Under-the-ACA-Updated-Findings. Published February 2017. Accessed May 2, 2017.

33. KFF. State Health Insurance Marketplace Types, 2017. http://kff.org/health-reform/state-indicator/state-health-insurance-marketplace-types/?currentTimeframe=0&sortModel=%7B%22colId%22:%22Location%22,%22sort%22:%22asc%22%7D. Published January 1, 2017. Accessed March 29, 2017.

34. Williamson A, Antonisse L, Tolbert J, Garfield R, Damico A. ACA coverage expansions and low-income workers (issue brief). June 10, 2016. The Kaiser Family Foundation.

Retrieved March 29, 2017, from http://kff.org/report-section/aca-coverage-expansions-and-low-income-workers-issue-brief/.

35. Collins SR, Gunja MZ, Doty MM, Beutel S. *How the Affordable Care Act has improved Americans' ability to buy health insurance on their own.* 2017. The Commonwealth Fund. http://www.commonwealthfund.org/~/media/files/publications/issue-brief/2017/feb/1931_collins_biennial_survey_2016_ib.pdf. Accessed March 29, 2017.

36. Weiss A, Long SK, Ramos C, Coughlin T. *Federally Qualified Health Centers' importance in the safety net continues as Affordable Care Act implementation moves ahead.* Urban Institute Health Policy Center. 2016. http://hrms.urban.org/briefs/fqhc-importance-safety-net.pdf. Accessed March 13, 2017.

37. McMorrow S, Polsky D. *Insurance coverage and access to care under the Affordable Care Act.* University of Pennsylvania Access Brief. https://www.ncbi.nlm.nih.gov/pubmed/28080011. December 8, 2016. http://ldi.upenn.edu/brief/insurance-coverage-and-access-care-under-affordable-care-act. Accessed March 14, 2017.

38. Holahan J, McMorrow S. *The widespread slowdown in health spending growth.* Robert Wood Johnson Foundation and Urban Institute. 2015. http://www.urban.org/sites/default/files/publication/48991/2000176-The-Widespread-Slowdown-in-Health-Spending-Growth-Implications-for-Future-Spending-Projections-and-the-Cost-of-the-Affordable-Care-Act-ACA-Implementation-1.pdf. Accessed March 16, 2017.

39. Warfield M, DiPietro B, Artiga S. *How has the ACA Medicaid expansion affected providers serving the homeless population.* The Kaiser Family Foundation. March 2016. http://files.kff.org/attachment/issue-brief-how-has-the-aca-medicaid-expansion-affected-providers-serving-the-homeless-population. Accessed March 14, 2017.

40. KFF. Compare proposals to replace the Affordable Care Act. The Kaiser Family Foundation. http://kff.org/interactive/proposals-to-replace-the-affordable-care-act/. Published March 24, 2017. Accessed March 29, 2017.

41. FamiliesUSA.org. *Work requirements in Medicaid: a bad idea.* FamiliesUSA. 2017. http://familiesusa.org/product/work-requirements-medicaid-bad-idea. Accessed March 18, 2017.

42. Jacobsen G, Neuman T. Turning Medicare into a premium support system. Kaiser Family Foundation. 2016. http://files.kff.org/attachment/issue-brief-Turning-Medicare-Into-a-Premium-Support-System-Frequently-Asked-Questions. Accessed March 18, 2017.

43. Commonwealth Fund (CF). *Essential facts about health reform alternatives: high-risk pools.* The Commonwealth Fund. 2017. http://www.commonwealthfund.org/~/media/files/publications/explainer/2017/mar/explainer_highrisk_pools.pdf. Accessed March 18, 2017.

44. Mulvaney M. America first: a budget blueprint to make America great again. https://www.whitehouse.gov/sites/whitehouse.gov/files/omb/budget/fy2018/2018_blueprint.pdf. Published March 13, 2017. Accessed March 14, 2017.

45. Jacobson L. Were the early 1960s a golden age for health care? *Politifact.* http://www.politifact.com/truth-o-meter/article/2012/jan/20/was-early-1960s-golden-age-health-care/. Published January 20, 2012. Accessed March 30, 2017.

46. Giving USA. 2015 was America's most generous year ever. https://givingusa.org/giving-usa-2016/. Published June 13, 2016. Accessed March 30, 2017.

47. Philanthropy Roundtable. Statistics on US giving. http://www.philanthropyroundtable.org/almanac/statistics/. Accessed March 30, 2017.

48. Clemans-Cope L, Holahan J, Garfield R. *Medicaid spending growth compared to other payers: a look at the evidence.* Kaiser Family Foundation; 2016. http://kff.org/report-section/medicaid-spending-growth-compared-to-other-payers-issue-brief/. Accessed March 18, 2017.

49. Office of the Assistant Secretary for Planning and Evaluation. Frequently asked questions related to the poverty guidelines and poverty. HHS. https://aspe.hhs.gov/frequently-asked-questions-related-poverty-guidelines-and-poverty#programs. Accessed April 26, 2017.

50. Fisher GM. The development and history of the poverty thresholds. *Social Security Bulletin.* 1992;55(4):3–14. https://www.ssa.gov/policy/docs/ssb/v55n4/v55n4p3.pdf. Accessed April 26, 2017.

51. Fisher GM. Mollie Orshansky: Author of the poverty thresholds. *Amstat News.* https://ww2.amstat.org/about/statisticiansinhistory/bios/OrshanskyMollie.pdf. Published September 2008. Accessed April 26, 2017.

52. Office of the Assistant Secretary for Planning and Evaluation. The development and history of the poverty thresholds—a brief overview. https://aspe.hhs.gov/history-poverty-thresholds. Published January 1997. Accessed April 26, 2017.

53. KFF. Poverty rate by race/ethnicity. Timeframe: 2015. http://kff.org/other/state-indicator/poverty-rate-by-raceethnicity/. Accessed April 28, 2017.

54. Keehan SP, Poisal JA, Cuckler GA, et al. National health expenditure projections, 2015–2025: Economy, prices, and aging expected to shape spending and enrollment. *Health Aff.* 2016;35(8):1522–1531. doi:10.1377/hlthaff.2016.0459

55. Mitchell EM. Concentration of health expenditures in the US civilian noninstitutionalized population, 2014. Agency for Healthcare Research and Quality. https://meps.ahrq.gov/data_files/publications/st497/stat497.pdf. Published November 2016. Accessed May 2, 2017.

56. Squires D, Anderson C. US health care from a global perspective: Spending, use of services, prices, and health in 13 counties. The Commonwealth Fund. http://www.commonwealthfund.org/~/media/files/publications/issue-brief/2015/oct/1819_squires_us_hlt_care_global_perspective_oecd_intl_brief_v3.pdf. Published October 2015. Accessed May 2, 2017.

57. Taylor LA, Tan AX, Coyle CE, Ndumele C, Bradley EH, et al. Leveraging the social determinants of health: What works? *PLoS ONE.* 2016;11(8):e0160217. doi:10.1371/journalpone.0160217.

58. Bradley EH, Canavan M, Rogan R, Talbert-Slagle K, Curry LA, et al. Variation in health outcomes: The role of spending on social services, public health, and health care, 2000–09. *Health Aff.* 2016;35(5):760–768. doi:10.1377/hlthaff.2015.0814.

59. Adler NE, Cutler DM, Fielding JE, Galea S, Satcher D, et al. Addressing social determinants of health and health disparities. *National Academy of Medicine's Vital Directions for Health and Health Care Initiative.* https://nam.edu/wp-content/uploads/2016/09/Addressing-Social-Determinants-of-Health-and-Health-Disparities.pdf. Published September 19, 2016. Accessed May 2, 2017.

A FINAL MUSE
ON SOLIDARITY WITH THOSE AT THE MARGINS

David Wendell Moller

Why are kings without pity for their subjects? Because they count on never being common human beings. Why are the rich so hard toward the poor? It is because they have no fear of being poor. . . .
—Jean-Jacques Rousseau, *Émile; or, On Education*[1]

In Shakespeare's *King Lear*, the King and two of his retainers are wandering aimlessly about in the throes of rejection, tribulations, and denouncement. He has given up the monarchy, fractured ties with his daughters, and is enduring the consequences of his own failed narcissism and related inability to love. Lear is descending inescapably into an abyss of madness, and despite being the former holder of great power, wealth, and the adulation that associates with nobility, he is now mostly isolated and suffering greatly. Tragically so: after all, this is a Shakespearean play!

During their journey, as an impending storm is adding to their worries, the three of them encounter a naked beggar. The King looks first at his companions, then at himself with his luxurious robes, then to the naked man, and proclaims:

> Is man no more than this? Consider him well. Thou owest the worm no silk, the beast no hide, the sheep no wool, the cat no perfume. **Ha! Here's three on's are sophisticated. Thou art the thing itself** [emphasis added].[2]

It may have been that, in his burgeoning insanity and separation from the trappings of privilege, the king was having an epiphany of self- and other-awareness, and coming to recognize that the trappings of royalty were just that—materialistic add-ons, a veneer of opulence that obscured the essence of that which makes us all human and binds us together. Lear's insight is synchronistic with Rousseau's observation; namely, that when affluence leads to a veil of grandiosity and omnipotence it enables a false and self-serving dichotomy between the rich and poor to emerge. In this dichotomy, the worldview of the rich and privileged does not lend itself to understanding or recognition that, despite their wealth, they ultimately share both a common humanity and universal experience of being human with those who are poor.

This book speaks against that self-serving mirage and seeks to affirm that the poor, marginalized, and sick share a core human essence with each of us. Unfortunately, for the most part, as a nation and as individuals we are not willing to recognize and honor that reality. There is a noticeable tendency to dismiss notions of a shared humanness with those living at the margins. In fact, it is not stretching too far to state that an obliviousness, lack of interest, and even disdain toward those who are poor and marginalized are widespread throughout the society. Our intent in this book is to become a voice for those who live, suffer, and die at the margins. The goal, simply stated, is to declare their humanity and nurture empathic understandings about who they are through story-telling, espousing a moral obligation for the broader society to recognize that humanity and advancing ways of responding to their needs in ways that enhances their dignity as human beings and relieves their sufferings throughout illness.

Any meaningful "walking of the walk" about the Judeo-Christian ethic, around which the notion of American exceptionalism and our political claim to specialness has been organized and promoted throughout our history, requires we do just that.

> In the context of urban poverty, people suffer greatly throughout life and life's end because of social exclusion and impaired opportunities.

The human suffering of living and dying at the fringes of society is illuminated by the stories of the Whites, J. W., Annie, the Wheelers, Cowboy, and so many others who live in inner-city poverty. They reveal how the circumstances of their lives degrade and dehumanize them and result in unnecessary hardship. In the context of urban poverty, people suffer greatly throughout life and at life's end because of social exclusion and impaired opportunities. In many ways, the capacity to fully realize their human potential is undermined by the obstacles that they face on a daily basis. In fact, for many who are born poor, the prospects for a healthy life are compromised from the moment of conception and birth. As we have been noting, these are people whose capability to live a healthy life is broken by racism, discrimination, stigmatization, hostility, and poverty; all factors that compromise cognitive, physical, emotional, social, and behavioral well-being. Simply put, living in poverty and being subjected to racism, even in its most covert expressions, constricts the capacity of the human being to flourish. It leads to instability and devolution in personal and community life, including the ability to cope with life's stressors in productive ways.

There is no secret that social injustice underlies many of the problems that populations who are challenged by racial and economic barriers face. As *Dancing with Broken Bones* reveals, there is real hardship that takes place at the intersection of race, poverty, and serious illness. For this reason, it is important to understand justice and injustice not merely as abstract moral principles. Rather, they must be recognized as major, causative factors in promoting unnecessary, and dare I say unconscionable, suffering for people in life and throughout dying.

The irony is that discrimination and disparity, despite some substantial efforts to address them through social and political activism, stand in stark contrast to the American ideals of freedom, equality, justice, and respect for life—qualities we like to celebrate as those that distinguish America from much of the rest of the world and make us who we are.

Perhaps the crucial question on a macro level is why and how such widespread socioeconomic and racial disadvantage are permissible or tolerable in a nation that prides itself on the ideals of equality and respect. The answers, to be sure, are complex and elusive. Our intent in this collaboration is not to try to answer those questions. Many gifted and thoughtful people are working on that. Our intent instead is to declare the harm of injustice to real people in daily life, elucidating how marginalization assaults their dignity and intensifies suffering both in life and while dying. It is also to advance a call to action to improve the health and illness experiences of those who are socially and economically disadvantaged through greater social awareness, improved capacity to care for their unique needs, and argue for more just distribution of resources to serve those needs.

> This, too, is our approach; deepening empathic understanding through the use of story-telling and story-listening.

A very useful framework for understanding the impact that inequity has on the lives of people can be found in the capabilities approach advanced by Martha Nussbaum.[3] In her view, there are certain key capabilities that promote human development and allow for our human potential to flourish. She identifies ten core capabilities, which include:

1. *Life.* The capacity to live to the end of a human life of normal length; of not dying prematurely.
2. *Bodily health.* Being able to have good health, including adequate nutrition and shelter.
3. *Bodily integrity.* Living free from fear of violence and assault; feeling free and safe to move from place to place.
4. *Senses, imagination, thought.* Being able to draw on the senses; having adequate education that informs and cultivates growth and development; having opportunities for pleasure and to avoid non-beneficial pain.
5. *Emotions.* The ability to establish healthy attachments to one's environment and other people in it; freedom from fear and anxiety.
6. *Practical reason.* Being able to form a conception of goodness and the ability to be an active planner in one's own future.
7. *Affiliation.* Being treated as a dignified being whose worth is equal to that of others.
8. *Other species.* Being able to live with concern for and in relation to animals, plants, and the world of nature.
9. *Play.* The ability to laugh, to recreate, and enjoy life.
10. *Control over one's environment.* The opportunity to own property and seek employment on an equal basis with all others.

It is instructive to think about these capabilities and how they play out for those who are born into, live, and die at the margins. Let's take Cowboy as an example and consider his life specifically in terms of these capabilities:

1. Did the circumstances of his life make it more or less likely he would die prematurely?
2. Did he have good health, including good nutrition and shelter?

3. Did he live free from fear of violence and assault?
4. Did his youthful experience allow for adequate education and promote his growth and development?
5. Did his formative experiences cultivate healthy attachments to others, including his own family?
6. Was he given the tools to become an active planner in shaping his own destiny?
7. Did his experiences in the Deep South as a multiracial boy confirm his equal worth and dignity as a human being?
8. Was he able to develop a concern for the environment and the world that surrounded him? (How would you explain his connection to his beloved Cowgirl? Was he capable of extending that concern to other animals? To people?)
9. Was his life joyful from birth on to death?
10. Did he experience equal opportunities throughout his life?

The answers, regrettably, are fairly straightforward and illuminate how deeply injured he was by the salient conditions of his life: racism and poverty. The answers to these questions are not reserved just for Cowboy. They would be similar in the life narratives of so many people throughout the landscape of urban and rural poverty in America. In many ways, the inescapable fact is that those who are born into economic disadvantage and racial marginalization have futures that are imperiled from the outset, and are not able to fulfill their human potential and maximize their potential for well-being.

Nussbaum's framework is especially useful in that it provides a method for understanding the circumstances of peoples' lives, not through clinical or intellectual detachment but with a certain amount of empathy for their suffering. In this regard, the capabilities approach directs us not towards arcane philosophical or moral principles. It guides us toward compassionate understanding of people who live lives fractured by injustice and disparity. Enhancing our understanding of real people and their struggles is central to advancing Nussbaum's goal of helping society to achieve greater justice. This, too, is our approach; deepening empathic understanding through the use of story-telling and story-listening. In this way, our overall goal is not academic. Rather, it is humanistic and pragmatic. We hope to inform and inspire by facilitating a more-personal engagement with the lives of people. For this reason, we seek to involve the emotions as well as the intellect as catalysts for both empathy and activism.

Our approach in presenting and discussing patient experiences is based on a recognition that it is important to understand who they are as human beings, including the social situations in which they live. It establishes cultural humility and proficiency as prerequisites in serving members of vulnerable populations and declares a need for social, healthcare, and policy reform if we are to adequately meet their needs.

So, for example, Richard Payne clearly establishes that the pain and suffering endured by Mr. Greene were a consequence of his being born an African-American male in the Deep South. His personal experience as a black man, as Richard describes it, was a product of structural racism. That is to say, it was shaped by prejudice and discrimination that were embedded directly in folkways, practices, and public policies that led to blocked opportunities that undermined his capability to fulfill his human potential and resulted in a lifetime of disempowerment. I have often observed that, in substantial ways, many

Americans still turn a blind eye to racism's existence. Richard takes that observation one step further and notes that perhaps people even take a "pernicious" interest in the social disadvantages that afflict African Americans. He posits that systematic disenfranchisement of black people weakens them economically and politically and keeps them "in place," namely, stuck at the margins. This system protects the status quo, including the privileges that surround being white in America. In this regard, he argues that racism and discrimination may not just be a matter of indifference. They may actually, and perhaps this functions on a subconscious level, be desirable and protective of prevailing vested interests of the already privileged.

In any event, as Richard notes, "It is impossible to understand Mr. Green's illness experiences, and his reaction to them, without a sense of the institutionalized systems of racism that give rise to persistent poverty and the manifestations of health inequalities in our society." The result of institutionalized and cultural racism for J. W. was a life filled with struggle. He endured enormous poverty in the rural setting of his youth, faced restricted opportunities upon his migration to the Midwest, found adaptive coping by turning to risk-promoting behaviors as he ran the streets, and suffered death at an early age from prostate cancer.

Yet, as Richard emphasizes, this is not the entire story of Mr. Greene's life. Despite the disadvantages that weighed him down throughout his life and into illness, he found a way to cope and get along. His strong faith was not surprising, as religious belief is deeply embedded in the history of African-American culture. This faith was formed out of a response to living in extreme hardship and the historical realities of social and economic discrimination. It served as a protective armor during slavery, the era of lynchings, segregation, and so forth. It provided strength, support, and a sense of purpose to suffering, enabling people to survive earthly afflictions as they looked forward to great reward after life on this earth has ended.

People like Mr. Greene, the weak, the disadvantaged, the vulnerable, the discriminated against, endure profound violations of their intrinsic dignity as human beings. Yet, despite this harm, many are able to achieve a remarkable sense of equanimity in living and dying. In Mr. Greene's case, he was able to do this primarily through support from his religious beliefs, along with social support from his extended family; both of which are norms of cultural life in the African-American community.

The words of Richard Payne are an apt way to conclude our contemplation of the story of J. W. and his struggle to maintain dignity throughout a life whose circumstances continually assaulted his worth and undermined his capabilities to flourish:

> We honor his life, and the life of our collective humanity when we commit our emotional, intellectual and physical capabilities to address suffering in all forms (but especially when it is driven by the persistence of poverty in the wealthiest nation on earth) of our fellow human brothers and sisters.

As Betty Ferrell chronicles, there are two overwhelming messages that emerge from the end-of-life experience of Ms. Annie Dickens: gratitude and faith. In many ways, Ms. Dickens embodied the very definition of vulnerability, having lived a life filled with poverty and distressing events. Her final challenge emerged as she was actively dying in the county nursing home with overwhelming pain. There can be no doubt that Ms. Annie was suffering greatly throughout her illness. Her suffering was a consequence of and explainable by the pathophysiology of her disease and its unrelenting physical distress. However, despite her vulnerability, as Betty observes, she displayed great strength throughout dying. In particular, she evinced unwavering faith and sincere gratitude both of which became sources of resilience, enabling her to triumph over the physical tribulations of her disease. To draw upon the conceptualization of Ernest Becker discussed in Chapter 1, these qualities served as her own personal "hero system" over suffering and death. They allowed her to preside over her own dying with a majestic spirit.

In many important ways, her transcendence was assisted by palliative care "done right," as she received care which helped facilitate emotional, social, and spiritual well-being. The story of Annie prompts us to contemplate how one can remain so positive and spirit-filled while the body is literally being ravaged by pain. The answer with specific regard to Annie was that she maintained her dignity with conscious intent. She committed herself to dying in a fashion that would honor the God she deeply trusted. "I can't let Him down," she would often proclaim. For her, dying well was a sacred responsibility and she was determined not to let God down by allowing herself to feel negative emotions. One of the additional things that supported her in the effort to assert her personal dignity over the dying process was participating in the *Dancing with Broken Bones* project. She drew strength and sustenance from the opportunity to share her story and to share her faith with those who would hear it. It gave her meaning to know that people were interested in her story, and that helped, at least to some degree, to ease her suffering.

She thought about you quite a bit, I am sure: the careful reader who would hear her story one day. She trusted that you would not judge her harshly but rather would view her with respect, perhaps even honor. In fact, I believe that is true of all the patients who shared their stories with us.

Robin Franklin observes that Mrs. Angel lived much of her life under a dark cloud. But she never lost her capacity for love and kindness. It is quite remarkable how some human beings are able to maintain an essential goodness in the midst of circumstances that injure them deeply. Rachel Diamond also describes the injuries of Mrs. Angel's life, commenting specifically on how it was shaped by betrayal. Her capabilities to thrive as a person were insulted not just by being born poor, but by her husband who abused her and the physician who dismissed the seriousness of that abuse. While the culture may have had a different view of domestic violence during that time than it does presently, the harmful impact of abuse on victims is never variable. It caused as much trauma to the mind, body, and spirit back then as it does today. So, her life from early stages was shaped by experiences of tragic losses and betrayals that sometimes led to feelings of internal conflict and anger. As Robin aptly describes, "She suffered more than most."

Yet, somehow Mrs. Angel did not succumb to anger or hatred. Instead, she sought ways in which she could assert some control over her destiny. She found that in being a good mother. Her lifelong involvement with a faith community and her faith in God also helped to sustain her. In many ways her life was unfair. Yet faith gave her strength to endure. Her commitment to being a good mother kindled a capacity for softness, kindness, and love. Remarkably, those qualities flourished throughout her life despite the harsh circumstances that confronted her.

Tim Quill identifies lost opportunities for addressing the sufferings that surrounded the end-of-life experience of Mrs. Angel. We have noted that hospice and palliative care have been demonstrated to improve quality of life and ease suffering throughout dying. He argues that meaningful involvement of palliative care throughout her battle with cancer could have made a positive difference. For example, inadequate conversations between her doctors and herself led to feelings of frustration and mistrust. Skilled end-of-life conversations would have led to a different result. In addition, as palliative care is in essence interdisciplinary, he notes that her spiritual needs would have been assessed and hopefully addressed in a meaningful fashion. Instead, she awaited the promised visit from her minister with a sense of abandonment and, once again, the theme of betrayal and letdown loomed large in her life. As Tim insightfully notes:

> There are no simple answers to these complex issues raised when poverty, serious illness, and alienation collide, but despite the associated chaos and losses there can also be opportunity for healing and coming together as was experienced by [Mrs. Angel's] family.

His point is that the stories of the poor are not simple, but complicated; and, despite the injustice and enormous struggles of their lives, empathic, skilled care can provide an opportunity for healing and transcendence.

Perhaps there is no greater tribute that can be offered to Mrs. Angel than that expressed by the words of Rachel, Robin, and Tim: "We wish we had met her. . . ."

The difference that palliative care, uniquely tailored for vulnerable populations, can make is chronicled in the chapter by Richard Gunderman and Greg Gramelspacher. They emphasize that palliative care for the dying poor is not primarily medical care. They affirm that it is important that care for marginalized populations be informed by understandings about patients' lives outside the hospital. Factors in their economic, social, and cultural backgrounds not only shape their views and responses to life: they also deeply influence how patients view illness, perceive the care they receive, trust or mistrust the system in which it is delivered, and how they make decisions about their care.

In some ways, surviving the hardships of living in poverty on a daily basis creates a resilience and hardiness that "toughens" people. In this regard, the poor may "kick and scream" less than the more affluent when they receive a bad clinical diagnosis. These are folks who face setbacks and catastrophes as a matter of course. They are used to bad things happening. So a life-threatening diagnosis with a poor prognosis may become one more setback and tragedy to deal with. Thus, the hardships of living poor may actually generate a certain toughness and stamina that equip patients and families to cope with the strain of serious illness.

A key to establishing successful end-of-life initiatives for inner-city poor is building trust through cultural humility and proficiency. In order to maximize achievement of these qualities, it is important to understand patient life outside the hospital. Patients and families come from very different worlds than their inner-city providers. In order to develop empathic understandings of who they are, it is essential to gain some appreciation of where they come from. Many are "economically terminal" and live in social chaos, both of which can easily undermine empowerment and effective decision-making in life and throughout an illness. Social estrangement during serious illness can exacerbate feelings of vulnerability, and the poor and homeless are especially isolated. Lack of financial or personal resources strains the ability to meet basic needs. When this happens, things for patients and loved ones can become turbulent. As a result, they may, at times, become nonadherent with treatment and be perceived as difficult and angry. These reactions must be understood in terms of the context of their lives and the difficulties they are trying to manage. A lack of understanding about their circumstances can easily lead to negative judgments and compromised care.

I often ask myself if I were faced with the problem of incessant bills, constant financial worry, unreliable transportation, unrelenting social and personal chaos in my life, and difficulty getting to the hospital or clinic, what kind of mood I might be in upon arrival. Probably not the best! Then, I imagine myself as an inpatient in the safety-net hospital, with a seemingly endless parade of caregivers asking me questions, and wondering who my "real" doctor is. I would have to think that feelings of abandonment and isolation might result as I lay in the hospital bed pondering things. Being sick is tough enough without things being made worse by feelings of isolation and disconnection.

A major point that Richard and Greg make is illuminated by the title of their chapter, "Dying Poor Needn't Mean Dying Poorly: Insights from a Safety-Net Hospital Palliative Care Program." They show how the dedication of professionals in their safety-net hospital, along with collaboration with the local community, led to the establishment of a palliative care program that is sustainable and a 'game changer' for the lives of people it cares for. They show what a positive difference palliative care "done right" can make in serving the most vulnerable among us.

However, when palliative care is absent or functioning poorly, the opposite prevails—namely, suffering is worsened. The story of Mr. and Mrs. Wheeler reveals that situation. As Robert Arnold laments, the life of the Wheelers was difficult enough before they got seriously ill. After the onset of their respective illnesses, however, their suffering got much worse. They descended into an abyss of frustration, anger, and chaos that kept eating away at their lives. Their dominant view of the world and the healthcare system they were dependent upon was filled with perceptions of injustice and mistreatment. They correspondingly became suspicious and distrusting. Their despair was so palpable that Bob Arnold literally was overwhelmed with moral distress, and he himself became "frustrated—angry—overwhelmed" by what the Wheelers had endured.

Bob, as Greg and Richard also do, shows that a better way in dying can be found in high-quality palliative care programs. He targets the miscommunication that surrounded both Carl and Evelyn Wheeler's illness experiences as being symptomatic of a broken system. The structural issues that underlie inadequate communication run deep, and include factors related to health illiteracy, chaotic patterns of doctor–patient relationships, suboptimal skill in having difficult conversations among providers, inadequate training around cultural competence, a reimbursement system that does not reward or support time-consuming conversations about end-of-life issues, and a lack of understanding of the challenges faced by patients in their daily lives.

While poor communication near the end of life can affect patients and families across all economic strata, its impact is intensified among the poor who are disenfranchised and mistrusting to start with. For this reason, developing skills in effective and empathic communication is critical to providing good care to those living at the margins. Again, building trust is a core competency, and this requires compassionate listening and development of mindful understandings of who patients and families are outside of the health system.

> Empathic, skilled care can provide the opportunity for healing and transcendence.

An important take-home lesson offered by Bob is that if palliative and hospice services were integrated into the illness experience of the Wheelers, some of their despair and anger would have been eased, and some sense of peace and dignity would have been possible. Simply, their lives would not have been so miserable.

If the Wheelers' story is, in part, a consequence of "failed palliative and hospice care," the narrative of Cowboy reveals the impact that supportive care delivered with cultural humility and competence can have in facilitating dignity and helping patients achieve tranquility in dying. His story shows how a life that started grimly can end most peacefully.

The team met Cowboy where he was as a person, putting into action the reminder by Shirley Otis-Greene that palliative care is best done in the community. It was the outreach of the team in venturing to the cave and attentively listening to his story that generated empathic understandings. There was so much in Cowboy's life that let him down. Two of the institutions that Americans like to define as the bedrock of our society failed to live up to their advertised promises for him. These were family and religion. His family system clearly betrayed him and became the foundation of mental instability and social estrangement. Not surprisingly, he passed the legacy of harm they inflicted on him onto his own children, perpetuating the cycle of abuse and neglect. Religion provided little support as he navigated life as an outlier. He felt a sense of abandonment, not by God, but by the ministers who "rejected him a long time ago." It was his own personal resilience and creative capacity, often fueled by anger and suspicion, that enabled him to survive and perhaps even thrive in a certain sense. The palliative care team figured all of the unique historic and present-day circumstances of his life into their relationship with him. The team met him where he was as a human being, and that made all the difference throughout his final months of life (Figure 15.1).

Ultimately, it was the indelible imprint of rural poverty and racism that shaped who Cowboy was and the manner in which he lived life. He was able to achieve peace near the end precisely because the palliative care team understood and responded to his unique biography as a person. They recognized that he was profoundly marginalized by class and racial barriers and did not judge him in his behaviors because they came to appreciate how life had harmed him. As Terry Altilio observes, "The clinicians who assisted Cowboy through this last chapter of his life attribute the outcome to the 'redemptive power of love' and 'mindful presence.'" As she says, it ultimately was their skills in cultural humility and empathic understanding that enabled the team to serve Cowboy in exemplary fashion.

A major take-home lesson that emerges from his story is that effective palliative care must extend beyond the clinical, medical model. It must involve focus on the unique qualities of the person's cultural background; the deeply ingrained socioeconomic factors

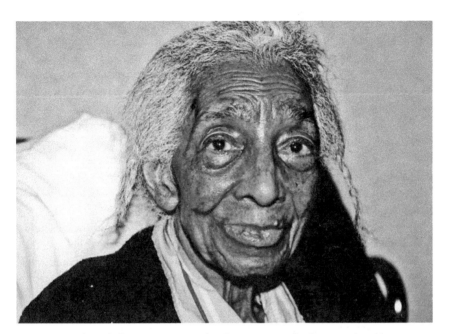

FIGURE 15.1 The soul of a nation is measured in the ways we care for the most vulnerable among us.

that impact their lives. In this way, quality care must reach beyond focus on the body and the medical narrative. It must pay attention to the myriad factors that render people marginalized and vulnerable, caring for them as persons, not just patients. Once again, it is important to emphasize that this approach requires cultural humility and proficiency. These skills are components of what Shirley describes as community-based palliative care. This approach enables more complete understanding of who patients and their loved ones are. And, as Terry persuasively notes, this model is more likely to bridge the divide that separates inner-city patients from their providers and facilitate more-trusting relationships. The result of expanding the focus of palliative care into the community is that the care that is delivered will be more complete and in touch with patient needs.

Ken and Virble played by the rules but the deck was stacked against them. They worked hard and lived from paycheck to paycheck, never finding a way to escape the control of poverty. So throughout their lives they struggled mightily, not only suffering their illnesses but also enduring illness and death among their children. As Christian Sinclair describes, the healthcare system failed them both. In no small part, this was because they were indigent and lacking financial and personal resources. He notes that the care they received was not only not the best, it was troubling in many ways. In his words, they "had the nursing-home experience many people dread. Both of them were left to sit in their own soiled sheets for hours at a time, unable to help each other. Afraid to speak up and advocate for themselves, they continued to suffer these indignities. . . ." As he observes, their story reflects a failure of the healthcare system and resulted in a total undermining of respect and dignity. Their situation was severe. And it is startling to recognize this assault on their human dignity took place in the most affluent country in the world.

Once again, the theme of inadequate conversations about the end of life appears in the narrative. Instead of seizing the opportunity to discuss the benefits of hospice care once Ken decided to forgo chemotherapy, all that the oncology fellow offered was a return-to-clinic appointment. Not only was this interaction with the physician clinically suboptimal, Ken perceived his demeanor as being impatient and dismissive. It focused on the disease exclusively and did not tend to his needs as a person; a person who was alarmed, vulnerable, and disempowered. Regrettably, not only did that encounter fail to establish appropriate goals of care or goals of life, Ken walked away feeling that the doctor was rushed and "rude," offering all of us a challenge to disagree with his assessment by exclaiming, "Tell me you think he wasn't rude."

It is hard read the narrative of Ken and Virble and not come to the conclusion that they were salt-of-the earth, good people. They were devoted spouses. They worked hard. They were law-abiding. They raised their children with love and rarely complained. What was their reward? A lifetime of hardship of living in poverty coupled with inexcusable indignity at the end of life, which included: experience with a health system that was unresponsive to their needs, inadequate communication with doctors, excremental assault in the nursing home, the inability to pay for Ken's funeral, disrespectful treatment during the viewing service, and an impersonal and hurried graveside service at Ken's burial. What a sad and sorry way to come to the end of life and a 43-year marriage.

In short, the story of Ken and Virble declares the essential goodness of who they were as human beings. It also illuminates a dark side of American life, exposing the cruelty that comes from poverty along with the equally egregious consequences of societal indifference to the suffering of people who live in it. All I can say is: Shame on all of us that they suffered as they did!

Our collaboration in this book asserts that we have a moral obligation to improve the end-of-life experience for the marginalized. It is rooted in the belief that social justice requires that palliative and hospice care be especially attuned to the ethical principles of fairness and equity. Our goal is to enhance understanding of the authenticity and humanity that reside within many of the people who live and die at the margins. We emphasize that empathic understandings of how real people are beleaguered because of poverty and racism must remain a cornerstone of the effort to improve end-of-life care. In this regard, we believe that telling their stories is essential in facilitating more effective strategies for addressing their needs.

In important ways, the willingness or unwillingness to commit to reducing disparities in both living and dying reflects the core moral character of a society. The degree to which we are not willing to meaningfully address disparities and remain indifferent to the plight of the marginalized suggests something kind of disturbing. On the other hand, the more we actively seek to address inequities and social injustice, the more aligned we are with the ideals of American life. With this being said then, to the extent to which the hospice and palliative care movements, and the healthcare professions in general, commit to practices in cultural humility and competency, we will be better positioned to serve the most vulnerable among us and advance our ideals as a society.

> In important ways, the willingness or unwillingness to commit to reducing disparities in both living and dying reflects the core moral character of a society.

Diane Meier and Stacie Sinclair make a compelling case for rethinking American priorities with specific regard to the implications of government policy for the lives of the poor. As they note, in significant part, the lives and deaths of the patients in *Dancing with Broken Bones* reflect a failure in public policy. In part, this failure is related to an absence of political will to tackle the problems of disparity and injustice.

They begin by discussing how patient and family experiences that are described in the book reflect some modest successes of policy and societal concern. Safety-net hospitals (now often referred to as "America's Essential Hospitals") exist in many urban areas. Despite constant problems of being under-resourced, their presence shows some commitment to caring for the poor, and the poor do have someplace they can turn to when they get sick. Various government programs designed as a buffer against extreme destitution, such as Medicaid and CHIP, are intended to assist the poor in their struggles. The very existence of hospitals, community health clinics, and supportive government services means that the poor are not entirely abandoned and disregarded. That said, however, and consistent with the themes which run throughout this book, Diane and Stacie observe how the needs of the poor remain grossly unattended and, in reality, their sufferings are minimally addressed by present-day policies and their associated programs of support. Their analysis concludes by observing that America's sense of duty to promote opportunity for those excluded by poverty and racism pales in comparison to the effort exerted towards nurturing economic growth among more affluent sectors of the population.

As Amos Bailey accurately describes, the poor are underserved throughout life and near life's end. The life of the poor is challenged by the daily grind of poverty which makes living "difficult, exhausting, and dangerous." The poor's lives are burdened by unhealthy behaviors, excess morbidity, and early death. But, he also advises that there are strategies and programs, such as found in The Balm of Gilead, that can be designed to meet their unique needs and ease their struggles and maximize their wellbeing. This requires both societal and professional commitment, however. A willingness, as Tammy Quest and Kimberly Cursteen put it, to venture into the trenches and stand with and fight for the most vulnerable among us. Increased investment of societal resources will need to underpin any serious effort in this regard. An increased commitment towards enhanced cultural humility and skills in cultural competence among healthcare providers is also essential. And Tammy and Kimberly are correct in their observation that "sacrifice" is required if entrenchment, solidarity, and caring partnerships in serving the underserved is to become normative. But, as this book argues, if society and healthcare providers are willing to make the effort, end-of-life experience for marginalized populations will be transformed.

The unavoidable point is that the basic human worth of the poor is often overlooked and even dismissed in the prevailing social, economic, and political climate. Each of the collaborators in this book shows how this disparagement results in real harm for real people. They posit that the patients described in *Dancing with Broken Bones,* and others like them, deserve better. In doing so, they challenge us directly to think about some very hard questions:

- Did Cowboy deserve to grow up free from the abuse of racial hatred and the burden of tenant farming that is directly traceable to the American institution of slavery?
- Did Mr. Greene deserve to be born into a society that did not punish him for being a black person?
- Should Mr. White have been rewarded with a pension and adequate health care for 25 years of loyal service as an employee?
- Why was Mrs. Angel betrayed so frequently throughout her life? Did she do anything to bring that upon herself?
- Was it fair, after years of working in the healthcare industry, that an injury sustained while doing his job exacerbated an already precarious financial position and led to tremendous burden for Mr. Noble and his family?
- Why do we, in the richest country in the world, tolerate the degradation and indignities that the Whites encountered in the county nursing home? How can we accept the Whites, and others like them, lying uncared for in their own excrement? What does this say about our society?

As we think about the issues that surround these circumstances, a final and especially perturbing two-part question arises:

- Were the human capabilities of these people, and many others who live at the economic and social fringes, greatly undermined from the beginning and throughout their lives because of the afflictions of poverty and racism?
- Why are the circumstances that these patients lived in tolerated in a society that prides itself as a beacon of virtue and moral decency?

I must declare that these situations are allowed to persist because of a general indifference toward the lives and sufferings of those who live and die at the margins. Our democratic heritage along with the claims of American exceptionalism require a deeper commitment to fulfilling the fundamental needs of these human beings. For this reason, I wonder if we are failing in our own vision of ourselves as a society.

In the last speech he gave, Hubert Humphrey noted that "the moral test of government is how that government treats those who are in the dawn of life, the children; those who are in the twilight of life, the elderly; those who are in the shadows of life; the sick, the needy and the handicapped." The stories of the patients and families in *Dancing with Broken Bones* affirm that, in some egregious ways, American society is failing that test. People who live and die at the margins suffer hardship and indignity most would not accept for themselves or their loved ones. Their stories reveal that in some profound ways American society is failing the moral test of which Humphrey spoke.

In this vein, I must finish by asking each reader to ponder how this sobering reality casts a dark stain on the soul of our nation and how we can come together in solidarity to improve upon it.

REFERENCES

1. Rousseau JJ. *Emile; or, on education.* New York: Simon and Schuster; 1979.
2. Shakespeare W. *King Lear.* Act 3, Scene 4. New York: Basic Books. 2005.
3. Nussbaum M. Capabilities and social justice. *International Studies Review.* Summer 2002;4(2):123–135.

INDEX

Figures, tables, and boxes are indicated by an italic *f, t,* and *b* following the page number.